GASTROENTEROLOGY AND HEPATOLOGY

The Comprehensive Visual Reference

GASTROENTEROLOGY AND HEPATOLOGY

The Comprehensive Visual Reference

series editor
Mark Feldman, MD

Southland Professor and Vice Chairman
Department of Internal Medicine
University of Texas Southwestern
　Medical Center at Dallas

Chief, Medical Service
Veterans Affairs Medical Center
Dallas, Texas

volume 1
The Liver

volume editor
Willis C. Maddrey, MD, MACP

Executive Vice President for Clinical Affairs
University of Texas
Southwestern Medical Center at Dallas
Dallas, Texas

With 20 contributors

Churchill Livingstone
Developed by Current Medicine, Inc.
Philadelphia

Current Medicine

400 Market Street
Suite 700
Philadelphia, PA 19106

Managing Editor	*Lori J. Bainbridge*
Development Editors	*Kelly Streeter and Raymond Lukens*
Editorial Assistant	*Jennifer Rosenblum*
Indexer	*Maria Coughlin*
Art Director	*Paul Fennessy*
Design and Layout	*Robert LeBrun*
Illustration Director	*Ann Saydlowski*
Illustrators	*Sue Ann Fung-Ho, Wieslawa Langenfield, Beth Starkey, Larry Ward, Lisa Weischedel, and Gary Welch*
Typesetting Director	*Colleen Ward*
Production	*David Myers and Lori Holland*

The liver/volume editor, Willis C. Maddrey.
     p. cm. – (Gastroenterology and hepatology; v. 1)
  Includes biliographical references and index.
  ISBN 1-878132-78-4 (hardcover)
  1. Liver–Diseases–Atlases. I. Maddrey, Willis C. II. Series.
  [DNLM: 1. Liver Diseases–atlases. WI 17 G257 1996]
RC846.L53 1996
616.3'62–dc20
DNLM/DLC
for Library of Congress   95-22343
                                 CIP

Library of Congress Cataloging-in-Publication Data
ISBN 1-878132-78-4

Printed in Singapore by Imago Productions (FE) Pte Ltd.

10 9 8 7 6 5 4 3

DISTRIBUTED WORLDWIDE BY CHURCHILL LIVINGSTONE, INC.

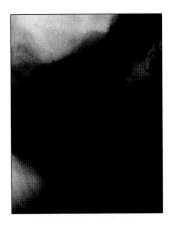

Series Preface

In recent years dramatic developments in the practice of gastroenterology have unfolded, and the specialty has become, more than ever, a visual discipline. Advances in endoscopy, radiology, or a combination of the two, such as endoscopic retrograde cholangiopancreatography and endoscopic ultrasonography, have occurred in the past 2 decades. Because of advanced imaging technology, a gastroenterologist, like a dermatologist, is often able to directly view the pathology of a patient's organs. Moreover, practicing gastroenterologists and hepatologists can frequently diagnose disease from biopsy samples examined microscopically, often aided by an increasing number of special staining techniques. As a result of these advances, gastroenterology has grown as rapidly as any subspecialty of internal medicine.

Gastroenterology and Hepatology: The Comprehensive Visual Reference is an ambitious 8-volume collection of images that pictorially displays the gastrointestinal tract, liver, biliary tree, and pancreas in health and disease, both in children and adults. The series is comprised of 89 chapters containing nearly 4000 images accompanied by legends. The images in this collection include not only traditional photographs but also charts, tables, drawings, algorithms, and diagrams, making this collection much more than an atlas in the conventional sense. Chapters are authored by experts selected by one of the eight volume editors, who carefully reviewed each chapter within their volume.

Disorders of the gastrointestinal tract, liver, biliary tree, and pancreas are common in children and adults. *Helicobacter pylori* gastritis is the most frequent bacterial infection of humans and is a risk factor for peptic ulcer disease and gastric malignancies. Colorectal carcinoma is the second leading cause of cancer mortality in the United States, with nearly 60,000 deaths in 1990. Pancreatic cancer resulted in an additional 25,000 deaths. Liver disease is also an important cause of morbidity and mortality, with more that 25,000 deaths from cirrhosis alone in 1990. Gallstone disease is also common in our society, with increasing reliance on laparoscopic cholecystectomy in symptomatic individuals. Inflammatory bowel diseases (ulcerative colitis, Crohn's disease) are also widespread in all segments of the population; their causes still elude us.

The past few decades have also witnessed striking advances in the therapy of gastrointestinal disorders. Examples include "cure" of peptic ulcer disease by eradicating *H. pylori* with antimicrobial agents, healing of erosive esophagitis with proton pump inhibitor drugs, remission of chronic viral hepatitis B or C with interferon-α2b, and hepatic transplantation for patients with fulminant hepatic failure or end-stage liver disease. Therapeutic endoscopic techniques have proliferated that ameliorate the need for surgical procedures. Endoscopic advances include placement of peroral endoscopic gastrostomy tubes for nutritional support, insertion of stents in the bile duct or esophagus to relieve malignant obstruction, and the use of injection therapy, thermal coagulation, or laser therapy to treat bleeding ulcers and other lesions, including tumors. *Gastroenterology and Hepatology: The Comprehensive Visual Reference* will cover these advances and many others in the field of gastroenterology.

I wish to thank a number of people for their contributions to this series. The dedication and expertise of the other volume editors—Willis Maddrey, Rick Boland, Paul Hyman, Nick LaRusso, Roy Orlando, Larry Schiller, and Phil Toskes—was critical and most appreciated. The nearly 100 contributing authors were both creative and generous with their time and teaching materials. Special thanks to Abe Krieger, President of Current Medicine, for recruiting me for this unique project and to his talented associates at Current Medicine, especially Kelly Streeter who served as developmental editor.

The images contained in this 8-volume collection are available in print as well as in slide format, and the series is soon being formatted for CD-ROM use. All of us who have participated in this ambitious project hope that each of the 8 volumes, as well as the entire collection, will be useful to physicians and health professionals throughout the world involved in the diagnosis and treatment of patients of all ages who suffer from gastrointestinal disorders.

Mark Feldman, MD

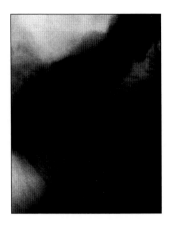

Volume Preface

The emergence of present day hepatology has resulted largely from the incorporation of often spectacular advances gathered from many diverse fields of medical science into the study of the liver. The pace of progress is quickening. A generation of ideas has a faster turnover rate than ever before. Clinicians need regular reminders of where we are, how we got here, and what more needs to be done. In less than a half century, hepatology has become a recognized and established discipline. Contributions from clinical chemistry and histopathology, and the development of effective imaging techniques have provided a scaffold on which to build. Armed with hope, a new generation of clinicians committed themselves to become hepatologists.

Hepatology experienced an extraordinary boost when the major viruses that affect the liver were identified. We cannot overestimate the importance of the contributions of modern virology to hepatology. The development of specific tests to identify hepatitis B, hepatitis D, and hepatitis C had a major impact on the understanding of those disorders gathered under the heading of chronic hepatitis. Within the past 2 decades, chronic viral hepatitis has been established as the leading cause worldwide of chronic inflammation of the liver. With the recognition that chronic hepatitis is the major precursor to the development of cirrhosis, it has become widely accepted that chronic viral hepatitis is one of, if not the most, important causes of cirrhosis. The natural histories of chronic hepatitis B, chronic hepatitis B with superimposed hepatitis D, and chronic hepatitis C markedly differ. The availability of highly specific tests to identify and quantitate the virus has added greatly to our understanding of the

natural history of those factors that affect outcomes. The discoveries first of hepatitis B and subsequently hepatitis A have been followed by the creation of effective vaccines. The remarkable opportunities offered by the advent of hepatitis B vaccines will undoubtedly be realized in the reduction or even elimination of one of the major disorders affecting mankind. It is hoped that progress in the prevention of hepatitis B and hepatitis A will soon be followed by the development of a vaccine to prevent another major worldwide disease—hepatitis C.

Occurring within the same time frame are the defining events that led to the development of liver transplantation. In less than 2 generations, liver transplantation has moved from a concept to a series of early successes and now is accepted as therapy. Along the way, much has been learned about the pathogenesis of the major complications of liver diseases and more effective means to either recognize the complications, prevent them, or if needed, treat them.

Eliminating patients with chronic viral hepatitis from the pool of patients who have evidence of chronic hepatic inflammation, along with the development of highly specific tests identifying autoimmune hepatitis, has increased the confidence and validity of long-term clinical trials in these disorders. Among the unusual causes of chronic hepatitis are the occasional individuals who have Wilson's disease. Furthermore, reactions from several therapeutic drugs have been established to cause patterns of hepatic damage and follow courses that closely mimic chronic hepatitis of other etiologies.

The recognition of the importance of antimitochondrial antibodies and the diagnosis of primary biliary cirrhosis opened the way to separate this disorder from other conditions characterized by chronic cholestasis. Once primary biliary cirrhosis was defined, natural history studies became more meaningful. Models that accurately predict the course of primary biliary cirrhosis were developed and proved relevant to clinical practice. As in other disorders, the time to proceed to liver transplantation for a patient with primary biliary cirrhosis is in that window between the time hepatitis reserve has been lost to a near critical level and before the development of complications that may further reduce the chances for patient survival.

In *Liver*, the reader is introduced (or reintroduced) to many concepts. Each chapter stands on its own yet is related to the others in remarkable ways. Several chapters deal with the major manifestations of liver disease, providing up-to-date reviews of jaundice, portal hypertension, hepatic encephalopathy, ascites, hepatorenal syndrome, and spontaneous bacterial peritonitis. Several modern therapeutic approaches have improved the chances of affected patients. The spectrum of manifestations of hepatitis—viral, autoimmune, and drug-induced—is interwoven throughout the book. In addition, there is a comprehensive discussion of the problems attendant to the development of acute liver failure. The various causes of acute and chronic hepatitis are covered in depth. Hepatitis B and hepatitis C receive individual attention in separate chapters as well as frequent mention throughout the remainder of the volume as befits the importance of these conditions for the hepatologist.

The spectrum of drug-induced liver disease and the mechanisms by which drug-related liver injuries develop (and can be detected or prevented) is discussed. Alcohol-induced liver disease, surely the most important drug-related liver disorder,

is fully described. Liver disease caused by copper and iron receive special attention as do those disorders predominantly affecting the hepatic vasculature or the parenchyma in the form of abscesses or cysts. Tumors of the liver, once considered therapeutically hopeless, are carefully described with emphasis on recently acquired information regarding the roles of hepatitis B, hepatitis C, iron, and environmental toxins in the pathogenesis. In addition, in the chapter regarding tumors there is a status report evaluating the roles of hepatic resection and transplantation as treatments. It is fitting that the last chapter of the book is devoted to liver transplantation, because liver transplantation is the treatment of choice when other approaches fail.

The format of this atlas is visual images supported by relatively brief text. Useful tables, charts, diagrams, and photomicrographs bring to the fore concepts regarding liver diseases in a way that is informative and memorable. The chapters are constructed like well-prepared lectures, interweaving basic concepts with results of clinical observations and clinical trials. The contributors are all hepatologists with considerable clinical experience who have made their topics relevant and accessible.

It has been a pleasure to work with the contributors in the creation of this new approach to education. There are many strides forward recorded in these pages. Considering what has been accomplished in the field of hepatology in only a few years, we can surely look to the future with hope and anticipation of greater advances yet to come.

Willis C. Maddrey, MD, MACP

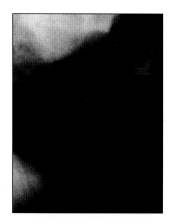

Contributors

Ignacio Aiza
Fellow, Department of Hepatology
University of Miami
Miami, Florida

Bruce R. Bacon
Professor of Internal Medicine
Director, Division of Gastroenterology and Hepatology
Department of Internal Medicine
Saint Louis University School of Medicine
St. Louis, Missouri

David Bernstein
Assistant Professor
Department of Medicine
University of Miami
Miami, Florida

Laurence Blendis
Professor, Department of Medicine
University of Toronto
The Toronto Hospital
Toronto, Ontario
Canada

Joseph R. Bloomer
Professor, Department of Medicine
University of Minnesota
University of Minnesota Hospital and Clinic
Minneapolis, Minnesota

Robert S. Brown, Jr.
Clinical Instructor
Department of Medicine
University of California, San Francisco
Attending Physician
Liver Transplantation Program
University of California Medical Center
San Francisco, California

Peter C. Buetow
Assistant Professor
Department of Radiology and Nuclear Medicine
Uniformed Services University of Health Sciences
Bethesda, Maryland
Chief, Gastrointestinal Radiology
Armed Forces Institute of Pathology
Washington, D.C.

Harold O. Conn
Professor of Medicine (Emeritus)
Department of Internal Medicine
Yale University School of Medicine
New Haven, Connecticut
Department of Veterans Affairs Medical Center
West Haven, Connecticut

Albert J. Czaja
Professor, Department of Medicine
Mayo Medical School
Consultant in Gastroenterology
Rochester, Minnesota

Adrian M. Di Bisceglie
Professor, Department of Internal Medicine
St. Louis University School of Medicine
St. Louis, Missouri

Anastacio Hoyumpa
Professor of Medicine
Department of Medicine
Division of Gastroenterology and Nutrition
University of Texas Health Sciences Center
San Antonio, Texas

Raymond S. Koff

Professor of Medicine
Department of Medicine
University of Massachusetts
Worcester, Massachusetts
Chairman, Department of Medicine
Metrowest Medical Center
Framingham, Massachusetts

Ann M. Kools

Assistant Professor
Department of Medicine
University of Minnesota
Minneapolis, Minnesota
St. Paul Ramsey Medical Center
St. Paul, Minnesota

John R. Lake

Associate Professor
Department of Medicine
University of California, San Francisco
Medical Director
Liver Transplantation Program
University of California Medical Center
San Francisco, California

William M. Lee

Professor, Department of Internal Medicine
University of Texas Southwestern Medical School
Dallas, Texas

Charles S. Lieber

Professor, Department of Medicine and Pathology
Mount Sinai School of Medicine
Director, GI-Liver Program and Alcohol Research
    and Treatment Center
Veterans Affairs Medical Center
Bronx, New York

Milton G. Mutchnick

Professor, Department of Medicine
Wayne State University
Director, Division of Gastroenterology
Harper Hospital
Detroit, Michigan

Steven Schenker

Professor and Division Chief
Department of Medicine
The University of Texas Health Science Center
    at San Antonio
San Antonio, Texas

Eugene R. Schiff

Professor of Medicine
Chief of Hepatology
University of Miami School of Medicine
Chief, Hepatology Section
Department of Veterans Affairs
Miami Medical Center
Miami, Florida

Florence Wong

Senior Research Fellow
The Toronto Hospital
Toronto, Ontario
Canada

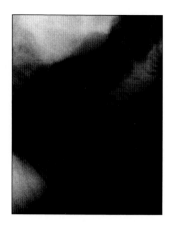

Contents

Chapter 13

Tumors of the Liver

ADRIAN M. DI BISCEGLIE

PETER C. BUETOW

Chapter 14

Liver Transplantation

ROBERT S. BROWN, JR.

JOHN R. LAKE

Chapter

1

Jaundice

ANN M. KOOLS
JOSEPH R. BLOOMER

Jaundice has long been of interest to the physician, and to the patient as well, because it is a visible manifestation of disease. Indeed, two of the four humors of Hippocrates were related to bile pigments [1]. Bilirubin, which is the principal component of bile pigments, is the end product of the catabolism of the heme moiety of hemoglobin and other hemoproteins. When bilirubin is produced in excessive amounts, or when hepatic excretion of bilirubin into bile is defective, the concentration of bilirubin in the blood and tissues increases. Jaundice is recognized if the accumulation of bilirubin in the sclerae and skin is of sufficient quantity to be visible. Generally this recognition occurs when serum bilirubin levels exceed 2.0 to 3.0 mg/dL.

After 1800 years, the following ancient description of icterus (jaundice) cannot be improved:

> *"If a distribution of bile, either yellow, or like the yolk of an egg, or like saffron, or of a dark-green colour, takes place from the viscus, over the whole system, the affection is called Icterus..."*
>
> From the extant works of Aretaeus, the Cappadocian (circa 200 A.D.)

Because jaundice is caused by an abnormality in bilirubin metabolism, understanding the steps of bilirubin formation and excretion is helpful in defining the reason for jaundice in the individual patient. After its formation by heme catabolism, bilirubin is transported from plasma to the intestine in discreet stages [2]. These stages are 1) the uptake of bilirubin from plasma, where it is bound to albumin, by the hepatocyte; 2) the conversion of bilirubin within the hepatocyte to a water-soluble compound by conjugation with glucuronic acid; 3) the transport of conjugated bilirubin across the bile canalicular membrane; and 4) the flow of bile through the biliary system into the intestine.

Information regarding the individual steps of bilirubin metabolism has collected slowly over time and is still incomplete. Perhaps one of the most important clinical observations occurred during World War I when Hijmans van den Bergh and coworkers used the diazo reaction to demonstrate the presence of a direct- and indirect-reacting fraction of bilirubin in serum [1]. The direct-reacting fraction was present in excess amounts when there was impaired bile formation or bile flow. Subsequently, in 1956, three groups of investigators demonstrated that the direct-reacting fraction is bilirubin conjugated with glucuronic acid [3–5]. The mechanism by which bilirubin is formed from heme was not characterized until 1968, when the enzyme responsible for this process, microsomal heme oxygenase, was described [6]. Proteins that bind bilirubin within the hepatocyte cytosol were described in 1969 [7], but there still remains some uncertainty about their precise role in bilirubin transport. In the 1970s, studies with radiolabelled bilirubin were used to examine the kinetics of bilirubin uptake from plasma and indicated that this uptake occurs by a facilitated transport system [8], but the transport process or processes have yet to be identified

precisely. The mechanism by which conjugated bilirubin is transported across the canalicular membrane has been difficult to study for technical reasons. Recent information suggests that there is an ATP–dependent system involved in this process which has been named the *multispecific organic anion transporter* [9].

Although several features of hepatic bilirubin transport remain incompletely defined, it is clear that bilirubin conjugation plays a critical role in the process. Thus, bilirubin metabolism can be divided into preconjugation and postconjugation phases, and an abnormality in bilirubin metabolism, which causes jaundice, can be classified as either unconjugated or conjugated hyperbilirubinemia. This classification is of significant help to the physician evaluating the patient with jaundice. This chapter reviews the steps of bilirubin metabolism and uses the classification of unconjugated and conjugated hyperbilirubinemia to describe those entities that cause jaundice.

■ BILIRUBIN METABOLISM

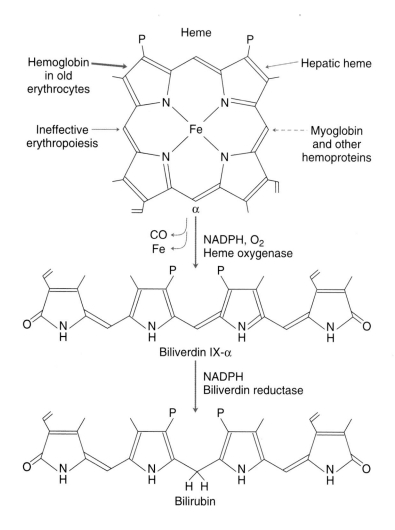

FIGURE 1-1.

Formation of bilirubin from heme. Approximately 80% of the daily bilirubin production is derived from the catabolism of hemoglobin in senescent erythrocytes that are destroyed in the reticuloendothelial system. The remainder results mainly from the degradation of hepatic heme and hemoproteins, of which the cytochromes P-450 are quantitatively the most important. A small fraction of bilirubin production occurs as a consequence of ineffective erythropoiesis and the degradation of myoglobin and other hemoproteins in the body. In the process of heme catabolism, heme dissociates from globin or other apoproteins, and the enzyme microsomal heme oxygenase catalyzes the cleavage of the tetrapyrrole ring at the α-methene bridge, causing the equimolar release of one molecule of iron and one molecule of carbon monoxide. Microsomal heme oxygenase is present in reticuloendothelial cells, macrophages, and hepatic parenchymal cells, the sites of bilirubin production. Biliverdin, a green pigment, is formed by this reaction. Biliverdin is subsequently reduced to bilirubin IX-α by the cytosolic enzyme biliverdin reductase, which is abundantly present in the cells where bilirubin is formed. NADPH—reduced nicotinamide-adenine-dinucleotide phosphate.

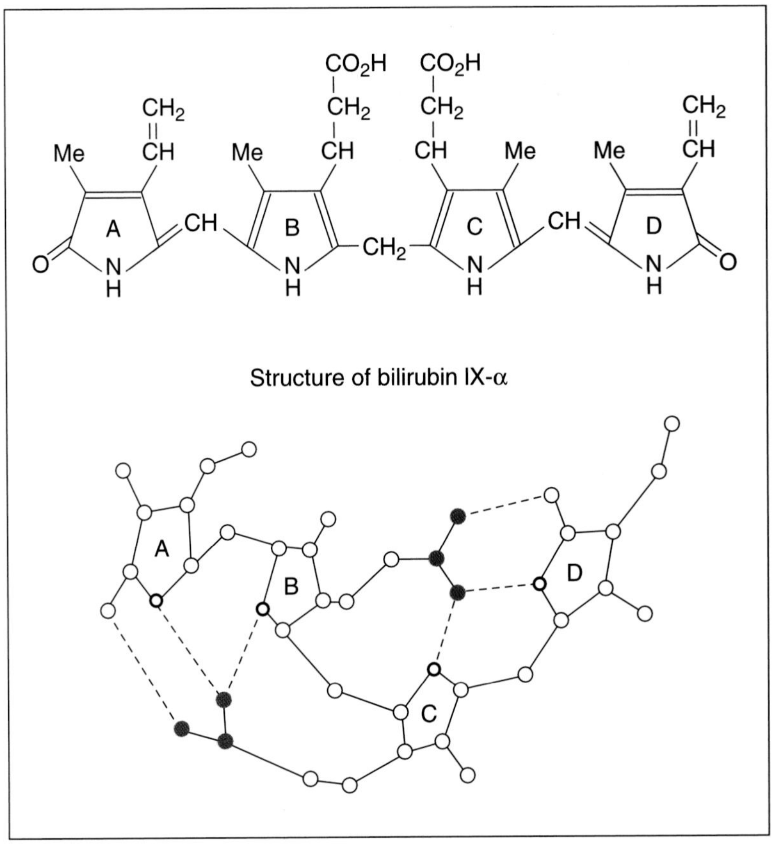

FIGURE 1-2.

Structure of bilirubin IX-α

Structure of bilirubin IX-α (unconjugated bilirubin) in physiologic solution. The conventional linear tetrapyrrole structure of unconjugated bilirubin is shown in the upper portion of the figure. In its native confirmation, however, the molecule is folded upon itself because of hydrogen bonding between each of the propionic side chains and the CO and NH groups of the opposite half of the molecule. This bond holds the molecule in a rigid three dimensional confirmation and causes it to be poorly soluble in aqueous solution at physiologic pH levels.

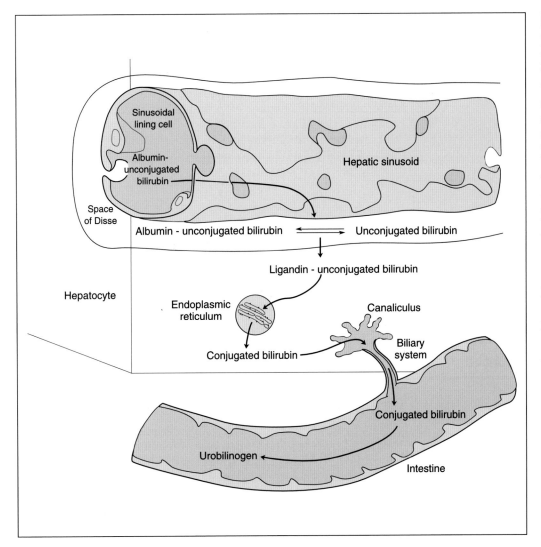

FIGURE 1-3.

Pathway of bilirubin excretion. Because of its poor solubility in physiologic aqueous solution, unconjugated bilirubin circulates in the blood as a noncovalent complex with albumin. The pores in the hepatic sinusoids are sufficiently large so that the bilirubin-albumin complex readily diffuses to the plasma membrane of the hepatocyte as blood flows through the liver. It is there unconjugated bilirubin dissociates from albumin and enters the cytosol. This dissociation occurs by facilitated transport. Within the hepatocyte cytosol, unconjugated bilirubin is bound to the protein ligandin (glutathione-S-transferase). The bilirubin molecule is subsequently conjugated with one or two molecules of glucuronic acid by the enzyme uridine diphosphate-glucuronyl transferase, which is located in the interior of the endoplasmic reticulum, and conjugated bilirubin is excreted across the canalicular membrane into bile. Conjugated bilirubin remains largely intact during passage through the biliary tract and the small intestine, but it is degraded by colonic bacteria to a series of tetrapyrroles that are collectively termed *urobilinogen*. These compounds partially account for the color of stool. A portion of urobilinogen is absorbed and excreted in bile; less than 2% is excreted in urine under normal circumstances. (*From* Bloomer [10]; with permission.)

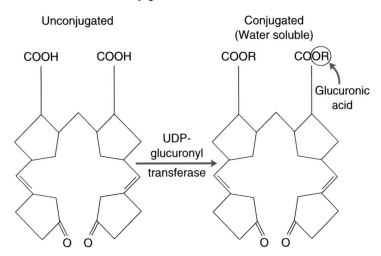

Conjugation of bilirubin

Unconjugated

Conjugated
(Water soluble)

FIGURE 1-4.

Bilirubin IX-α is conjugated with glucuronic acid at one or both of its propionic acid side chains. This conjugation of bilirubin significantly increases the water solubility of the molecule and allows it to be excreted in aqueous solutions, such as bile or urine. Bilirubin diglucuronide constitutes over 90% of the bilirubin conjugates in normal human bile. Another process that increases the water solubility of unconjugated bilirubin is photoisomerization, in which exposure of the molecule to light of wavelength 425 to 475 nm changes the configuration of the double bonds adjacent to the outer pyrrole rings. This effect of photoisomerization is the basis for the use of phototherapy in jaundiced infants to prevent kernicterus.

■ MEASUREMENT OF BILIRUBIN IN SERUM

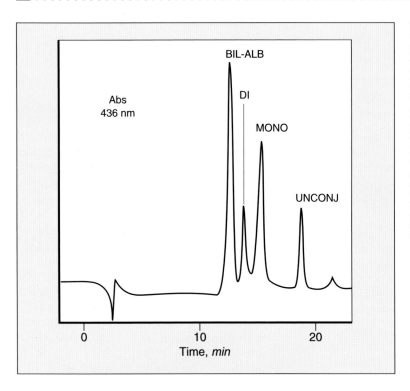

FIGURE 1-5.

Forms of bilirubin in serum. The bilirubin fractions in serum may be separated by high-performance liquid chromatography and measured by their absorbance (Abs) at 436 nm. In normal individuals serum bilirubin is almost exclusively in the form of unconjugated bilirubin (UNCONJ). When hepatic bilirubin clearance is impaired, monoconjugated bilirubin (MONO) and diconjugated bilirubin (DI) may also be detected. A fourth fraction in which bilirubin is covalently bound to albumin (BIL-ALB) may also be detected when the hepatic excretion of conjugated bilirubin is impaired. The BIL-ALB fraction is not detected in normal individuals, neonates with physiologic jaundice, or in patients with unconjugated hyperbilirubinemia caused by hemolysis or Gilbert's syndrome. (From Weiss *et al.* [11]; with permission.)

TABLE 1-1. SERUM BILIRUBIN MEASUREMENT

FORM	REACTION WITH DIAZO REAGENTS
Bilirubin monoglucuronide	Direct reacting
Bilirubin diglucuronide	Direct reacting
Bilirubin-albumin covalent complex	Direct reacting
Unconjugated bilirubin	Indirect reacting

Total serum bilirubin – direct-reacting fraction = indirect-reacting fraction

TABLE 1-1.

The most commonly used approach to quantitate serum bilirubin concentration is based on the van den Bergh reaction, in which bilirubin and its conjugates are diazotized to form azo pigments, which are then measured spectrophotometrically. The violet color that develops immediately when diazotized sulfanilic acid is added to serum is called the direct-reacting fraction of serum bilirubin. Bilirubin monoglucuronide, bilirubin diglucuronide, and bilirubin covalently bound to albumin give a direct reaction. When alcohol or some other accelerant is then added to the mixture, the color increases further because of the reaction of unconjugated bilirubin with diazotized sulfanilic acid. This method thus yields values for direct-reacting bilirubin and the total bilirubin concentration. The difference between the two is designated as the indirect-reacting fraction of bilirubin and is equated with the unconjugated bilirubin concentration.

TABLE 1-2. JAUNDICE

Unconjugated Hyperbilirubinemia

A. Increased bilirubin production
  1. Hemolysis
    a. Erythrocyte abnormality (*eg*, hereditary spherocytosis, G-6-PD deficiency)
    b. Extracellular abnormality (*eg*, hypersplenism, immunohemolytic anemia)
  2. Ineffective erythropoiesis (*eg*, thalassemias)
  3. Hematoma breakdown
B. Decreased hepatic bilirubin clearance
  1. Neonatal hyperbilirubinemia
  2. Fasting
  3. Gilbert's syndrome
  4. Crigler-Najjar syndromes

Conjugated Hyperbilirubinemia

A. Intrahepatic disorder
  1. Hepatocellular disease of any cause (*eg*, viral hepatitis)
  2. Cholestatic disease of any cause (*eg*, primary biliary cirrhosis)
  3. Metabolic disorder
    a. Dubin-Johnson syndrome
    b. Rotor syndrome
    c. Benign recurrent intrahepatic cholestasis
    d. Cholestasis of pregnancy
B. Extrahepatic disorder
  1. Biliary tract pathology (*eg*, tumor or stricture)
  2. Pancreatic pathology (*eg*, carcinoma)

TABLE 1-2.

Classification of jaundice according to the serum bilirubin measurement. Jaundice may be detected clinically when the serum bilirubin concentration exceeds 2.0 to 3.0 mg/dL. In this situation the separate quantitation of the serum unconjugated bilirubin concentration (indirect-reacting fraction) and conjugated bilirubin concentration (direct-reacting fraction) can be used to classify jaundice into two general categories that direct further evaluation. Conjugated hyperbilirubinemia is diagnosed when the direct-reacting fraction of serum bilirubin is increased. Because the diazo reaction does not precisely separate conjugated bilirubin from unconjugated bilirubin, some direct-reacting bilirubin will be measured even in normal individuals. Thus conjugated hyperbilirubinemia is present if the direct-reacting fraction of serum bilirubin exceeds 0.3 mg/dL when the total serum bilirubin level is below 2.0 mg/dL or is greater than 15% of the total serum bilirubin concentration when the level exceeds 2.0 mg/dL. Pure unconjugated hyperbilirubinemia is the diagnosis when the direct-reacting fraction of serum bilirubin is normal and the indirect-reacting fraction exceeds 1 mg/dL. The unconjugated bilirubin level may also be increased in those disorders that cause conjugated hyperbilirubinemia (*eg*, hemolysis from hypersplenism in cirrhosis).

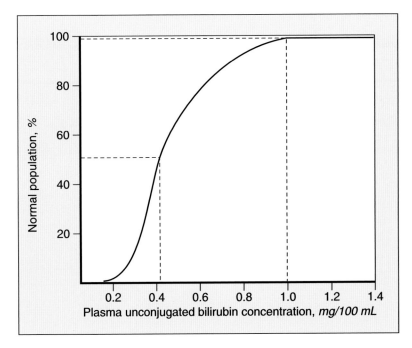

FIGURE 1-6.

Cumulative distribution curve for the plasma (serum) unconjugated bilirubin concentration in a normal population. Based on calculations made from experimental measurements of plasma bilirubin turnover and hepatic bilirubin clearance using a lognormal function, 99% of the normal population will have a serum unconjugated bilirubin concentration below 1 mg/dL. The *dashed lines* indicate the bilirubin concentrations corresponding to the 50th and 99th cumulative percentiles of the normal population. (*From* Bloomer *et al.* [12]; with permission.)

Causes

TABLE 1-3. EVALUATION OF HEMOLYSIS AS CAUSE OF UNCONJUGATED HYPERBILIRUBINEMIA

GENERAL TESTS	SPECIFIC TESTS
Blood smear	Hemoglobin electrophoresis
Erythrocyte indices and reticulocyte count	G-6-PD Assay
Haptoglobin level	Coombs' test
Lactic dehydrogenase level	Osmotic fragility test
Bone marrow examination	Ham's test

TABLE 1-3.

A hemolytic state must be considered when evaluating the patient with unconjugated hyperbilirubinemia. Determining the erythrocyte indices and reticulocyte count, evaluating the peripheral blood smear, and measuring a haptoglobin level will usually determine if a hemolytic state is present. If the tests are positive, more specific studies are done to determine the cause of the hemolysis. If the studies are negative, the unconjugated hyperbilirubinemia is caused by impaired hepatic bilirubin clearance. When the serum unconjugated bilirubin concentration exceeds 3.5 mg/dL, hepatic bilirubin clearance is usually impaired irrespective of whether hemolysis is present or not.

TABLE 1-4. UNCONJUGATED NEONATAL HYPERBILIRUBINEMIA

Physiologic neonatal hyperbilirubinemia
  Peak bilirubin level at day 5
  Level >10 mg/dL in 23% of infants caused by a combination of functional immaturity in bilirubin clearance, increased bilirubin production, and intestinal absorption of unconjugated bilirubin
Hyperbilirubinemia associated with breast feeding
  Peak bilirubin level at 10 to 20 days
  Inhibitor of bilirubin conjugation in maternal breast milk
Transient familial neonatal hyperbilirubinemia
  Peak bilirubin level within 4 days
  May cause kernicterus
  Inhibitor of bilirubin conjugation in maternal serum

TABLE 1-4.

Unconjugated hyperbilirubinemia is a common phenomenon in the neonate; it is called *physiologic jaundice of the newborn*. The cause is multifactorial. In two uncommon conditions, the unconjugated bilirubin level may reach a much higher value in the neonate because of the presence of an inhibitor of bilirubin conjugation in breast milk or in maternal serum. Kernicterus may occur in the latter situation, and exchange transfusion and phototherapy may be necessary. For situations other than that of the firstborn infant, taking the history is helpful in identifying these conditions.

TABLE 1-5. CHARACTERISTICS OF GILBERT'S SYNDROME AND CRIGLER-NAJJAR SYNDROME

	GILBERT'S SYNDROME	CRIGLER-NAJJAR SYNDROME TYPE I	CRIGLER-NAJJAR SYNDROME TYPE II (ARIAS)
Serum bilirubin, *mg/dL*	Usually 1.0–5.0	Usually >20	Usually 10–20
Bilirubin UDP–glucuronyl transferase	50% of normal	0	10% of normal
Bile bilirubin conjugates			
Monoglucuronide	40%	0	95%
Diglucuronide	60%	0	5%
Kernicterus	No	Yes	Rare
Inheritance	Autosomal dominant?	Autosomal recessive	Autosomal dominant?
Response to phenobarbitol	Yes	No	Yes

TABLE 1-5.

Unconjugated hyperbilirubinemia is the principal biochemical abnormality in patients with Gilbert's and the Crigler-Najjar syndromes. Gilbert's syndrome is a common condition, estimated to occur in 5% to 10% of the population, in which mild unconjugated hyperbilirubinemia results from a combination of diminished hepatic uptake of unconjugated bilirubin and a deficiency in bilirubin conjugation. Prognosis is excellent. In the Crigler-Najjar syndrome, however, the absence or marked deficiency of bilirubin UDP-glucuronyl transferase causes much higher levels of unconjugated hyperbilirubinemia, and in type 1 is usually associated with death in infancy or early childhood from kernicterus. Phenobarbital administration lowers the serum bilirubin level in both Gilbert's and type II Crigler-Najjar syndromes, but has no effect in type I Crigler-Najjar syndrome.

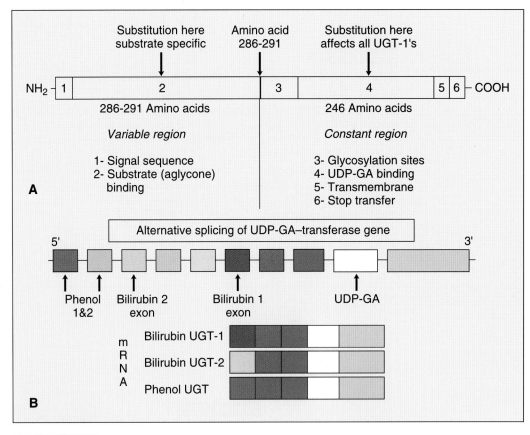

terminal half of the molecule (regions 3 to 6). Region 2 of the variable amino-terminal half of the peptide contains the aglycone substrate binding site, which is unique for each type of UGT. **B**, The scheme of the super gene for the UGT family, with each box representing an exon and the connecting lines representing the intervening introns. The 6-kB downstream segment of the gene contains four conserved exons that code the constant carboxyl-terminal half of each UGT, including the UDP-glucuronic acid (UDP-GA) binding site. Mutations here cause abnormal function of all UGT in this subclass. The 104-kB upstream segment of the gene contains six exons, four of which code the unique regulatory aglycone-binding sites of one of the UGT in the subclass. The substrate specificity of each UGT is determined by translational splicing of the unique exon coding for that substrate binding region with the four constant downstream exons of the gene. Mutations in the upstream region usually affect conjugation only of the specific substrates of the UGT coded by the mutated gene. Mutations in the *UGT* gene are responsible for the unconjugated hyperbilirubinemia that occurs in both Gilbert's and the Crigler-Najjar syndromes. UGT-1—UGT, family 1; UGT-2—UGT, family 2. (*From* Tiribelli and Ostrow [13]; with permission.)

FIGURE 1-7.

Schematic structure of UDP-glucuronyl transferase (UGT) peptides and messenger RNA (mRNA). **A**, All UGT peptides have the same amino acid sequence in the carboxy-

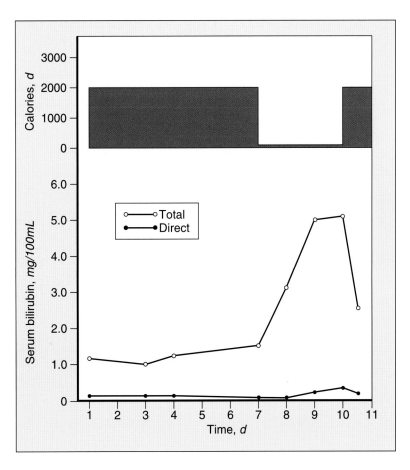

FIGURE 1-8.

Effect of reduced caloric intake on the serum bilirubin level in Gilbert's syndrome. Reduced caloric intake may cause a significant increase in the serum unconjugated bilirubin level in patients with Gilbert's syndrome. This increase also occurs, although to a lesser degree, in normal individuals. In this particular case, the diet on days 7 to 9 supplied only 30 calories. Following refeeding, the serum bilirubin level rapidly returned to its prefasting level. The reciprocal relationship between caloric intake and the level of serum bilirubin is one reason for the fluctuation in serum bilirubin. The precise mechanism by which caloric intake affects the serum bilirubin level has not been defined. (*From* Felsher *et al.* [14]; with permission.)

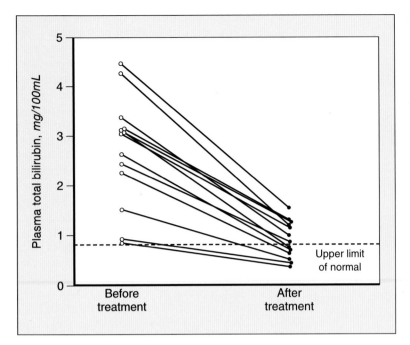

FIGURE 1-9.

Effect of phenobarbital administration on plasma bilirubin in Gilbert's syndrome. In this study, 13 patients with Gilbert's syndrome were given 180 mg/d of phenobarbital for 2 weeks. In each case, the plasma bilirubin level fell significantly. This reduction was evident as early as 2 to 3 days after treatment was begun; this lowering was maintained as long as the medication was continued. Reduction in the plasma bilirubin level was associated with, and was thought to be the result of, an increase in hepatic bilirubin UDP-glucuronyl transferase activity. (*From* Black and Sherlock [15]; with permission.)

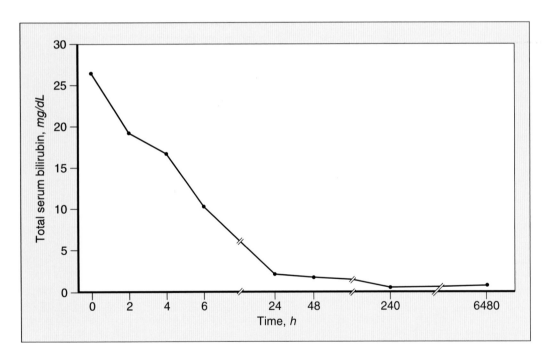

FIGURE 1-10.

Liver transplantation in the Crigler-Najjar syndrome. A neurologically normal 3-year-old girl with type I Crigler-Najjar syndrome was successfully treated with orthotopic liver transplantation. Preoperatively, phenobarbital therapy and phototherapy had not significantly lowered the serum bilirubin level. UDP-glucuronyl transferase activity in the patient's liver was not detectable. Following liver transplantation, the serum bilirubin concentration decreased to normal levels. Hours 0 and 6 indicate the start and completion of transplantation in this patient, respectively. Liver transplantation thus offers an effective method for treating this condition, which otherwise leads to death caused by kernicteric brain injury. (*From* Kaufman *et al.* [16]; with permission.)

CONJUGATED HYPERBILIRUBINEMIA

Evaluation

TABLE 1-6. CAUSES OF CONJUGATED HYPERBILIRUBINEMIA

BILIARY OBSTRUCTION	PARENCHYMAL LIVER DISEASES/CHOLESTASIS	METABOLIC DISORDERS
Choledocholithiasis	Viral hepatitis	Cholestatic jaundice of pregnancy
Malignancies	Alcoholic hepatitis	
Choledochal cyst	Cirrhosis (any etiology)	Dubin-Johnson syndrome
Bile duct stricture	Sepsis	Rotor's syndrome
Biliary atresia	Drugs	

TABLE 1-6.

The site of impairment that causes conjugated hyperbilirubinemia may be located variously from the hepatocyte to the distal common bile duct. Gallstones, carcinoma of the pancreas, and cholangiocarcinoma account for most cases of extrahepatic bile duct obstruction in adults, whereas biliary atresia is an important consideration in the jaundiced infant. Parenchymal liver diseases such as alcoholic hepatitis, primary biliary cirrhosis, and viral hepatitis, among others, cause jaundice by interfering with bile formation or bile flow in the small intrahepatic biliary ducts and ductules. Some cases of conjugated hyperbilirubinemia result from metabolic disorders. Cholestasis of pregnancy is a relatively common cause. Dubin-Johnson and Rotor's syndrome are rarer disorders in which conjugated hyperbilirubinemia is caused by a defect in the transport of conjugated bilirubin across the bile canalicular membrane.

TABLE 1-7. EVALUATION OF THE PATIENT WITH CONJUGATED HYPERBILIRUBINEMIA

ESSENTIAL FOR DIAGNOSIS	ANCILLARY AIDS TO CONFIRM CLINICAL SUSPICION
Age of patient	Liver/biliary ultrasound
History	CT
Physical examination	Nuclear medicine imaging
Liver chemistries	ERCP/PTC
	Liver biopsy

TABLE 1-7.

Evaluation of the jaundiced patient begins with a thorough clinical evaluation and routine liver chemistries. If conjugated hyperbilirubinemia is present, the clinical differential between extrahepatic obstruction and an intrahepatic process can usually be narrowed based on the history, physical examination, and liver chemistries. Ancillary studies for further evaluation of the jaundice are based on the clinical suspicion. Ultrasonography is accurate for imaging the gallbladder and extrahepatic bile ducts and is the test of choice when such disorders are suspected. The liver parenchyma can also be evaluated for tumors, cysts, and altered parenchymal density caused by fat or fibrosis. Ultrasound has the additional advantage of being relatively inexpensive and readily available. Computed tomography (CT) is an excellent means of evaluating the hepatic parenchyma and better visualizes the pancreas than ultrasonography. Nuclear medicine imaging is helpful in suspected biliary atresia. Cholangiography is the criterion standard for evaluating the biliary ducts. A cholangiogram can be obtained endoscopically through endoscopic retrograde cholangiopancreatography (ERCP) or through a percutaneous transhepatic cholangiogram (PTC). Therapeutic maneuvers to relieve biliary obstruction can often be done at the same time. Finally, liver biopsy in cases of suspected parenchymal disease may be the means to establish a diagnosis.

TABLE 1-8. BIOCHEMICAL PATTERNS IN LIVER DAMAGE

	HEPATOCELLULAR NECROSIS	CHOLESTASIS
Transaminase	8–200x*	1–8x
Alkaline phosphatase	1–3x	3–10x

* Times upper limit of normal

TABLE 1-8.

Pattern of liver chemistry abnormalities in the differential diagnosis of the jaundiced patient. The hepatocellular picture of injury implies that hepatocyte injury or death causes release of enzymes into the serum. High levels of serum transaminase over 1000 U/L occur in viral hepatitis, hepatic ischemia, drug hepatitis, and toxin exposure. Large increases in serum alkaline phosphatase with mildly elevated serum transaminases occur in disorders which are termed *cholestatic disorders*. The high levels of alkaline phosphatase are caused by increased synthesis of the enzyme and regurgitation into the serum. However, some disorders may present with a mixed picture so that classification by this scheme is not always possible.

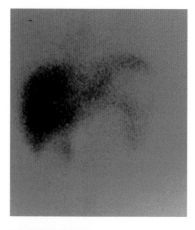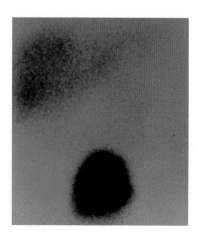

TABLE 1-9. ETIOLOGY OF JAUNDICE IN PREGNANCY

FIRST AND SECOND TRIMESTERS	THIRD TRIMESTER
Gallstones	Cholestasis of pregnancy
Viral hepatitis	Preeclampsia
Alcoholic liver disease	HELLP syndrome
Cholestasis of pregnancy	Acute fatty liver
Hyperemesis gravidarum	Gallstones
	Viral hepatitis

FIGURE 1-11.

Nuclear medicine scan in biliary atresia. Biliary atresia commonly presents within the first few months of life. Liver chemistries are elevated in a cholestatic pattern. Any portion of the biliary tree may be atretic, but in the most common form, the entire biliary tree (including the gallbladder) is fibrotic. Ultrasound may demonstrate an absent gallbladder. Hepatobiliary scintigraphy reveals good uptake of the isotope by the liver but no excretion into the biliary tree or bowel. Delayed excretion of isotopes may occur in neonatal hepatitis or partial obstruction so that caution must be used in interpreting the results of the nuclear imaging scan. The diagnosis of biliary atresia must be made promptly because cirrhosis develops quickly. Surgical correction is usually performed with a hepatic portoenterostomy (Kasai procedure). In cases where surgery is not successful or not possible, liver transplantation is the preferred treatment, and biliary atresia accounts for most liver transplantations in children. (*From* Majd *et al.* [17]; with permission.)

TABLE 1-9.

Jaundice during the first and second trimesters of pregnancy is often caused by the same illnesses to which a young woman may be susceptible if she is not pregnant. Accordingly, viral hepatitis, alcoholic liver disease, and biliary obstruction account for most cases. More rarely, patients with hyperemesis gravidarum develop jaundice for unknown reasons. Cholestasis of pregnancy may present during the first or second trimesters, although it more typically occurs in the third. Jaundice in the third trimester of pregnancy is more likely related to the pregnancy itself. Preeclampsia, the HELLP (Hemolysis, Elevated Liver enzymes, and Low Platelets) syndrome, and fatty liver of pregnancy are parts of a spectrum of toxemic liver involvement. They must be identified promptly because delivery of the infant is usually indicated to resolve these potentially fatal problems.

TABLE 1-10. CHOLESTASIS OF PREGNANCY

PATIENT CHARACTERISTICS	FEATURES
Personal history	Oral contraceptives
Family history	Common
Onset	Third trimester usually
Clinical features	Jaundice and pruritus
Liver histology	Cholestasis
Maternal outcome	Good
Fetal outcome	Increased premature delivery
	Increased stillbirths

TABLE 1-10.

Cholestasis of pregnancy typically begins during the third trimester, but it can present at any time during pregnancy. Patients often have had similar episodes with previous pregnancies or with oral contraceptive use. A family history of jaundice or pruritus during pregnancy is present in up to 50% of patients. The etiology is believed to be estrogen mediated. Liver histology shows cholestasis without other abnormalities, but biopsy is rarely necessary for the diagnosis. As far as the patient is concerned, this condition is benign and resolves after delivery of the infant. An increase in premature delivery and stillbirths has been reported, so cholestasis of pregnancy should be considered an increased risk for the fetus, however.

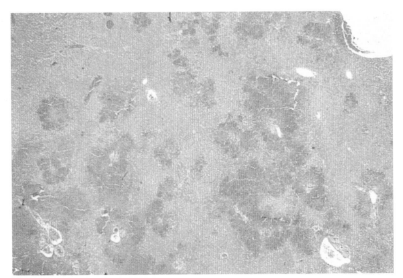

FIGURE 1-12.

Liver biopsy in the HELLP (Hemolysis, Elevated Liver enzymes, and Low Platelets) syndrome. Preeclampsia is characterized by hypertension, proteinuria, and edema. The addition of seizures defines eclampsia. Patients with preeclampsia or eclampsia have intense vasospasms that are thought to damage the vascular epithelium and result in platelet or fibrin deposition. Many women have mild liver involvement. The HELLP syndrome is a severe subset of this condition. Transaminases are often in the range of 200 to 400 U/L; the bilirubin is elevated. On liver histology, fibrin is deposited along the sinusoids, portal and periportal hemorrhage is present, and ischemic necrosis of hepatocytes is seen. If necrosis becomes confluent, hematomas may form beneath the capsule and rupture spontaneously. Treatment is aimed at controlling the hypertension and assessing the fetal lung maturity. Immediate delivery of the infant is indicated if either mother or infant shows signs of deterioration. (*From* Klatskin and Conn [18]; with permission.)

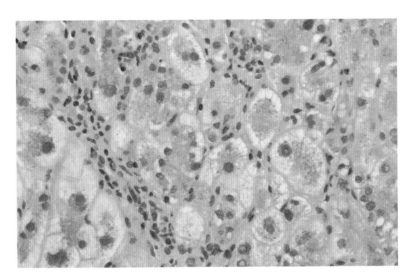

FIGURE 1-13.

Liver biopsy in fatty liver of pregnancy. Acute fatty liver of pregnancy is a rare disorder of the third trimester in which the hepatocytes become infiltrated with microvesicular fat in a pattern similar to that seen in Reye's syndrome. The incidence is estimated at 1/13,000 deliveries and is more common in primigravidas. The cause is unknown but may be an abnormality in lipid metabolism or mitochondrial function. Liver histology reveals microvesicular fat in a centrilobular distribution. The fat is primarily in the form of triglycerides and free fatty acids. Patients present with nausea, malaise, fatigue, and mild abdominal distress. Jaundice follows several weeks later. Renal dysfunction is a frequent complication. Prognosis is poor with maternal and fetal mortality rates at about 50%. Most authorities recommend prompt delivery of the infant once this entity is recognized because survival rates of both infant and mother are improved.

TABLE 1-11. DIAGNOSIS OF EXTRAHEPATIC OBSTRUCTION

EVALUATION	FALSE POSITIVE, %	FALSE NEGATIVE, %	SENSITIVITY, %	SPECIFICITY, %	OVERALL ACCURACY, %
Clinical (n = 50)	24	5	95	76	84
Ultrasonography (n = 49)	7	45	55	93	78
CT (n = 47)	7	37	63	93	81
Nuclear medicine scanning (n = 41)	12	59	41	88	68

TABLE 1-11.

In this 1983 study comparing modalities to diagnose extrahepatic bile duct obstruction [19], the clinical evaluation including history, physical examination, and liver chemistries was accurate. Combining the clinical evaluation with ultrasonography and requiring either or both to be positive raised both the sensitivity and specificity. Computed tomography (CT) had results similar to those in ultra-sonography. Nuclear medicine scanning produced an unacceptably high number of false negatives. Thus in the jaundiced patient, an experienced clinician is usually able to form an accurate opinion as to the likelihood of extrahepatic bile duct obstruction based on the clinical examination and liver chemistries.

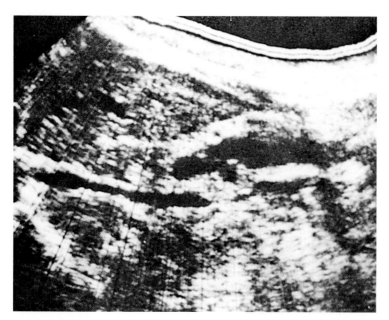

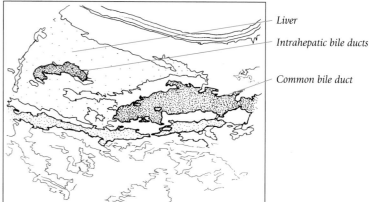

Liver

Intrahepatic bile ducts

Common bile duct

FIGURE 1-14.

Ultrasonography in extrahepatic biliary destruction. Dilation of the ducts suggests obstruction distally. Gallstones commonly lodge at the narrowest point of the common bile duct near the ampulla of Vater. Carcinoma of the head of the pancreas causes obstruction because the distal common bile duct passes through the head of the pancreas. Unfortunately, technical considerations often prevent more specific information than that the bile duct is dilated. The air contained in the duodenum obscures visual-ization of the distal common bile duct and the pancreas. Even if a gallstone is present, ultrasound will detect it only about 10% of the time. Similarly, a mass in the head of the pancreas may be missed because of the overlying bowel gas. A problem of greater concern is that a stone may be present in the common bile duct without dilation of the duct. If the clinical suspicion is high, a cholangiogram is warranted to exclude possible obstruction more definitively.

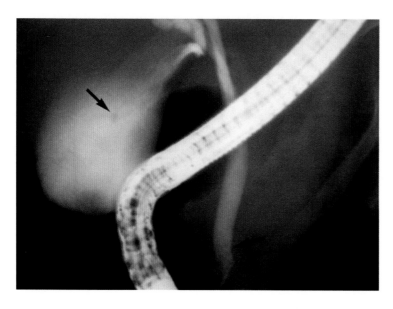

FIGURE 1-15.

Endoscopic retrograde cholangiopancreatography (ERCP) in extrahepatic biliary obstruction. ERCP is a technique for performing cholangiograms and pancreatograms using a side-viewing endoscope specifically adapted for this procedure. A small cannula is advanced into the ampulla of Vater, contrast is injected, and fluoroscopic images are recorded. Gallstones appear as radiolucent areas. Once stones are identified, an attempt is made to remove the stones by cutting the sphincter of Oddi and extracting the stones. ERCP with sphincterotomy and stone extraction may be sufficient therapy in elderly or frail patients with gallbladder in situ, because only 10% to 15% of patients develop biliary colic or cholecystitis after the procedure. In this photograph of a cholangiogram obtained at ERCP, tiny gallstones (*arrow*) are present in the gallbladder and the common bile duct.

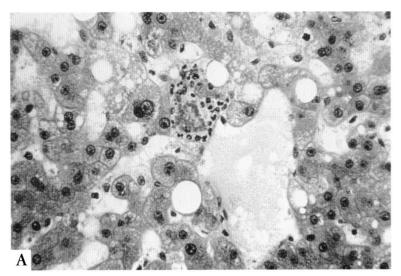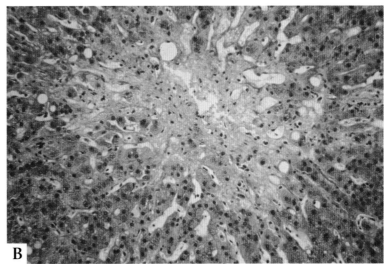

FIGURE 1-16.

Liver biopsy in alcoholic hepatitis. Alcoholic hepatitis is a common cause of jaundice in adults. Even if the patient denies alcohol consumption, one is suspicious of alcoholism if liver chemistries' results reveal moderate elevations of the transaminases with an aspartate aminotransferase that is two or more times greater than the alanine aminotransferase. Coupled with an elevated γ-glutamyl transpeptidase level and an elevated erythrocyte mean corpuscular volume, alcohol is the probable cause. If the diagnosis remains in doubt, liver biopsy may be indicated. Alcoholic hepatitis has a characteristic, although not pathognomonic, appearance. Marked fatty infiltration is usually present. Ballooning degeneration of hepatocytes is seen with Mallory hyalin often present in a centrilobular location (**A**). Mallory hyalin appears to be composed of intermediate filaments of the microtubular apparatus. Polymorphonuclear cell infiltration often occurs in association with Mallory hyalin. Finally, fibrosis may be present. In the earliest stage, fibrosis begins around the central vein (central hyaline sclerosis) (**B**).

TABLE 1-12. JAUNDICE RELATED TO DRUGS

HEPATOCELLULAR PATTERN	CHOLESTATIC PATTERN	MIXED PATTERN
Isoniazid	Chlorpromazine (Geneva Pharmaceuticals, Broomfield, CO)	Sulfonamides
Methyldopa	Erythromycin estolate	
Acetaminophen	Anabolic steroids	

TABLE 1-12.

Medications being taken should always be reviewed when evaluating the jaundiced patient. This table provides some examples of medications that have caused jaundice. Careful inquiry into use of over-the-counter medications, health foods, and nontraditional remedies, such as folk medicines, is important. Components of herbal teas such as germander or comfrey have caused liver disease and jaundice in unsuspecting patients. If in doubt as to whether a medication, health food, or remedy is causing the jaundice, the best course is to stop the suspected medication and follow-up with the patient. Improvement in liver chemistries is usually seen in 1 to 2 weeks if the discontinued medication is the offending agent.

TABLE 1-13. ETIOLOGY OF JAUNDICE IN THE CRITICALLY ILL PATIENT

HEPATOCELLULAR PATTERN	CHOLESTATIC PATTERN	HYPERBILIRUBINEMIA ONLY	MIXED PATTERN
Liver ischemia	Parenteral nutrition	Transfusions Hematoma Hemolysis	Multiple coincidental factors
			Sepsis
Congestive heart failure	Sepsis	Sepsis	
Drugs	Drugs	Drugs	Drugs

TABLE 1-13.

The differential diagnosis of jaundice in the critically ill patient is different from that of a patient presenting to the clinic with jaundice as the primary complaint [20]. Most often the critically ill patient has several reasons to be jaundiced. A careful history and physical examination are useful but most important is a careful review of the patient's hospital course. Particular attention should be directed to surgical procedures and the intraoperative course, episodes of hypotension, sepsis, medications, transfusions, evidence of heart failure, and feeding route. Any of these factors, alone or in combination, can cause jaundice. The jaundice is usually a marker of the severity of the underlying illness and not a sign of liver failure. Treatment is supportive and if the patient recovers from the primary illness, the jaundice will clear.

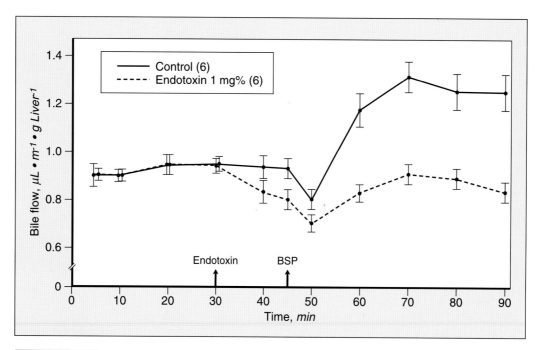

FIGURE 1-17.

Jaundice during infection. Jaundice can occur in the course of nonhepatic infection, particularly in children. The infection may be anywhere in the body and is frequently caused by gram-negative organisms. Bacteremia is common but not necessary for jaundice to develop. The bilirubin is predominantly conjugated, and the levels of alkaline phosphatase and transaminases are normal or only mildly elevated. Liver biopsy is rarely necessary but if performed reveals intrahepatic cholestasis with little hepatocyte necrosis. As the infection clears, the jaundice resolves with no long-term sequelae. The exact mechanism by which infection causes jaundice is not clear. Endotoxin has been implicated as one cause. Studies with isolated rat livers demonstrate decreased bile salt–independent bile flow when endotoxin is infused. In this experiment, bacterial lipopolysaccharide was added to the perfusate and 15 minutes later, sulfobromophthalein (an organic anion excreted by the liver into bile) was added. When exposed to endotoxin, decreased bile flow and sulfobromophthalein excretion occurred. (*From* Utili *et al.* [21]; with permission.)

TABLE 1-14. BILIRUBIN LOAD IN TRANSFUSIONS AND HEMATOMAS

Transfusion	250 mg bilirubin/U blood
Hematoma	2500 mg bilirubin/500 mL

TABLE 1-14.

Under normal circumstances, the liver readily excretes the additional bilirubin load resulting from a blood transfusion or a hematoma. In a critically ill patient, poor perfusion of the liver, sepsis, medications, and other factors may impair the liver's ability to excrete excess bilirubin. Approximately 10% of transfused erythrocytes are nonviable at the time of transfusion and will be destroyed quickly. The bilirubin produced from these cells or erythrocytes in a hematoma may cause jaundice in the critically ill patient.

TABLE 1-15. CHARACTERISTICS OF DUBIN-JOHNSON SYNDROME AND ROTOR'S SYNDROME

	DUBIN-JOHNSON SYNDROME	ROTOR'S SYNDROME
Serum bilirubin (mg/dL)	Usually 2.0–5.0	Usually 2.0–5.0
Conjugated fraction	>50%	> 50%
Serum bile acid level	Normal	Normal
Liver appearance	Black	Normal
Liver histology	Normal except for dark pigment granules, predominantly in centrilobular distribution	Normal
Urinary coproporphyrin	Normal or mild increase in total; isomer I > 80%	Marked increase in total; isomer I < 80%
Inheritance	Autosomal recessive	Autosomal recessive

TABLE 1-15.

These disorders are associated with conjugated hyperbilirubinemia, resulting from abnormalities in hepatocellular transport of conjugated bilirubin into bile. The liver in both conditions is histologically normal except for the presence of dark pigmented granules in the hepatocytes of the patient with Dubin-Johnson syndrome, predominantly in centrilobular areas. The pigment is related to melanin, but the mechanism by which it accumulates has not been determined. In Rotor's syndrome, there is no pigment accumulation. Both conditions are benign, and therapy is not required.

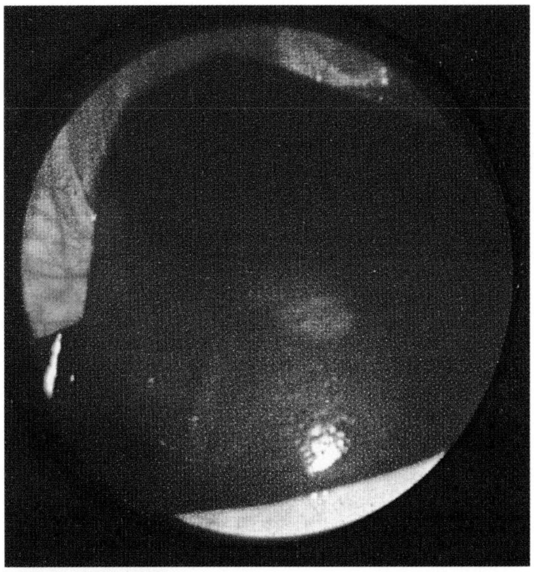

FIGURE 1-18.

Liver in the Dubin-Johnson syndrome. This illustration shows the black left lobe of the liver in a patient with the Dubin-Johnson syndrome. The surface of the liver is smooth. In the upper left of the figure are the ligamentum teres and the falciform ligament. (*From* Beck [22]; with permission.)

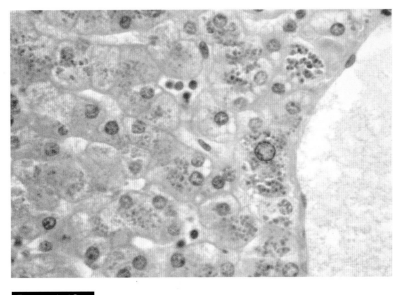

FIGURE 1-19.

Liver histology in the Dubin-Johnson syndrome. The black appearance of the liver in the Dubin-Johnson syndrome is caused by the presence of dark pigment granules in hepatocytes, predominantly located in centilobular areas. The pigment is related to melanin.

TABLE 1-16. PROGNOSTIC VALUE OF SERUM BILIRUBIN LEVEL

CONDITION	LEVEL INDICATING POOR PROGNOSIS
Alcoholic cirrhosis	>3 mg/dL
Primary biliary cirrhosis	>5 mg/dL
Fulminant hepatic failure	>18 mg/dL
Alcoholic hepatitis	>20 mg/dL

TABLE 1-16.

Prognostic value of the serum bilirubin level. In addition to its use in the evaluation and follow-up of patients with hepatobiliary disorders, the serum bilirubin level provides prognostic information in some disorders. This information is helpful when deciding on the therapeutic management for these patients. The serum bilirubin level has been used for a long time in staging patients with alcoholic cirrhosis to predict surgical mortality [23]. Together with the prothrombin time, it has also been used to predict those patients with alcoholic hepatitis who may have a fatal outcome [24]. Similarly, it has been used in patients with fulminant hepatic failure [25]. Finally, the serum bilirubin level has been used for predicting the prognosis of patients with primary biliary cirrhosis and primary sclerosing cholangitis in order to decide on the timing of liver transplantation. The Mayo Clinic has developed a scoring system by which the serum bilirubin level and other factors can be entered into a formula that predicts the survival of these patients at different intervals [26,27].

REFERENCES AND RECOMMENDED READING

1. Watson CJ: Historical review of bilirubin chemistry. In *Chemistry and Physiology of Bile Pigments*. Edited by Berk PD, Berlin NI. Washington, DC: US Government Printing Office; 1977:3–16.

2. Berk PD, Noyer C: Bilirubin metabolism and the hereditary hyperbilirubinemias. *Semin Liver Dis* 1994, 14:321–394.

3. Schmid R: Direct-reacting bilirubin, bilirubin glucuronide, in serum, bile and urine. *Science* 1956, 124:76–77.

4. Billing BH, Cole PG, Lathe GH: The excretion of bilirubin as a diglucuronide giving the direct van den Bergh reaction. *Biochem J* 1957, 65:774–784.

5. Talafant E: Properties and composition of bile pigment giving a direct diazo reaction. *Nature* 1956, 178:312.

6. Tenhuren R, Marver HS, Schmid R: The enzymatic conversion of heme to bilirubin by microsomal heme oxygenase. *Proc Natl Acad Sci U S A* 1969, 61:748–755.

7. Levi AJ, Gatmaitan Z, Arias IM: Two hepatic cytoplastic protein fractions, Y and Z, and their possible role in the hepatic uptake of bilirubin, sulfobromophthalein, and other anions. *J Clin Invest* 1969, 48:2156–2167.

8. Scharschmidt BF, Waggoner JG, Berk PD: Hepatic organic anion uptake in the rat. *J Clin Invest* 1975, 56:1280–1292.

9. Onde Elferink RPJ, Ottenhoff R, Liefting W, *et al.*: Hepatobiliary transport of glutathione and glutathione conjugates in rats with hereditary hyperbilirubinemia. *J Clin Invest* 1989, 84:476–483.

10. Bloomer JR: Jaundice—why it happens—what to do. *Med Times* 1979, 107:43–52.

11. Weiss JS, Gautam A, Lauff JJ, *et al.*: The clinical importance of a protein-bound fraction of serum bilirubin in patients with hyperbilirubinemia. *N Engl J Med* 1983, 309:147–150.

12. Bloomer JR, Berk PD, Howe RB, Berlin NI: Interpretation of plasma bilirubin levels based on studies with radioactive bilirubin. *JAMA* 1971, 218:216–220.

13. Tiribelli C, Ostrow JD: New concepts in bilirubin chemistry, transport and metabolism: Report of the second international bilirubin workshop, April 9-11, 1992, Trieste, Italy. *Hepatology* 1993, 17:715–736.

14. Felsher BF, Rickard D, Redeker AG: The reciprocal relation between caloric intake and the degree of hyperbilirubinemia in Gilbert's syndrome. *N Engl J Med* 1970, 283:170–172.

15. Black M, Sherlock S: Treatment of Gilbert's syndrome with phenobarbitone. *Lancet* 1970, 1:1359–1362.

16. Kaufman SS, Wood RP, Shaw BW Jr, *et al.*: Orthotopic liver transplantation for type I Crigler-Najjar syndrome. *Hepatology* 1986, 6:1259–1262.

17. Majd M, Reba RC, Altman RP: Hepatobiliary scintigraphy with ^{99m}Tc PIPIDA in the evaluation of neonatal jaundice. *Pediatrics* 1981, 67:140–145.

18. Klatskin G, Conn HO: *Histopathology of the Liver*, vol 11. New York: Oxford University Press; 1993.

19. O'Connor KW, Snodgrass PJ, Swonder JE, *et al.*: A blinded prospective study comparing four current noninvasive approaches in the differential diagnosis of medical versus surgical jaundice. *Gastroenterology* 1983, 84:1498–1504.

20. Kools AM, Bloomer JR: Jaundice in the ICU: A bedside approach. In *Perspectives in Critical Care*, vol. 2. Edited by Cerra FB. St. Louis: Quality Medical Publishing; 1989:165–177.

21. Utili R, Abernathy CO, Zimmerman HJ: Studies on the effects of *E. coli* endotoxin on canalicular bile formation in the isolated perfused rate liver. *J Lab Clin Med* 1977, 89:471–482.

22. Beck K: *Color Atlas of Laparoscopy*. Philadelphia: WB Saunders; 1984:213.

23. Child CG III, Turcotte J: *The Liver and Portal Hypertension*. Philadelphia: WB Saunders; 1965.

24. Maddrey WC, Boitnott JK, Bedine MS, *et al.*: Corticosteroid therapy of alcoholic hepatitis. *Gastroenterology* 1978, 75:193–199.

25. O'Grady JG, Alexander GJM, Hayllar KM, Williams R: Early indicators of prognosis in fulminant hepatic failure. *Gastroenterology* 1989, 97:439–445.

26. Dickson ER, Grambsch PM, Fleming TR, *et al.*: Prognosis in primary biliary cirrhosis: Model for decision making. *Hepatology* 1989, 10:1–7.

27. Dickson ER, Murtaugh PA, Wiesner RH, *et al.*: Primary sclerosing cholangitis: Refinement and validation of survival models. *Gastroenterology* 1992, 103:1893–1901.

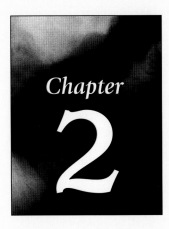

Chapter 2

Acute Viral Hepatitis

RAYMOND S. KOFF

This collection of figures and tables focuses on the subject of acute viral hepatitis, an area of continuing expansion of knowledge and change. Each of the five known agents of human viral hepatitis—hepatitis A virus, hepatitis B virus, hepatitis C virus, hepatitis D virus, and hepatitis E virus—is described in some detail and the natural history of the diseases with which they are associated is defined. The genomic structure of the nucleic acid of these agents, the epidemiologic features of infection, the serologic characteristics of each infection, and where available, immunoprophylaxis are described.

TABLE 2-1. THE HUMAN HEPATITIS VIRUSES

FEATURE	HAV	HBV	HCV	HDV	HEV
Family	Picornavirus	Hepadnavirus	Flavivirus	Satellite	Alpha-like supergroup
Genome	RNA	DNA	RNA	RNA	RNA
Virion size, *nm*	27	42	55	35	32
Enveloped	No	HBsAg	Yes	HBsAg	No
Enteric transmission	Yes	No	No	No	Yes
Carrier state	No	Yes	Yes	Yes	No
Chronic hepatitis	No	Yes	Yes	Yes	No

TABLE 2-1.

Human hepatitis viruses. The five known agents of viral hepatitis belong to distinct, and unrelated, classes of viruses. Four of the five viruses (hepatitis A virus [HAV], hepatitis C virus [HCV], hepatitis D virus [HDV], and hepatitis E virus [HEV]) are RNA–containing viruses whereas the fifth virus, hepatitis B virus (HBV), is a DNA–containing agent. The two nonenveloped agents, HAV and HEV, are characteristically transmitted through enteric routes of spread, and neither is associated with a carrier state of chronic hepatitis. In contrast, the enveloped viruses (HBV, HDV, and HCV) may lead to persistent infection and chronic hepatitis. HBsAg—hepatitis B surface antigen.

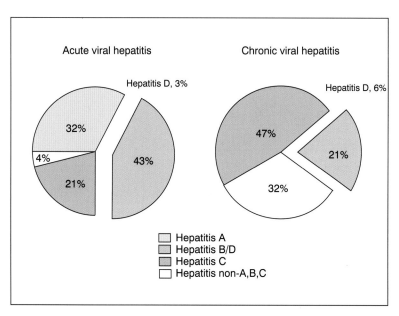

FIGURE 2-1.

Acute and chronic viral hepatitis proportioned by agent. These figures provide an overview of the relative contributions of each of the agents to acute and chronic viral hepatitis in the United States. Hepatitis E is not shown in the acute hepatitis pie chart because only a handful of cases of this imported infection are reported annually in the United States. The etiology of the small proportion of cases of acute hepatitis, labeled non-A,B,C, remains uncertain. As shown in the chronic viral hepatitis diagram, hepatitis A plays no role. Non-A,B,C is considerably more prevalent in chronic than acute hepatitis, but just as in the case of acute hepatitis, the responsible agent or agents remains to be identified. (*Adapted from* Alter and Hadler [1]; with permission.)

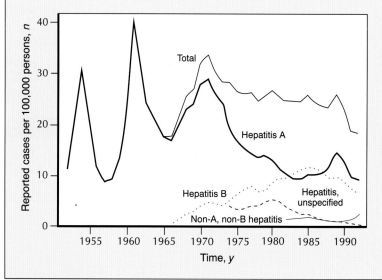

FIGURE 2-2.

Acute hepatitis in the United States from 1952 to 1992. Viral hepatitis has been a reportable disease in the United States for over 4 decades. Although reporting is incomplete, asymptomatic infections are infrequently identified, and serologic testing is a relatively recent innovation, reported rates probably are a reasonable reflection of trends over time. The peaks shown for 1954, 1961, and 1971, and the minor blip for 1989 are believed to represent epidemics of hepatitis A. Based on attempts to correct for under-reporting and asymptomatic infections, the Centers for Disease Control and Prevention estimated that about 130,000 hepatitis A virus infections occurred in 1992. (*Adapted from* McQuillan *et al.* [2]; with permission.)

Hepatitis A

Virus

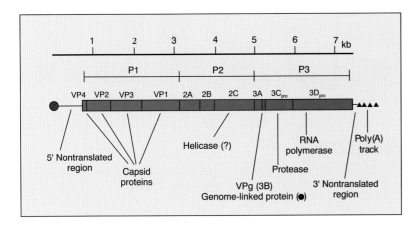

FIGURE 2-3.

Hepatitis A virus (HAV). The HAV genome is 7.4-kb long. A 5′ nontranslated region precedes the open reading frame that encodes a large polyprotein that is cleaved into capsid (structural) proteins (virion polypeptides [VP]), labeled VP4 to VP1, and nonstructural proteins (P), the P2 and P3 regions. It is believed that the HAV capsid contains 60 copies of VP1 to VP3. VP4 has been difficult to demonstrate; it may be an internal VP. Among the nonstructural proteins are a protease, an RNA polymerase, and possibly a helicase. A genome-linked protein, VPg (3B), has also been reported in the nonstructural area. At the 3′ end, a short nontranslated region is followed by a poly(A) track. (*Adapted from* Brown *et al.* [3]; with permission.)

Serology

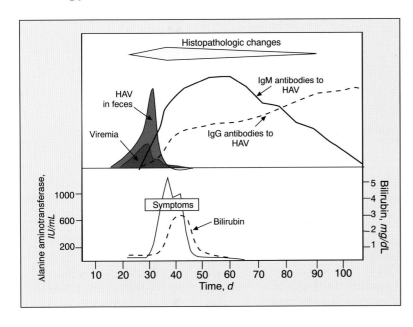

FIGURE 2-4.

Hepatitis A virus (HAV) serologic events. Fecal shedding of HAV is first seen during the latter half of the incubation period, before the development of histopathologic changes in the liver, and reaches a peak with the onset of symptoms and elevation of the alanine aminotransferase levels. Viral shedding declines rapidly thereafter and is often absent within a week after the onset of symptoms. Viremia is usually short-lived. Immunoglobulin M (IgM) antibodies to HAV appear concomitant with the onset of symptoms, reach peak levels within several weeks, and may disappear at 3 to 6 months. In contrast, immunoglobulin G (IgG) antibodies to HAV, the neutralizing, protective antibody, reaches peak levels during the convalescent phase and decline slowly over many decades. (*Adapted from* Brown *et al.* [3]; with permission.)

Epidemiology

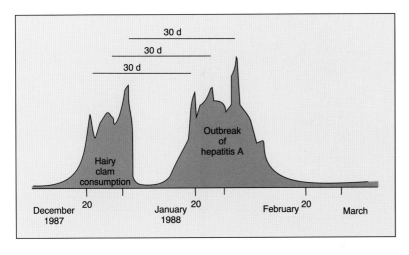

FIGURE 2-5.

Incubation period of hepatitis A virus. This very graphic demonstration of the 30-day incubation period of hepatitis A is drawn from an analysis of the interval between hairy clam consumption and the onset of illness during an extraordinarily large outbreak in Shanghai in 1988. Over 290,000 cases were estimated to have occurred. (*From* Hu *et al.* [4]; with permission.)

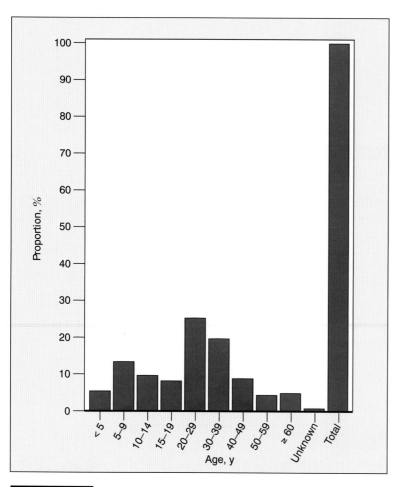

FIGURE 2-6.

Cases of hepatitis A virus (HAV)—proportion by age. Among reported cases of HAV in the United States for 1992, a bimodal age distribution was observed with peaks in the 5- to 9-year-old group and in the 20- to 29-year-old group. In earlier years, HAV was predominantly a disease of children below age 15. The evolution into a bimodal pattern with a predominance in the young adult age group suggests a changing prevalence of infection and susceptibility (*see* Fig. 2-11). (*Adapted from* McQuillan *et al.* [2]; with permission.)

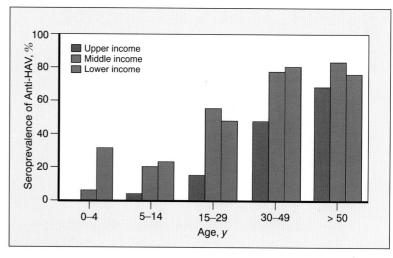

FIGURE 2-7.

Infection with hepatitis A virus (HAV) by age and socioeconomic level. The relationship of age and socioeconomic class to seroprevalence of HAV infection was analyzed in Corpus Christi, Texas in 1967. In the randomly selected population studied, antibodies to HAV (Anti-HAV) were present in 44% of the total group, a figure higher than the present estimate of 32% for a representative sample of the United States, as studied in 1988 to 1991. As anticipated, seroprevalence increased proportionately with increasing age and was lowest, within each age group, in the upper income groups. (*Adapted from* McQuillan *et al.* [2]; with permission.)

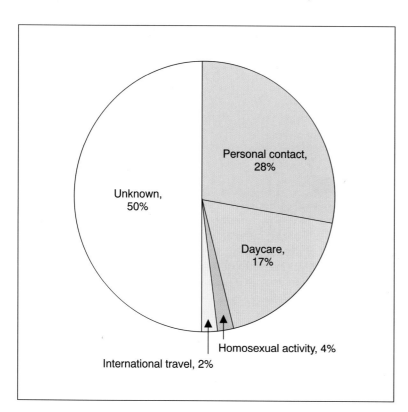

FIGURE 2-8.

Risk factors of acute hepatitis A virus infection. This diagram demonstrates results of an analysis of certain risk factors (sources of exposure) associated with hepatitis A in cases reported in four sentinel counties of the United States in 1992. Personal contact, usually with an infected household contact, was found in 28% of cases and an association with a day care center in 17%. Homosexual activity and international travel were less important factors. As shown, no risk factors could be identified in half of the cases. (*Adapted from* McQuillan *et al.* [2]; with permission.)

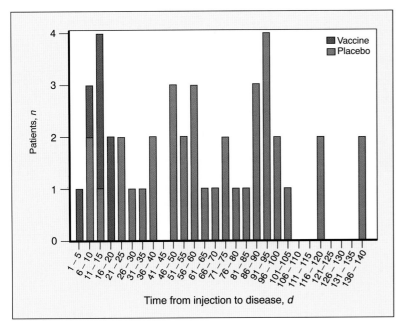

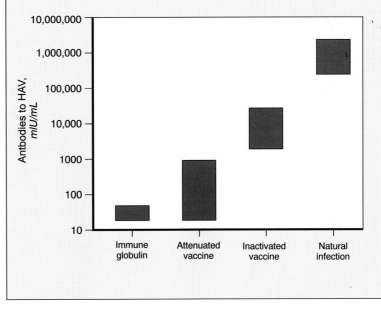

FIGURE 2-9.

Vaccine against hepatitis A virus (HAV). During a summer outbreak of HAV among children in a Hasidic Jewish community in upstate New York, a single dose of a formalin-inactivated HAV vaccine or a placebo was given to 1037 seronegative, healthy children (half received vaccine and half received placebo). As shown in this figure, during the first 20 days after vaccination, seven clinical cases of HAV occurred in the vaccinated group and three cases occurred in the placebo group. Thereafter, no clinical cases of HAV occurred in the vaccinated group. These observations indicate that an inactivated HAV vaccine is highly protective against clinically apparent HAV. (*Adapted from* Werzberger *et al.* [5]; with permission.)

FIGURE 2-10.

Serum levels of antibodies against hepatitis A virus (HAV). Although the absolute level of antibodies to HAV necessary for protection from infection is not established, it seems probable that levels in excess of 10 to 20 mIU/mL, a range of values seen after injection of immune globulin, are protective. As shown here, antibodies to HAV levels reach very high levels following natural infection. Levels after administration of inactivated HAV vaccines are lower, but exceed by several fold those reported to be induced by attenuated vaccine preparations. It is presumed that the higher the level of antibodies to HAV, the longer the duration of protection will be. (*Adapted from* Lemon and Stapleton [6]; with permission.)

FIGURE 2-11.

Impact of declining hepatitis A infections. The seroprevalence of hepatitis A, as determined by measuring antibodies to hepatitis A virus, was studied in the northern region of Spain from 1986 to 1987 and again in 1992. **A,** Seroprevalence rates declined for each age group studied. **B,** As anticipated, reported cases of hepatitis A also fell in this geographic region. **C,** Most importantly, the mean age of patients with serologically confirmed hepatitis A rose from 15.5 to 20.1 years. These observations indicate that in this region, as the infection rate declines, susceptibility increases and the age of infected patients also rises. Because increasing age at time of hepatitis A acquisition is associated with an increased frequency of symptomatic and clinically severe disease, it seems likely that morbidity will increase over time. (*Adapted from* Perez-Trallero *et al.* [7]; with permission.)

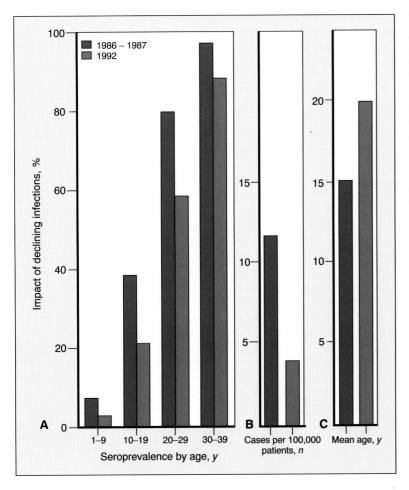

TABLE 2-2. IMMUNOPROPHYLAXIS OF HEPATITIS A: IMMUNE GLOBULIN VS INACTIVATED HAV VACCINE

FEATURE	IMMUNE GLOBULIN	INACTIVATED HAV VACCINE
Derived from blood	Yes	No
Acquisition of Anti-HAV	Passive	Active
Preferred injection site	Deltoid	Deltoid
Peak Anti-HAV level	Low	High, approaching level in natural infection
Preexposure efficacy	Yes	Yes
Duration of protection	2–3 months	>6–10 years
Postexposure efficacy	Yes, if given within 2 weeks of exposure	Possibly, but limited data
Cost	$	$$$

TABLE 2-2.

Immune globulin, used for passive immunoprophylaxis of hepatitis A virus (HAV) infection for nearly 50 years, is a relatively inexpensive blood product that provides good preexposure protection and some postexposure protective efficacy if give early after exposure [8]. Unfortunately, peak antibodies to HAV (Anti-HAV) levels are low and the passively acquired antibodies disappear and protection wanes after a few months. In contrast, the more costly inactivated HAV vaccine induces Anti-HAV production which may reach levels similar to those seen after natural infection. Preexposure protective efficacy is excellent [9], and based on Anti-HAV levels it is likely that protection may last for years. Whether the inactivated HAV vaccine is effective in postexposure settings requires further study.

Hepatitis E

Virus

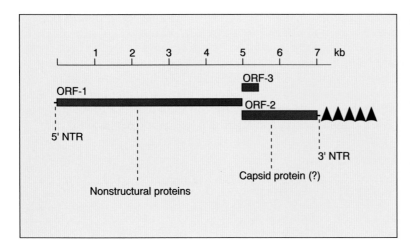

FIGURE 2-12.

Genome of hepatitis E virus (HEV). The HEV genome is 7.5 kb in length. A very short 5' nontranslated region (NTR) precedes the initial open reading frame (ORF-1) that encodes nonstructural HEV proteins. A helicase, RNA polymerase, protease, and methyltransferase are believed to be included among these proteins. The second open reading frame (ORF-2) appears to encode the major capsid protein and an epitope recognized by antibodies in convalescent sera. A third, smaller open reading frame (ORF-3) overlaps the others and also may encode an epitope that induces antibodies in infected individuals. (*Adapted from* Brown *et al.* [3]; with permission.)

Serology

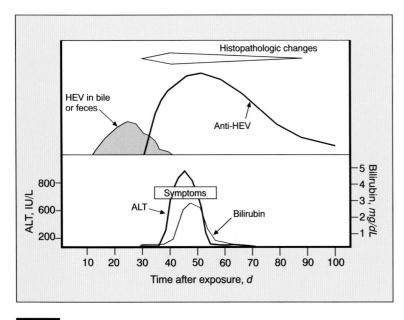

FIGURE 2-13.

Serologic events in hepatitis E virus (HEV) infection. Although information on the subject is very limited, the incubation period of HEV is, as shown here, approximately 40 days. HEV particles may appear in bile and then feces during the second half of the incubation period. Fecal HEV shedding may peak before the onset of jaundice or during the first week after the onset of jaundice. HEV disappears rapidly; it has not been identified in stool samples obtained 8 to 15 days after the onset of jaundice. Antibodies to HEV (Anti-HEV) have been found in sera taken during the acute phase. Although levels of Anti-HEV appear to decline during the late convalescent phase, the duration of detectable Anti-HEV remains uncertain. ALT—alanine aminotransferase. (*Adapted from* Brown *et al.* [3]; with permission.)

Epidemiology

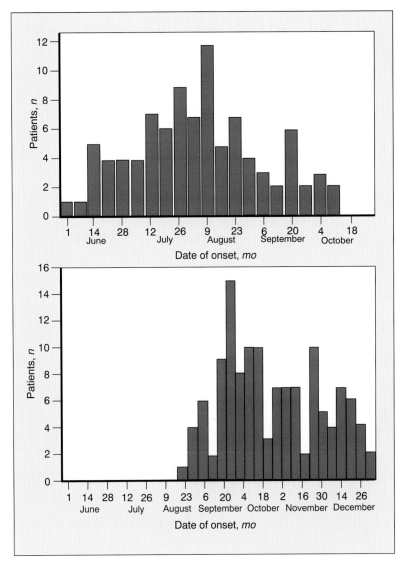

FIGURE 2-14.

Epidemic curve of hepatitis E virus (HEV). This figure represents
the epidemic curve of HEV cases in two rural villages in Mexico,
reported from 1986 to 1987. Attack rates of icteric hepatitis were
similar in both communities, 5% and 6%, and both outbreaks
lasted about 5 months. Epidemiologic studies suggested a strong
association with water in the first outbreak (*top*) but not in the
second outbreak (*bottom*). These outbreaks were the first reported
occurrence of enterically transmitted non-A, non-B hepatitis (HEV-
like particles were identified by immune electron microscopy in
stool specimens) in the Americas. (*Adapted from* Velazquez *et al.*
[10]; with permission.)

Hepatitis B

Virus

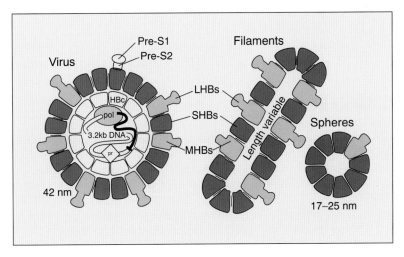

FIGURE 2-15.

Hepatitis B virus (HBV) particles. This schematic diagram shows
the 42-nm HBV particle, tubular filaments, and spherical particles
composed of the HBV envelope proteins, which also appear in the
circulation of HBV–infected individuals. The envelope of intact
HBV contains the so-called small (SHBs), middle-sized (MHBs),
and large (LHBs) envelope proteins (hepatitis B surface antigen
[HBsAg]). Although the filaments contain similar proportions of
these proteins, the spheres contain less of the large protein. The
small protein of HBsAg is specified by the *S* gene, the middle
protein by *S* and *Pre-S2*, and the large protein by *S*, *Pre-S1*, and
Pre-S2. The *S*, *Pre-2*, and *Pre-S1* domains are shown on the LHBs
of the HBV particle. The 3.2-kb DNA, HBV DNA polymerase (pol),
and a primase protein (pr) are shown within the capsid (HBc).
(*Adapted from* Gerlich [11]; with permission.)

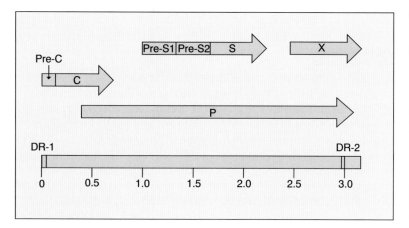

FIGURE 2-16.

Hepatitis B virus (HBV) open reading frames (ORF). In this diagram, the four overlapping HBV ORFs have been presented in a linear rendition; the genome is usually depicted in a circular model. The Pre-S and S ORFs encode the hepatitis B surface antigen proteins, the X ORF encodes a protein that is a transcriptional transactivator, the P ORF encodes the DNA polymerase and primase, and the Pre-C and C ORFs encode hepatitis B core antigen and hepatitis B e antigen. The direct repeat sequences, DR-1 and DR-2, are also shown. (*Adapted from* Yoffe and Noonan [12]; with permission.)

TABLE 2-3. HBV mRNA TRANSCRIPTS

LENGTH, *kb*	FUNCTION
3.5	HBV DNA replication; expression of precore/core and HBV polymerase
2.4	Expression of Pre-S1, Pre-S2, and HBsAg
2.1	Expression of Pre-S2 and HBsAg
0.7	Expression of X protein

TABLE 2-3.

Hepatitis B virus (HBV) messenger RNA (mRNA) transcripts. A number of HBV mRNA transcripts have been identified through studies of the replication of the virus and replicative intermediates. HBsAg—hepatitis B surface antigen.

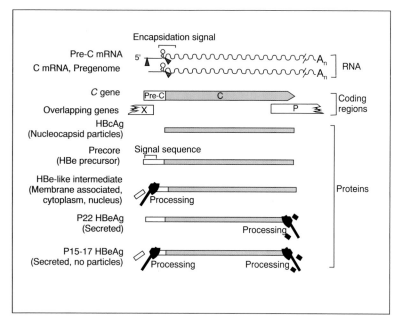

FIGURE 2-17.

Precore and core messenger RNA (mRNA) transcripts, open reading frames, and products. This schematic diagram illustrates the production of hepatitis B core antigen (HBcAg) and hepatitis B e antigen (HBeAg). The HBcAg is used in the production of hepatitis B virus (HBV) nucleocapsid particles. Part of the signal sequence on the precore protein is cleft off to form HBeAg intermediates, which are further processed by proteolytic cleavage to form the secreted, nonparticulate HBeAg proteins. HBeAg is an imperfect marker of active HBV replication; in HBV precore mutant strains, replication may occur in the absence of detectable HBeAg. HBe—hepatitis B e. (*Adapted from* Miska and Will [13]; with permission.)

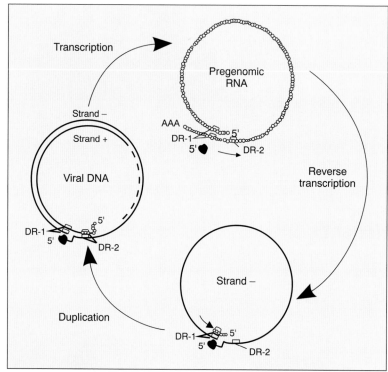

FIGURE 2-18.

Replication of hepatitis B virus (HBV). This simplified depiction of HBV replication nonetheless highlights the key steps of the complex process. A pregenomic RNA, larger than a genome, is transcribed from the minus strand of HBV DNA in the HBV in nucleocapsid particles. Through reverse transcription of the pregenomic RNA, a nascent minus strand of HBV DNA is produced. This strand then serves as a template for the synthesis of the plus strand of DNA. DR—direct repeat. (*Adapted from* Bova *et al.* [14]; with permission.)

Hepatitis B mutants

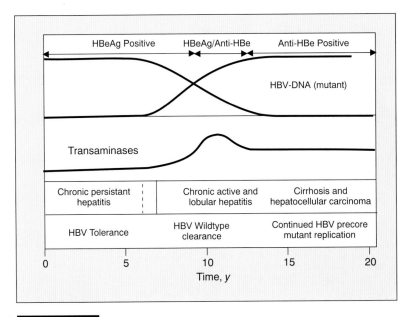

FIGURE 2-19.

Hepatitis B e antigen (HBeAg)–negative mutant hepatitis B virus (HBV). The emergence of the HBeAg–negative (precore) mutant is shown here schematically. After years of active replication of the wild-type HBV, with the presence of HBeAg, and mild chronic hepatitis, the precore mutant emerges and may dominate the natural history of HBV infection. HBeAg is lost, antibodies to HBeAg (Anti-HBe) become detectable, mutant HBV replication continues, and the sequelae of cirrhosis and hepatocellular carcinoma may become evident. (*Adapted from* Carmen *et al.* [15]; with permission.)

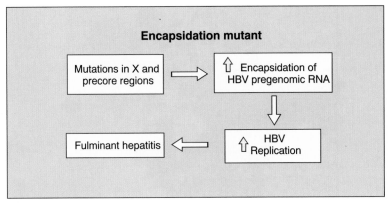

FIGURE 2-20.

Encapsidation mutant of hepatitis B virus (HBV). Among the many HBV mutants that have been identified in the past few years, the so-called encapsidation mutant has received considerable attention because of a possible association with fulminant HBV. Limited observations suggest that this HBV variant arises as a consequence of mutations in the X and precore regions. As a result, encapsidation of HBV pregenomic RNA is more efficient than normal, leading to increased HBV replication, which in turn leads to fulminant hepatitis. (*Adapted from* Hasegawa *et al.* [16]; with permission.)

Natural history

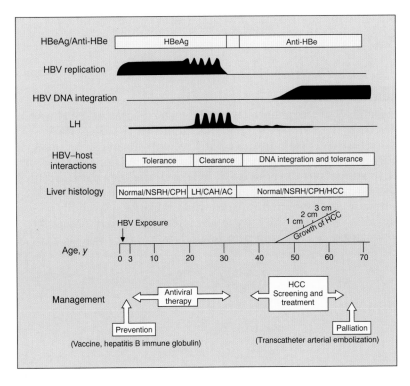

FIGURE 2-21.

Natural history of hepatitis B virus (HBV) infection. The natural history of HBV infection in individuals who acquire infection early in life, in the absence of immunoprophylaxis, is depicted in this schematic. During the early period after HBV acquisition, replication is high, hepatitis B e antigen (HBeAg) is present, and liver histology may be normal or show mild chronic hepatitis. Antiviral therapy at this point may alter the natural history of the disease. In its absence, over a period of time, HBV replication may diminish, HBeAg may disappear, and hepatic inflammation may increase. Eventually, HBV DNA genomic or subgenomic integration into the host hepatocyte may occur. Over many years, especially in patients who develop cirrhosis, hepatocellular carcinoma (HCC) may develop. AC—active cirrhosis; Anti-HBe—antibodies to HBeAg; CAH—chronic active hepatitis; CPH—chronic persistent hepatitis; LH—lobular hepatitis; NSRH—nonspecific reactive hepatitis. (*Adapted from* Chen [17]; with permission.)

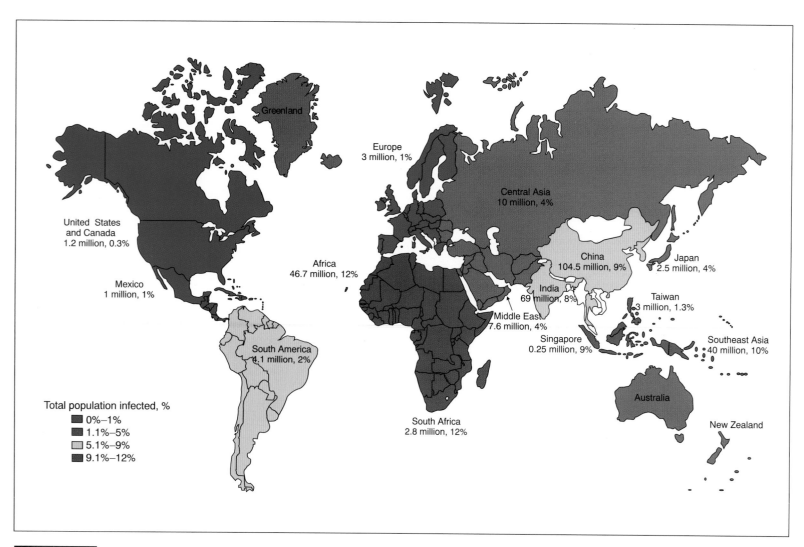

FIGURE 2-22.

Hepatitis B virus (HBV) worldwide. Chronic HBV infection is believed to affect close to 300 million people throughout the world. The prevalence of the hepatitis B surface antigen carrier state varies widely from area to area and even within the same country. None-theless, very high carrier rates have been identified in sub-Saharan Africa, in Southeast Asia, and in China. In addition to persistent infection, a very large proportion of the population of these regions has been exposed to HBV and infected by this virus. However, in contrast to the carriers, these individuals have successfully cleared the virus and resolved the infection. (*Adapted from* Hamilton and Gross [18]; with permission.)

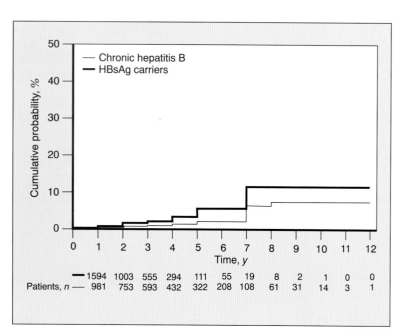

FIGURE 2-23.

Hepatitis B surface antigen (HBsAg) clearance. Clearance of HBsAg has been studied in Asian patients identified as either HBsAg carriers or as HBsAg–positive patients with chronic hepatitis B. HBsAg clearance in asymptomatic HBsAg carriers appears to occur at an annual rate of about 0.8%. HBsAg clearance in patients with chronic hepatitis B is slightly lower, that is, at a rate of about 0.5% annually. As shown in this figure, the cumulative probability of clearing HBsAg is greater in the asymptomatic carriers. (*Adapted from* Liaw *et al.* [19]; with permission.)

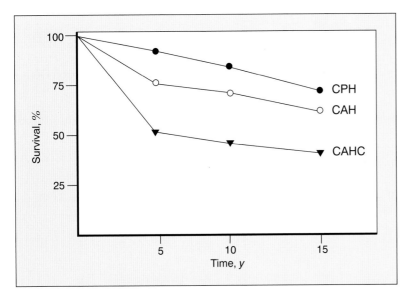

FIGURE 2-24.

Survival in chronic hepatitis B. This figure shows long-term survival data for 379 patients with chronic hepatitis B identified in research done at Stanford University. Patients were classified into three groups based on initial histologic assessment: chronic persistent hepatitis (CPH), chronic active hepatitis (CAH), and chronic active hepatitis with cirrhosis (CAHC). The marked differences in survival rates at 5, 10, and 15 years of follow-up indicate that histologic classification has prognostic value. (*Adapted from* Weissberg *et al.* [20] and Ladenheim *et al.* [21]; with permission.)

Epidemiology

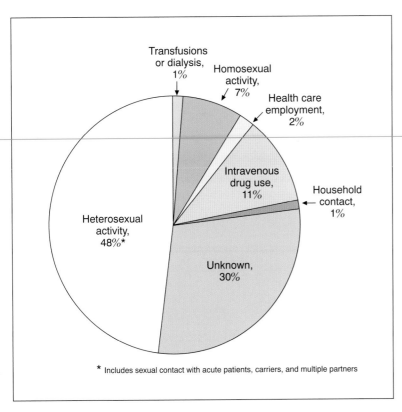

FIGURE 2-25.

Risk factors for infection with hepatitis B virus (HBV). This diagram depicts an analysis of risk factors (sources of exposure) associated with HBV in cases reported in four sentinel counties of the United States in 1992. The importance of sexual activity as a probable source of infection is reflected in the very large proportion of cases in which patients had heterosexual contact with acute cases, HBV carriers, and multiple sex partners. Homosexual activity was reported in 7% of cases and intravenous drug use in 11%. A small percentage of patients reported blood transfusion, dialysis, health care employment, or nonsexual household contact with known HBV cases. In 30% of cases, however, no known risk factors could be identified. (*Adapted from* McQuillan *et al.* [2]; with permission.)

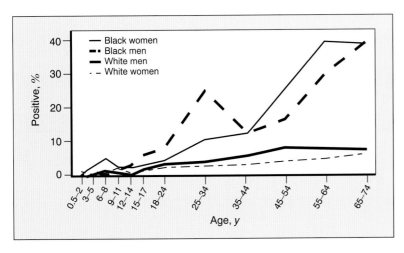

FIGURE 2-26.

Age-specific hepatitis B virus (HBV) prevalence in the United States, 1976 to 1980. The seroprevalence of HBV infection in a representative sample of the US population, collected during the period 1976 to 1980, is shown by race, age, and sex in this figure. HBV seroprevalence, indicating past or present infection, was 3% in the white population and 12% in the black population. Seroprevalence increased with increasing age, perhaps reflecting a cohort effect. Of considerable interest, however, with respect to sexual transmission, is the increased prevalence during the adolescent years. (*Adapted from* McQuillan *et al.* [2]; with permission.)

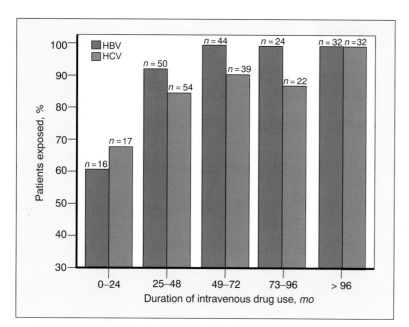

FIGURE 2-27.

Hepatitis B (HBV) and C viruses (HCV) in intravenous drug users. Intravenous drug users who share equipment are at high risk for both HBV and HCV. One of the risk factors in the acquisition of these infections is duration of behavior involving intravenous drug use. In the results of this Australian study, the seroprevalence of markers of HBV infection (hepatitis B surface antigen or antibodies to hepatitis B core antigen) and HCV infection (antibodies to HCV) increased with increasing months of intravenous drug use. As shown, after 8 years of drug use, all study subjects had markers for both infections. These observations indicate the high efficiency of transmission of these agents by sharing intravenous injection equipment. (*Adapted from* Bell *et al.* [22]; with permission.)

Immunoprophylaxis

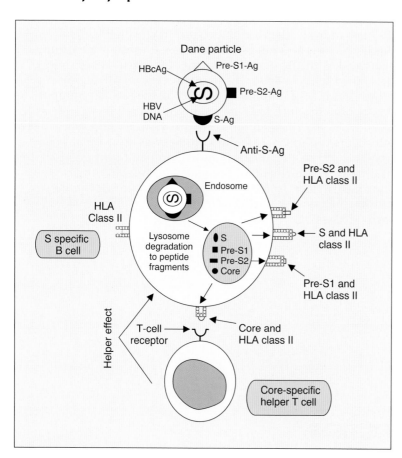

FIGURE 2-28.

Induction of antibodies to hepatitis B surface antigen (Anti-HBs). The complex interaction of hepatitis B virus (HBV) with the B and T lymphocyte, resulting in the production of Anti-HBs, is detailed in this figure. In this hypothetical model, the B cell expresses an immunoglobulin receptor for hepatitis B surface antigen (S-Ag) and captures HBV particles. Intracellular processing of the particles results in the release of degraded HBV proteins (S, Pre-S1, Pre-S2, and core) which bind to major histocompatibility complex class II molecules. These proteins are transported to the cell surface and are recognized by the hepatitis B core antigen (HBcAg)–specific helper T lymphocyte, which helps B cells produce Anti-HBs. (*Adapted from* Mondelli and Negro [23]; with permission.)

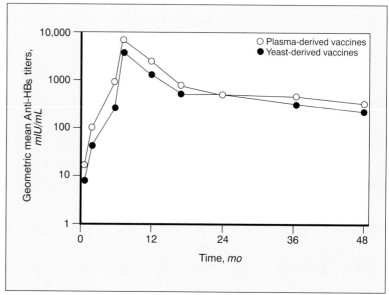

FIGURE 2-29.

Hepatitis B virus (HBV) vaccine–induced antibodies to hepatitis B surface antigen (Anti-HBs). HBV vaccines were originally produced by hepatitis B surface antigen (HBsAg)–positive plasma treated with chemicals (urea, pepsin, formaldehyde) to inactivate residual HBV. In contrast, the recombinant vaccines have been produced through genetic engineering: the S open reading frame of HBV DNA is incorporated into the DNA of a yeast cell. The cell then produces HBsAg which is used as the immunogen in the vaccine. In the results of the study illustrated here, peak levels of Anti-HBs produced after the conventional 0, 1, 6-month vaccination schedule were shown to be comparable for both plasma- and yeast-derived vaccines, and Anti-HBs persisted equally in recipients on follow-up through 48 months. (*Adapted from* Scheiermann *et al.* [24]; with permission.)

Hepatocarcinogenesis

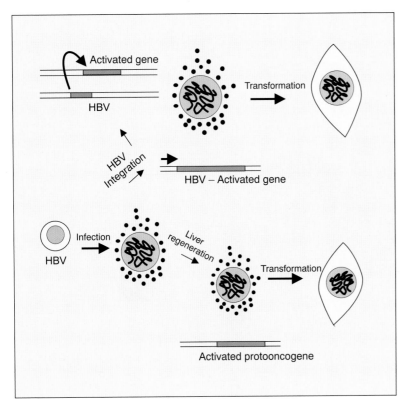

FIGURE 2-30.

Hepatitis B virus (HBV) and hepatocellular carcinoma. The precise mechanism by which persistent HBV infection leads to the development of hepatocellular carcinoma remains to be established. Two possible pathways leading to transformation of the hepatocyte into a malignant cell are shown in this diagram. In the upper pathway, it is postulated that integration of HBV genomic fragments may activate cellular growth genes, thereby resulting in malignant transformation of the hepatocyte. In the lower pathway, persistent infection may, through cycles of cell death and regeneration, activate cell protooncogenes, leading to malignant transformation. (*Adapted from* Buendia *et al.* [25]; with permission.)

Hepatitis D

Virus

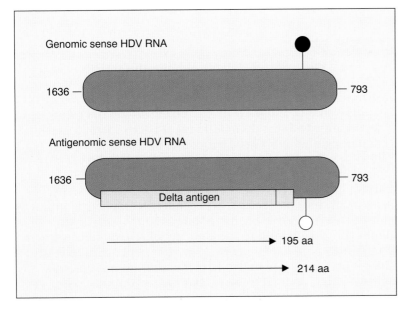

FIGURE 2-31.

Hepatitis D virus (HDV) genome. The HDV genome and antigenomic-sense HDV RNA are shown schematically in this figure. The antigenome is a genome-complementary, circular RNA molecule found in purified HDV particles and in larger quantities in HDV–infected hepatocytes. Both the genome of HDV and the antigenome contain self-cleavage sites. In the former, it is represented by a *closed circle* in the diagram. In the antigenome, the self-cleavage site is indicated by the *open circle*. The open reading frame coding for the HDV (delta) antigen has been identified on the antigenome. The smaller form of the HDV antigen is encoded by the region between nucleotides 1598 to 1010 whereas the large form extends to nucleotide 953. (*Adapted from* Polish *et al.* [26]; with permission.)

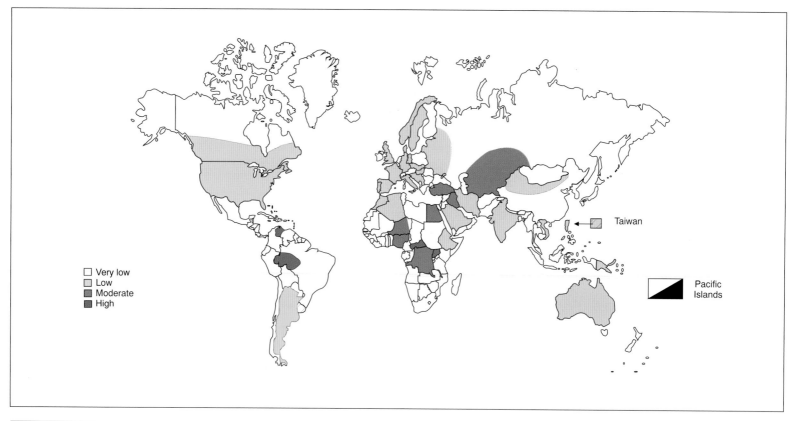

FIGURE 2-32.

Worldwide prevalence of hepatitis D virus (HDV). The prevalence of HDV infection varies greatly throughout the globe and may also vary enormously in different regions of the same country. Low prevalence rates have been identified in Southeast Asia and China. In contrast, foci of high antibodies to HDV prevalence have been found in several islands in the Pacific Ocean, in the Amazon basin and western Venezuela, in some parts of Central Africa, and in some sections of Eastern Europe. (*Adapted from* Polish *et al.* [26]; with permission.)

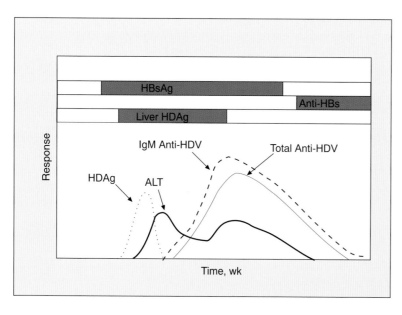

FIGURE 2-33.

Coinfection of hepatitis D (HDV) and hepatitis B (HBV) viruses. In HDV coinfection with HBV, serum HDV antigen (HDAg) may be detected shortly after or concurrently with the detection of hepatitis B surface antigen (HBsAg). HDAg disappears before or concomitantly with the disappearance of HBsAg. Seroconversion to immunoglobulin M (IgM) antibodies to HDV (Anti-HDV) follows the disappearance of HDAg. Immunoglobulin G (IgG) Anti-HDV may appear shortly after the IgM antibody. Both IgM and IgG Anti-HDV often disappear during convalescence. Occasionally the latter persists in declining titer for many months and may remain detectable for as long as 1 to 2 years. In a small number of patients with coinfection, the only detectable markers of HDV infection may be the early and transient appearance of isolated IgM Anti-HDV or the detection, during convalescence, of isolated IgG Anti-HDV. ALT—alanine aminotransferase; Anti-HBs—antibodies to HBsAg. (*Adapted from* Polish *et al.* [26]; with permission.)

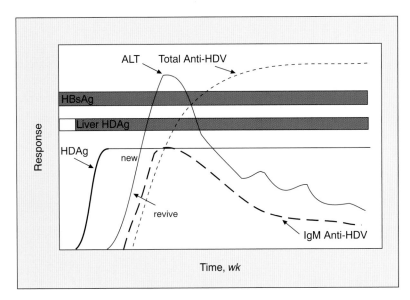

FIGURE 2-34.

Superinfection by hepatitis D virus (HDV). As shown in this schematic illustration of the serologic events in HDV superinfection of hepatitis B virus (HBV) (hepatitis B surface antigen [HBsAg]) carriers, a reduction in HBV replication is a regular feature of superinfection and leads to a diminution in the titer of circulating HBsAg or transient HBsAg nondetectability. Actual termination of the carrier state is an uncommon consequence of suppression of HBV replication by HDV. In contrast, in many instances, HDV infection becomes chronic, hepatitis D antigen (HDAg) remains detectable in the liver and occasionally in serum, and HBsAg levels return to pre-HDV infection levels. High titers of antibodies to HDV (Anti-HDV) are maintained in persistent HDV infection; the decline in immunoglobulin M (IgM) Anti-HDV level is very variable. ALT—alanine aminotransferase. (*Adapted from* Polish *et al.* [26]; with permission.)

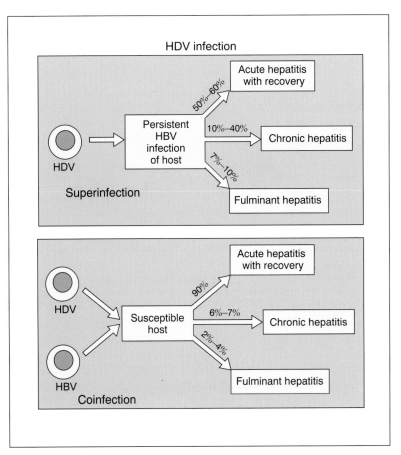

FIGURE 2-35.

Sequelae of hepatitis D virus (HDV). In general, the sequelae of HDV infection are more serious when superinfection of the host with persistent hepatitis B virus (HBV) infection occurs. As shown in the *upper panel*, superinfection is associated with a risk of chronic hepatitis in 10% to 40% of patients; fulminant disease is seen in 7% to 10%. In contrast, as shown in the *lower panel*, HDV and HBV coinfections are less often associated with grave outcomes. Only 6% to 7% coinfections lead to chronic hepatitis and only 2% to 4% end with fulminant hepatitis. (*Adapted from* Conjeevaram and DiBisceglie [27]; with permission.)

Virus

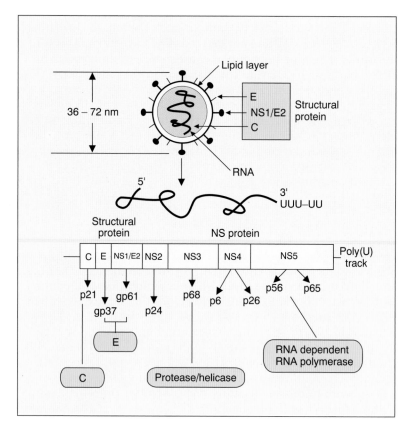

FIGURE 2-36.

Hepatitis C virus (HCV) particles and genome. This schematic diagram indicates that HCV is a positive sense, single-stranded RNA virus, with an estimated diameter of 36 to 72 nm. HCV is believed to represent a distinct genus in the *Flaviviridae* family. A viral envelope comprising a lipid layer and envelope proteins, surrounds a core (capsid) structure enclosing the viral nucleic acid. HCV RNA is 9.4 kb in length and consists of a 5'-nontranslated region, followed by core (C), envelope (E), and nonstructural (NS) protein encoding regions. The latter is followed by a short 3'-noncoding region with a poly(U) track at its end. Glycosylated (gp) and nonglycosylated (p) putative protein products of the structural and NS regions are shown. The NS protein products include a serine proteinase, helicase, and an RNA–dependent RNA polymerase. (*Adapted from* Esumi and Shikata [28]; with permission.)

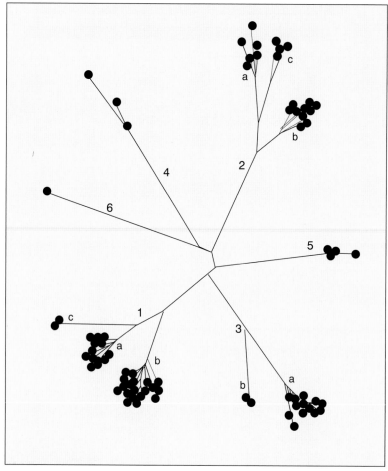

FIGURE 2-37.

Phylogenetic analysis of hepatitis C virus (HCV) genotypes and subtypes. HCV isolates have been reported to show considerable nucleotide sequence diversity, suggesting the existence of multiple genotypes. Within several of the genotypes, more closely related subtypes also have been identified. The phylogenetic analysis shown here, based on the nucleotide sequences derived from a part of the nonstructural region of the HCV genome, provides evidence for six major genotypes, labeled 1–6. Subtypes are given lower case letters. For example, as shown in the lower left corner, HCV 1 has three subtypes, 1a, 1b, and 1c. (*Adapted from* Simmonds *et al.* [29]; with permission.)

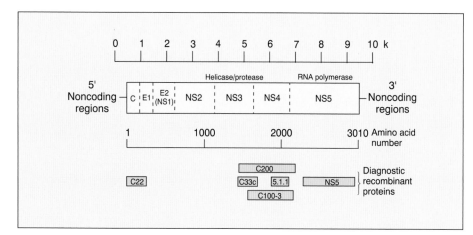

FIGURE 2-38.

Hepatitis C virus (HCV) genome and recombinant proteins. This schematic drawing shows the genomic organization of HCV, including, from left to right, the 5' nontranslated region, the core (C), envelope (E), and nonstructural regions (NS), and ending at the 3' nontranslated region. Below the genome are shown the recombinant proteins (C22 from the C region, C33c from NS3, C100-3 and 5.1.1 from NS4, and NS5 from the NS5 region) used diagnostically in the detection of antibodies to HCV. The protein C200 represents a fusion protein comprising C33c and C100-3. (*Adapted from* Garson and Tedder [30]; with permission.)

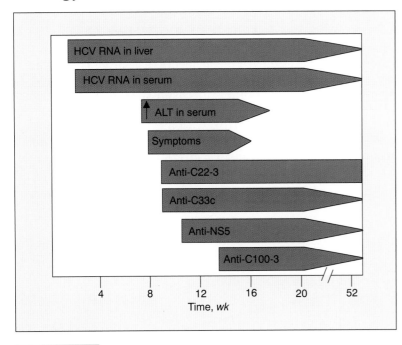

FIGURE 2-39.

Sequence of serological events in acute hepatitis C virus (HCV) infection. HCV RNA in liver and in serum appear to be the earliest markers of acute HCV infection, preceding the development of serum alanine aminotransferase (ALT) elevations, symptoms, or the appearance of antibodies to HCV (Anti-HCV). Some evidence exists that HCV RNA may persist for decades even if biochemical resolution of hepatitis occurs. Anti-C22-3 and Anti-C33c may be the first Anti-HCV antibodies to appear in HCV infection. Anti-NS5 appears somewhat later whereas Anti-C100-3 appears to be the last antibody to be detected in acute, self-limited infection. Limited data suggest that the titers of Anti-C33c, Anti-NS5, and Anti-C100-3 may decline, although levels of Anti-C22-3 may be maintained for a considerably longer period. (*Adapted from* Koff [31]; with permission.)

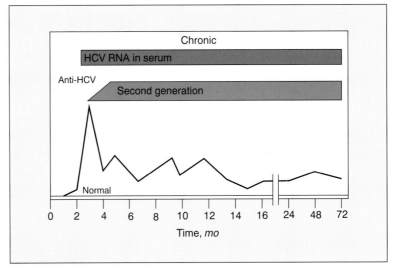

FIGURE 2-40.

Sequence of serologic events in chronic hepatitis C virus (HCV). As shown in this diagram of the serologic and biochemical events in chronic hepatitis associated with HCV, HCV RNA is detected consistently throughout the course of infection. HCV replication may be increased in advanced liver disease and may play a role in progression of disease. The second-generation assays for antibodies to HCV (Anti-HCV) (detecting antibodies to three or four HCV recombinant proteins) remain positive in affected patients for years. In a small number of patients, Anti-HCV levels may decline spontaneously or after treatment. Fluctuations in the serum levels of alanine aminotransferase appear to be a characteristic feature of chronic hepatitis caused by HCV and may reflect waves of hepatocellular inflammation and necrosis. The emergence of HCV neutralization escape mutants may be responsible but other ill-defined mechanisms also may play a role in these intermittent elevations of aminotransferase levels. (*Adapted from* Koff [31]; with permission.)

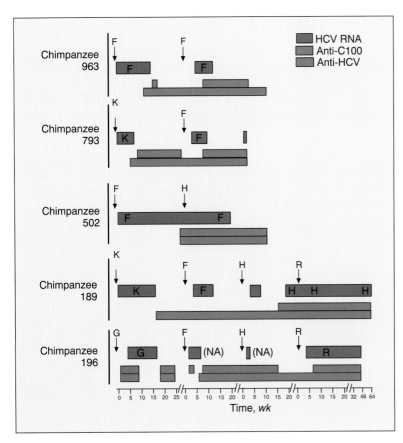

FIGURE 2-41.

Hepatitis C virus (HCV) cross-challenges in chimpanzees. These are the findings of multiple cross-challenge studies undertaken in chimpanzees inoculated with different HCV strains over a period of years. *Arrows* indicate the time of challenge with the strain of HCV indicated by the letter above the arrow. HCV RNA was measured by polymerase chain reaction, and both first- and second-generation assays for antibodies to HCV (Anti-HCV) were measured. All animals developed acute hepatitis following the first challenge and seroconverted as measured by first- or second-generation assays for Anti-HCV. HCV viremia was transient in four chimpanzees but persistent in one. Rechallenge of convalescent chimpanzees negative for HCV RNA at the time of rechallenge, in each instance, resulted in the appearance of the challenge strain of HCV RNA in serum and with histopathologic evidence of acute hepatitis. Serum alanine aminotransferase levels were lower during rechallenge hepatitis than during the primary HCV infection. In animals persistently infected with HCV, the challenge strain could not be detected in serum. Collectively these observations provide evidence for the lack of protective immunity against HCV reinfection. (*Adapted from* Farci and Purcell [32]; with permission.)

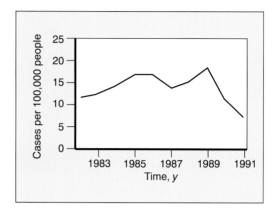

FIGURE 2-42.

Estimated incidence of acute hepatitis C virus (HCV) in the United States. The Centers for Disease Control and Prevention have estimated the incidence of acute viral hepatitis caused by HCV between 1982 and 1991. Based on data from their four sentinel county study and allowing for adjustments for underreporting, this figure suggests a greater than 50% decline in incidence after 1989. This decline is believed to reflect a decrease in blood-borne transmission (*see* Fig. 2-44). The Centers for Disease Control and Prevention has also estimated that an average of 150,000 HCV infections occurred annually in the United States during the past decade. (*Adapted from* McQuillan *et al.* [2]; with permission.)

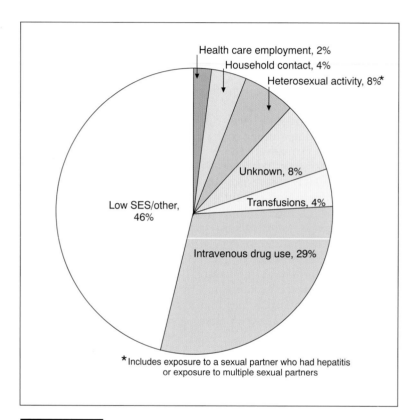

FIGURE 2-43.

Risk factors associated with acute hepatitis C virus (HCV). As shown in this diagram, based on data collected by the Centers for Disease Control and Prevention in their four sentinel county study in 1992, 29% of reported acute HCV infections were associated with intravenous drug use and 4% were associated with blood transfusion. Thus, a third of reported cases could be linked with bloodborne modes of transmission. Twelve percent could be linked with either heterosexual activity or household contact, which includes exposure to a sexual partner or household member with hepatitis or with exposure to multiple sexual partners. Health care employment was identified in 2% of cases. Although only 6% had no distinguishing risk factor or exposure history, nearly half of reported cases were in patients from low socioeconomic status (SES) levels or who reported so-called "high-risk" behaviors or contacts, but not in the 6 months before the onset of illness. The significance of low SES and high-risk indicators remains to be established. (*Adapted from* McQuillan *et al.* [2]; with permission.)

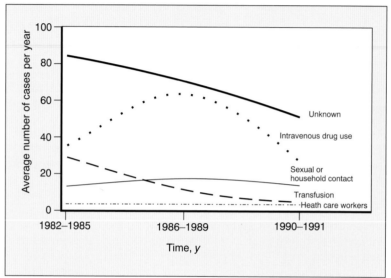

FIGURE 2-44.

Trends in reported cases of acute hepatitis C virus (HCV) in the United States. This figure depicts the changes in risk factors identified in the Center for Disease Control and Prevention's four sentinel county study between 1982 and 1991. Cases of acute HCV associated with intravenous drug use increased through 1989 and then declined dramatically. Transfusion as a risk factor declined significantly after 1985, prior to the introduction of surrogate testing of blood donors and the introduction of antibodies to HCV screening. Changes in the donor population resulting from self-exclusion of individuals with HIV risk factors may have been responsible. Health care workers accounted for a low and stable number of cases. Minor changes in the number of cases in which sexual or household contact was identified are shown. The continuing decline in cases without known risk factors during the past decade remains poorly understood. (*Adapted from* McQuillan *et al.* [2]; with permission.)

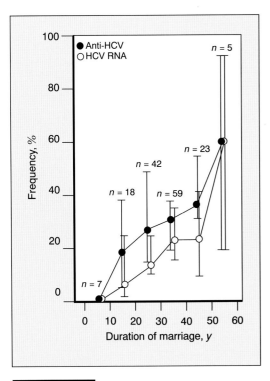

FIGURE 2-45.

Hepatitis C virus (HCV) infection in spouses of patients with chronic HCV–associated liver disease. Although early studies did not suggest that HCV could be efficiently transmitted sexually and some studies even failed to find any evidence of transmission, more recent data indicate that sexual transmission does occur. In this study from Japan, spouses of 154 patients with chronic hepatitis caused by HCV infection were tested for antibodies to HCV (Anti-HCV) and HCV RNA. Anti-HCV was found in 42 spouses (27%) whereas HCV RNA was detected in 25 (16%). As shown in this figure, HCV infection in spouses increased with duration of cohabitation: rates were 9% if married less than 30 years and 24% if married more than 30 years. HCV genotypes were identical in 24 of 27 spouses positive for HCV RNA. (*Adapted from* Akahane *et al.* [33]; with permission.)

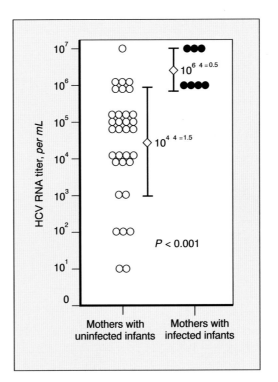

FIGURE 2-46.

Maternal-neonatal hepatitis C virus (HCV) transmission: role of maternal HCV titer. The frequency of maternal-neonatal transmission of HCV and risk factors favoring transmission have been studied in pregnant Japanese women found to be positive for antibodies to HCV by a second-generation enzyme immunoassay and to be HCV RNA positive. About 10% of the babies of viremic mothers became infected. Umbilical cord blood specimens were all negative for HCV RNA, thereby suggesting that in utero infection was not responsible. As shown in this figure, the seven infected mothers with infected infants had higher titers of HCV RNA than the mothers of infants in whom infection failed to occur. The infection rate was 50% in women with a titer of HCV greater than 10^6/mL. (*Adapted from* Ohto *et al.* [34]; with permission.)

TABLE 2-4. THE DECLINING FREQUENCY OF POSTTRANSFUSION HEPATITIS

TIME, y	CASES BY DIAGNOSIS, n			
	Hepatitis B	Non-A, non-B	Other	Total
1981–1982	222	434	318	974
1985–1986	166	401	276	843
1986–1987	141	353	190	684
1987–1988	108	194	113	415
1988–1989	68	163	139	370
1989–1990	126	208	152	486
1990–1991	135	112	147	394
1991–1992	83	75	153	311
1992–1993*	64	89	96	249
1993–1994	87	100	74	261

TABLE 2-4.

This table lists the numbers of cases of transfusion-associated hepatitis reported to the American Red Cross during the years between 1981 to 1994. The *asterisk* indicates that reporting categories were changed to hepatitis B, hepatitis C, hepatitis, other viral, hepatitis non-A, non-B, non-C, and hepatitis, unspecified. Although these data are limited by the retrospective nature of the reporting mechanism, they nonetheless suggest that all etiologic forms of transfusion-transmitted hepatitis are declining in frequency. (*Adapted from* Dodd [35]; with permission.)

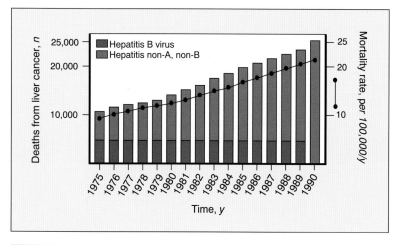

FIGURE 2-47.

Deaths from primary liver cancer (hepatocellular carcinoma) in Japan. During the 15-year period between 1975 and 1990, the number of deaths from liver cancer and the mortality rate for liver cancer increased dramatically in Japan. Although the number of liver cancer deaths related to hepatitis B virus (HBV) infection, based on hepatitis B surface antigen positivity, did not change over this time period, liver cancer deaths attributed to non-A, non-B hepatitis more than tripled. The overwhelming majority of these non-A, non-B hepatitis infections are believed to be caused by HCV and a large proportion of affected patients give a history of blood transfusion decades earlier. (*Adapted from* Okuda [36]; with permission.)

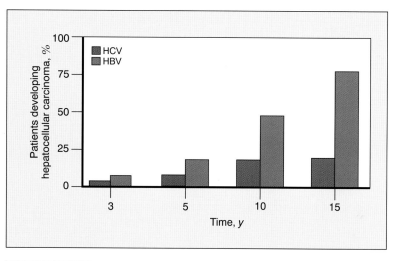

FIGURE 2-48.

Development of hepatocellular carcinoma in hepatitis B virus (HBV)–associated and hepatitis C virus (HCV)–associated cirrhosis. The data shown in this figure were collected during a prospective study of a large number of Japanese patients with cirrhosis caused by either HBV or HCV infection. The frequency of progression of cirrhosis to hepatocellular carcinoma increased with time, reaching 75% in HBV–related cirrhosis and 27% in HCV–related cirrhosis after 15 years of follow-up. The precise nature of the biologic differences that are responsible for these differences in carcinogenesis related to HBV and HCV (in the setting of cirrhosis) are ill-defined. (*Adapted from* Ikeda *et al.* [37]; with permission.)

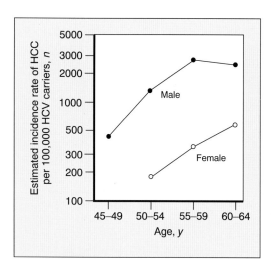

FIGURE 2-49.

Incidence of hepatocellular carcinoma (HCC) in hepatitis C virus (HCV) carriers. Osaka, Japan has been recognized as one of the highest risk regions for HCV–related HCC in the world. Based on second-gener-ation assays for antibodies to HCV (Anti-HCV), the prevalence of HCV RNA among volunteer blood donors in Osaka, the frequency of Anti-HCV among cases of HCC, and data from the Osaka Cancer Registry, estimates of the probability of developing HCC were drawn for HCV carriers and plotted by 5-year age groups for both males and females. The estimated HCC incidence was higher in males than females and peaked for males at ages 55 to 59, whereas no peak could be identified in females. The cumulative risk of developing HCC in 50-year-old male HCV carriers was 28% within the following 15 years; for female HCV carriers the risk was 6%. This gender difference remains poorly understood. (*Adapted from* Tanaka *et al.* [38]; with permission.)

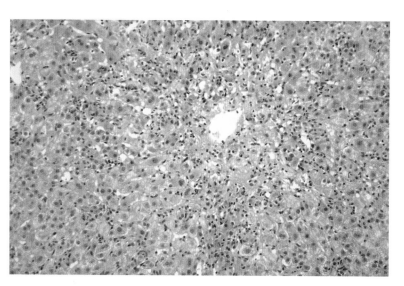

FIGURE 2-50.   **TYPICAL BIOPSY FINDINGS IN VIRAL HEPATITIS**

Diffuse hepatocellular necrosis with marked histiocytic reaction and infiltration with polymorphonuclear cells and mononuclear cells. Areas of necrosis and inflammation are intermingled. Hematoxylin and eosin. (*Courtesy of* Z. Goodman, Washington, D.C.)

■ REFERENCES AND RECOMMENDED READING

1. Alter MJ, Hadler SC: Delta hepatitis and infection in North America. In *Hepatitis Delta Virus*. Edited by Hadziyannis SJ, Taylor JM, Bonino F. New York: Wiley-Liss; 1993:243–250.

2. McQuillan G, Alter MJ, Everhart JE: Viral hepatitis. In *Digestive Diseases in the United States*. Edited by Everhart JE. Bethesda, MD: NIH; 1994:127–156.

3. Brown EA, Ticehurst J, Lemon SM: Immunopathogenesis of hepatitis A and E virus infections. In *Immunology of Liver Disease*. Edited by Thomas HC, Waters J. Dordrecht: Kluwer Academic Publishers; 1994:11–37.

4. Hu M, Kang L, Yao G: An outbreak of hepatitis A in Shanghai. In *Infectious Diseases of the Liver*. Edited by Bianchi L, Gerok W, Maier K-P, Deinhardt F. Dordrecht: Kluwer Academic Publishers; 1990:361–372.

5. Werzberger A, Mensch B, Kuter B, *et al.*: A controlled trial of a formalin-inactivated hepatitis A vaccine in health children. *N Engl J Med* 1992, 327:453–457.

6. Lemon SM, Stapleton JT: Prevention. In *Viral Hepatitis*. Edited by Zuckerman AJ, Thomas HC. Edinburgh: Churchill-Livingstone; 1993:61–79.

7. Perez-Trallero E, Cilla G, Urbieta M, *et al.*: Falling incidence and prevalence of hepatitis A in northern Spain. *Scand J Infect Dis* 1994, 26:133–136.

8. Winokur PL, Stapleton JT: Immunoglobulin prophylaxis for hepatitis A. *Clin Infect Dis.* 1992, 14:580–586.

9. Innis BL, Snitbhan R, Kuna sol P, *et al.*: Protection against hepatitis A by an inactivated vaccine. J Anna 1994, 271:1328–1334.

10. Velazquez O, Stetler HC, Avila C, *et al.*: Epidemic transmission of enterically transmitted non-A, non-B hepatitis in Mexico, 1986-1987. *JAMA* 1990, 263:3281–3285.

11. Gerlich W: Structure and molecular virology. In *Viral Hepatitis*. Edited by Zuckerman AJ, Thomas HC. Edinburgh: Churchill-Livingstone; 1993:83–113.

12. Yoffe B, Noonan CA: Progress and perspective in human hepatitis B virus research. *Prog Med Virol* 1993, 40:107–140.

13. Miska S, Will H: Hepatitis B virus C-gene variants. *Arch Virol* 1993, 8(suppl):155–169.

14. Bova R, Micheli MR, Nardiello S: Molecular biology of hepatocellular carcinoma and hepatitis B virus association. *Int J Clin Lab Res* 1991, 21:190–198.

15. Carmen WF, Thomas HC, Zuckerman AJ, Harrison T: Molecular variants. In *Viral Hepatitis*. Edited by Zuckerman AJ, Thomas HC, New York: Churchill-Livingstone; 1993:115–136.

16. Hasegawa K, Huang JK, Liang TJ: Enhanced viral replication of a hepatitis B virus mutant associated with an epidemic of fulminant hepatitis E [Abstract]. *Hepatology* 1993, 18:145a.

17. Chen D-S: Natural history of chronic hepatitis B virus infection: New light on an old story. *J Gastroenterol Hepatol* 1993, 8:470–475.

18. Hamilton J, Gross N: The huge bounty on a global killer. *Business Week* April 4, 1994:92,93–94.

19. Liaw Y-F, Sheen I-S, Chen T-J, *et al.*: Incidence, determinants and significance of delayed clearance of serum HBsAg in chronic hepatitis B virus infection: A prospective study. *Hepatology* 1991, 13:627–631.

20. Weissberg JI, Andres LL, Smith CI, *et al.*: Survival in chronic hepatitis B. An analysis of 379 patients. *Ann Intern Med* 1984, 101:613–616.

21. Ladenheim J, Yao F, Martin MC, *et al.*: Survival in chronic hepatitis B: A 15-year follow-up [Abstract]. *Hepatology* 1993, 18:119A.

22. Bell J, Batey RG, Farrell GC, *et al.*: Hepatitis C in intravenous drug users. *Med J Aust* 1990, 153:274–276.

23. Mondelli MU, Negro F: Immunobiology of hepatitis B and D virus infection. In *Immunology of Liver Disease*. Edited by Thomas HC, Waters J. Dordrecht: Kluwer Academic Publishers; 1994:39–55.

24. Scheiermann N, Gesemann M, Maurer C, *et al.*: Persistence of antibodies after immunization with a recombinant yeast-derived hepatitis B vaccine following two different schedules. *Vaccine* 1990, 8(suppl):S44.

25. Buendia MA, Paterlini P, Tiollais P, Brechot C: Liver Cancer. In *Viral Hepatitis*. Edited by Zuckerman AJ, Thomas HC. New York: Churchill Livingstone, 1993:137–164.

26. Polish LB, Gallagher M, Field HA, Hadler SC: Delta hepatitis: Molecular biology and clinical and epidemiological features. *Clin Microbiol Rev* 1993, 6:211–229.

27. Conjeevaram HS, DiBisceglie AM: Natural history. In *Viral Hepatitis*. Edited by Zuckerman AJ, Thomas HC. New York: Churchill-Livingstone, 1993:341–349.

28. Esumi M, Shikata T: Hepatitis C virus and liver disease. *Pathology International* 1994, 44:85–95.

29. Simmonds P, Holmes EC, Cha T-A, *et al.*: Classification of hepatitis C virus into six major genotypes and a series of subtypes by phylogenetic analysis of the NS-5 region. *J Gen Virol* 1993, 74:2391–2399.

30. Garson JA, Tedder RS: The detection of hepatitis C infection. *Rev Med Virology* 1993, 3:75–83.

31. Koff RS: Unit 3. *Viral Hepatitis*. Clinical Teaching Project, edn 2. Bethesda: American Gastroenterology Association, 1994.

32. Farci P, Purcell RH: Natural history and experimental models. In *Viral Hepatitis*. Edited by Zuckerman AJ, Thomas HC. New York: Churchill-Livingstone, 1993:241–267.

33. Akahane Y, Kojima M, Sugai Y: Hepatitis C virus infection in spouses of patients with type C chronic liver disease. *Ann Intern Med* 1994, 120:748–752.

34. Ohto H, Terazawa S, Sasaki N, *et al.*: Transmission of hepatitis C virus from mothers to infants. *N Engl J Med* 1994, 330:744–750.

35. Dodd RY: Hepatitis C, other types of non-B parenteral hepatitis and blood transfusion. In *Virological Safety Aspects of Plasma Derivatives*. Edited by Brown F. Basel: Karger, 1993, 81:35–40.

36. Okuda K: Liver cancer. In *Viral Hepatitis*. Edited by Zuckerman AJ, Thomas HC. New York: Churchill-Livingstone, 1993: 269–281.

37. Ikeda K, Saitoh S, Koida I, *et al.*: A multivariate analysis of risk factors for hepatocellular carcinogenesis: Prospective observations of 795 patients with viral and alcoholic cirrhosis. *Hepatology* 1993, 18:47–53.

38. Tanaka H, Hiyama T, Tsukuma H, *et al.*: Cumulative risk of hepatocellular carcinoma in hepatitis C virus carriers: Statistical estimations from cross-sectional data. *Jpn J Cancer Res* 1994, 85:485–490.

Chapter 3

Autoimmune Hepatitis

ALBERT J. CZAJA

Autoimmune hepatitis is an unresolving inflammation of the liver, characterized by autoantibodies in serum, hypergamma-globulinemia, and at least periportal hepatitis (piecemeal necrosis) on histologic examination [1]. It is the archetypal form of chronic hepatitis and has been the model that has fashioned the nomenclature, diagnostic strategies, treatment trials, and outcome analyses now applied to other forms of chronic hepatitis [2,3].

DIAGNOSIS BY EXCLUSION

There are no pathognomonic features of autoimmune hepatitis, and it remains a diagnosis that requires the exclusion of other similar conditions [1–3]. Hereditary (Wilson's disease, genetic hemochromatosis, and α_1-antitrypsin deficiency), drug-induced (oxyphenisatin, α-methyldopa, nitrofurantoin, and propyl-thiouracil toxicities), immunologic (primary biliary cirrhosis and primary sclerosing cholangitis), viral (chronic hepatitis C), and idiopathic (nonalcoholic steatohepatitis) diseases must be initially eliminated to ensure correct diagnosis [1]. Fortunately, this is usually accomplished by a careful review of clinical history, the performance of certain laboratory tests, and expert interpretation of liver biopsy tissue. Importantly, autoimmune hepatitis may have an acute, even fulminant, presentation and the conventional requirement for 6 months of disease activity to establish chronicity has been waived [4,5].

ETIOLOGY

The etiology of autoimmune hepatitis is unknown, but recent studies have emphasized the possibility of a viral origin [6–8]. Case reports have described the emergence of autoimmune hepatitis after acute hepatitis A and B virus infection; the disease has been reported in patients with HIV, and the measles virus genome has been found more frequently in peripheral blood cells of patients with autoimmune hepatitis than in control patients [9–12]. Serologic surveys in patients from regions highly endemic for hepatitis C virus (HCV) infection have suggested an etiologic relationship with this virus, and autoimmune hepatitis has been observed after interferon therapy in patients with chronic hepatitis B [6–8,13]. Importantly, the majority of patients with autoimmune hepatitis in the United States and the United Kingdom lack manifestations of viral infection. Early studies using first-generation immunoassays for HCV antibody detection were compromised by a high frequency of false-positive results [14–19]. Consequently, viral infection now appears to be a coincidental finding rather than an important cause of the disease in North America and Western Europe [20,21].

TREATMENT

Advances in molecular biology have facilitated the search for target autoantigens and investigative efforts have focused on the identification and characterization of a myriad of autoantibodies that might identify such antigens. The cytochrome monooxygenase, P450 IID6, has been proposed as an autoantigen recognized by antibodies to liver–kidney microsome type 1; asialoglycoprotein receptor is another candidate target autoantigen [22,23]. Autoantibodies that manifest exclusivity have been proposed as hallmarks of the disease, and subclassification schemes based on these markers have been used to identify pertinent pathogenic mechanisms [2].

The burgeoning battery of autoantibodies associated with the disease has generated confusing jargon. International efforts are now under way to standardize nomenclature and diagnostic requirements [4,24]. The concept of autoimmune hepatitis today is vastly different than that of 10 years ago, and it continues to evolve.

Prednisone alone or in combination with azathioprine continues to be the preferred treatment for patients with autoimmune hepatitis, but the limitations of these treatment regimens in establishing sustained remission and preventing eventual progression to cirrhosis are well recognized [1,25]. Additionally, drug-related complications diminish the net benefit–risk ratio of protracted therapy and also restrict the pursuit of ideal treatment endpoints [25]. Novel immunosuppressive agents are emerging from the transplantation arena. Similarly, cytoprotective agents that may either change the display of human leukocyte antigens on the hepatocyte surface, create a physical barrier against noxious or immunologic injury, or alter the microenvironment within the liver to reduce cytodestructive factors, have intuitive appeal in the management of this disease [25]. The stage is set to evaluate alternative therapies as principal regimens, additional options, or adjunctive treatments.

Clinicians can no longer be emboldened by perceptions that the diagnosis of autoimmune hepatitis is straightforward and the treatment standard. Current strategies require awareness of nomenclature, familiarity with diagnostic criteria, understanding of immunoserologic manifestations, and selection of confident treatment options.

BACKGROUND AND DIAGNOSTIC CRITERIA

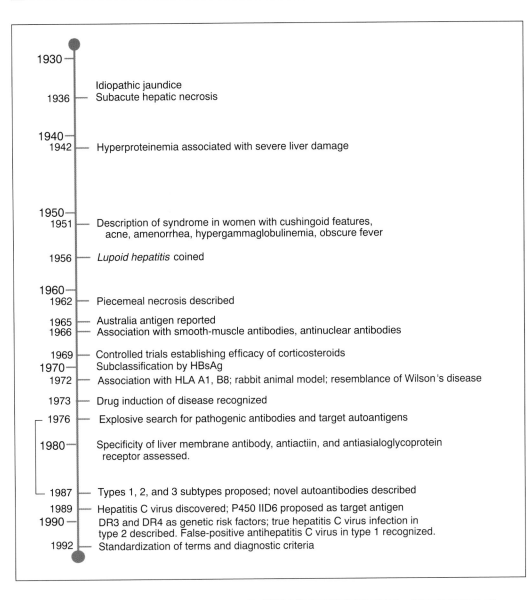

1930

1936 — Idiopathic jaundice
Subacute hepatic necrosis

1940
1942 — Hyperproteinemia associated with severe liver damage

1950
1951 — Description of syndrome in women with cushingoid features,
acne, amenorrhea, hypergammaglobulinemia, obscure fever

1956 — *Lupoid hepatitis* coined

1960
1962 — Piecemeal necrosis described

1965 — Australia antigen reported
1966 — Association with smooth-muscle antibodies, antinuclear antibodies

1969 — Controlled trials establishing efficacy of corticosteroids
1970 — Subclassification by HBsAg
1972 — Association with HLA A1, B8; rabbit animal model; resemblance of Wilson's disease

1973 — Drug induction of disease recognized

1976 — Explosive search for pathogenic antibodies and target autoantigens

1980 — Specificity of liver membrane antibody, antiactiin, and antiasialoglycoprotein
receptor assessed.

1987 — Types 1, 2, and 3 subtypes proposed; novel autoantibodies described

1989 — Hepatitis C virus discovered; P450 IID6 proposed as target antigen
1990 — DR3 and DR4 as genetic risk factors; true hepatitis C virus infection in
type 2 described. False-positive antihepatitis C virus in type 1 recognized.
1992 — Standardization of terms and diagnostic criteria

FIGURE 3-1.

Milestones in the emergence of autoimmune hepatitis as a disease entity. The syndrome was first described in 1951, and the term *lupoid hepatitis* was coined in 1956 to emphasize its autoimmune nature [2]. Piecemeal necrosis became the histologic hallmark for the disease in 1962, and the discoveries of hepatitis B surface antigen (HBsAg) in 1965 and hepatitis C virus in 1989 established by exclusion its independent nature [2,26]. The advances in molecular biology during the 1980s stimulated efforts to identify target antigens and pathogenic autoantibodies, and the 1990s heralded an era of international cooperation in standardizing terms and diagnostic criteria [4,24].

Autoimmune hepatitis

Definite diagnosis	Probable diagnosis
Piecemeal necrosis +/- Lobular hepatitis +/- Bridging necrosis	Piecemeal necrosis +/- Lobular hepatitis +/- Bridging necrosis
No biliary lesions	No biliary lesions
AST/ALT elevation	AST/ALT elevation
Normal serum α_1 antitrypsin, copper, ceruloplasmin	Abnormal copper and ceruloplasmin if Wilson's disease excluded
Gamma globulin or IgG >1.5 x normal	Any gamma globulin or IgG elevation
ANA, SMA, or LKM1 > 1:80	ANA, SMA, or LKM1 ≥ 1:40 Other autoantibodies Anti-HCV positive/RIBA negative
IgM Anti-HAV, HBsAg, IgM Anti-HBc, Anti-HCV negative	Alcohol (< 50g/d)
No active cytomegalovirus, Epstein-Barr virus	Previous blood/drug exposure
No blood/drug exposures	

FIGURE 3-2.

Diagnostic criteria for autoimmune hepatitis. The International Autoimmune Hepatitis Group met for the first time in Brighton, England, in June 1992. This panel formulated the criteria for a definite and probable diagnosis of autoimmune hepatitis [4]. The 6-month criterion of disease activity to establish chronicity was waived. Levels of significant hypergammaglobulinemia and autoantibody titer were described, and elimination factors were strictly defined [4]. Lobular hepatitis was accepted within the spectrum of the disease. Laboratory and histologic features of cholestasis precluded the definite diagnosis as did markers of true viral infection [4]. The criteria recognized the possibility of an acute, even fulminant, onset of the disease and permitted the diagnosis even in those patients without conventional immunoserologic markers [4]. ALT—alanine aminotransferase; ANA—antinuclear antibodies; Anti-HAV—antibodies to hepatitis A virus; Anti-HBc—antibodies to hepatitis B core antigen; Anti-HCV—antibodies to hepatitis C virus; AST—aspartate aminotransferase; HBsAg—hepatitis B surface antigen; IgG—immunoglobin G; IgM—immunoglobin M; LKM1—liver-kidney microsome type 1; RIBA—recombinant immunoblot assay; SMA—smooth muscle antibodies.

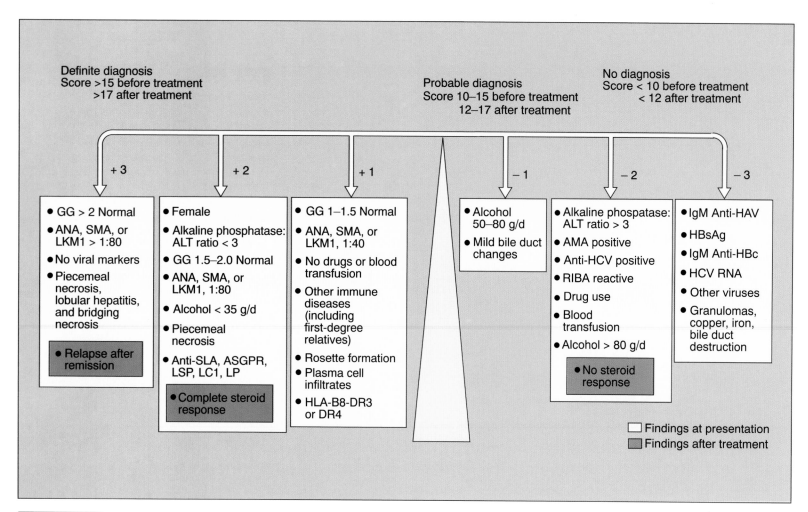

FIGURE 3-3.

Establishing the diagnosis of autoimmune hepatitis by a scoring system. A scoring system recognizes the multiplicity of findings that support the diagnosis of autoimmune hepatitis and the absence of individual pathognomonic or exclusionary features [4]. All features can be included in the formula, and the strength of the diagnosis can then be determined. Atypical or incompatible findings can be accommodated in the diagnosis, and scores based on response to corticosteroids allow treatment trials to support the diagnosis in patients with less pronounced features, mixed findings, or absent immunoserologic markers [4]. ALT—

alanine aminotransferase; AMA—antimitochondrial antibody; ANA—antinuclear antibodies; Anti-HAV—antibodies to hepatitis A virus; Anti-HBc—antibodies to hepatitis B core antigen; Anti-HCV—antibodies to hepatitis C virus; Anti-SLA—antibodies to soluble liver antigen; ASGPR—antibodies to asialoglycoprotein receptor; GG—gamma globulin; HBsAg—hepatitis B surface antigen; HCV—hepatitis C virus; IgM—immunoglobin M; LC1—liver cytosol type 1; LKM1—liver-kidney microsome type 1; LP—liver-pancreas; LSP—liver-specific protein; RIBA—recombinant immunoblot assay; SMA—smooth muscle antibodies.

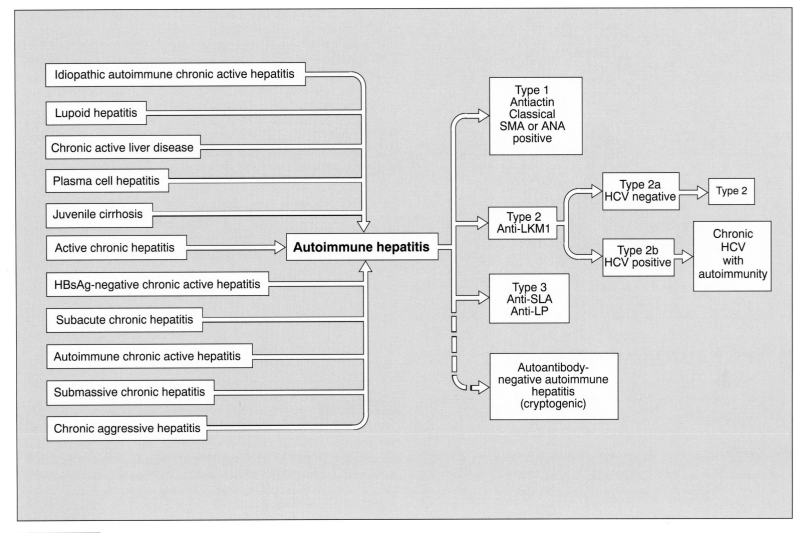

FIGURE 3-4.

Standardization of nomenclature and subclassification based on immunoserologic markers. The designation *autoimmune hepatitis* supersedes all previous terms implying chronicity, etiology, and activity [2,4]. Type 1 autoimmune hepatitis is characterized by the presence of smooth-muscle antibodies (SMA) or antinuclear antibodies (ANA) in serum [3,25]. Type 2 autoimmune hepatitis connotes the presence in serum of antibodies to liver–kidney microsome type 1 (Anti-LKM1) [3,25]. Patients with Anti-LKM1 may also have true hepatitis C virus (HCV) infection [27–30]. Those patients with Anti-LKM1 who do not have true HCV infection are designated as having type 2a autoimmune hepatitis, and those with true HCV

infection are classified as having type 2b autoimmune hepatitis [29,30]. Type 3 autoimmune hepatitis connotes seropositivity for antibodies to soluble liver antigen (Anti-SLA) [31]. Antibodies to liver–pancreas (Anti-LP) have also been proposed as markers of a type 3 autoimmune hepatitis [32]. Patients with all features of autoimmune hepatitis except seropositivity for conventional autoantibodies (cryptogenic chronic hepatitis) can be tentatively classified as having autoantibody-negative autoimmune hepatitis [2]. These patients typically respond to corticosteroid therapy [33]. HBsAg—hepatitis B surface antigen.

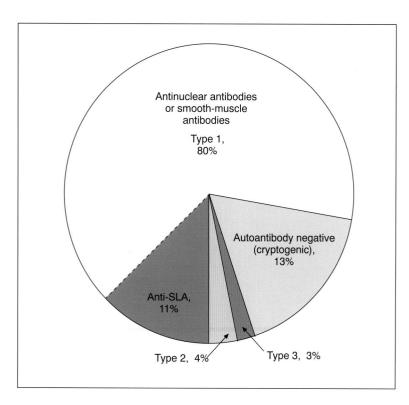

Figure 3-5.

Frequency of the different subtypes of autoimmune hepatitis in adults in the United States. Type 1 autoimmune hepatitis is the most common subtype [2,25]. Types 2 and 3 autoimmune hepatitis are very uncommon in American adults [34,35]. Autoantibody-negative autoimmune hepatitis (cryptogenic chronic hepatitis) is the second most common diagnosis. These patients may have escaped detection by conventional immunoserologic assays. Assessment for antibodies to soluble liver antigen (Anti-SLA) and antibodies to liver–pancreas may allow reclassification of these patients as autoimmune hepatitis in 18% and 33% of patients, respectively [32,35]. Unfortunately, 11% of patients with type 1 autoimmune hepatitis have Anti-SLA, and it is uncertain that these autoantibodies define a distinct subpopulation of patients [35].

◼ TYPE 1 AUTOIMMUNE HEPATITIS

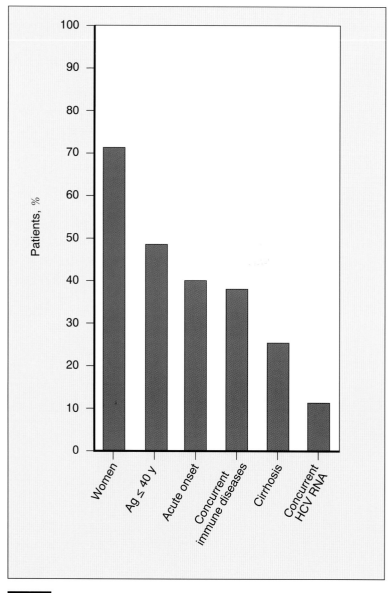

Figure 3-6.

Clinical features of type 1 autoimmune hepatitis. Forty percent of patients have an acute onset of symptoms [36]. These patients may be mistaken as having acute viral hepatitis and be denied expeditious therapy [5,36,37]. Fortunately, most of these patients have features such as hypoalbuminemia, thrombocytopenia, hypergammaglobulinemia, or ascites that indicate chronic liver disease [5]. Cirrhosis is demonstrated at presentation in 25% of patients, indicating that autoimmune hepatitis can have an indolent, aggressive, subclinical stage [5]. Indeed, an apparent acute onset of disease may actually reflect an exacerbation of subclinical chronic disease [5]. True hepatitis C virus (HCV) infection is present in no more than 11% of patients by polymerase chain reaction [16–18]. HCV infection is either an uncommon and unimportant etiologic factor or most likely a coincidental finding.

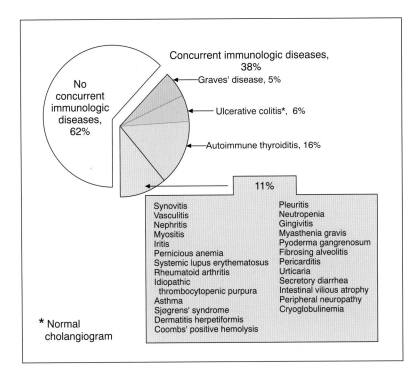

FIGURE 3-7.

Concurrent immunologic diseases in type 1 autoimmune hepatitis. Autoimmune thyroiditis is the most common associated immune disease [20,36,38]. The presence of ulcerative colitis does not compel the diagnosis of primary sclerosing cholangitis (PSC), but it does mandate the performance of cholangiography [39]. Forty-two percent of patients with type 1 autoimmune hepatitis and ulcerative colitis have cholangiographic features of PSC and recalcitrance to corticosteroid therapy [39]. Patients with concurrent immunologic diseases commonly have the HLA DR4 [38,40].

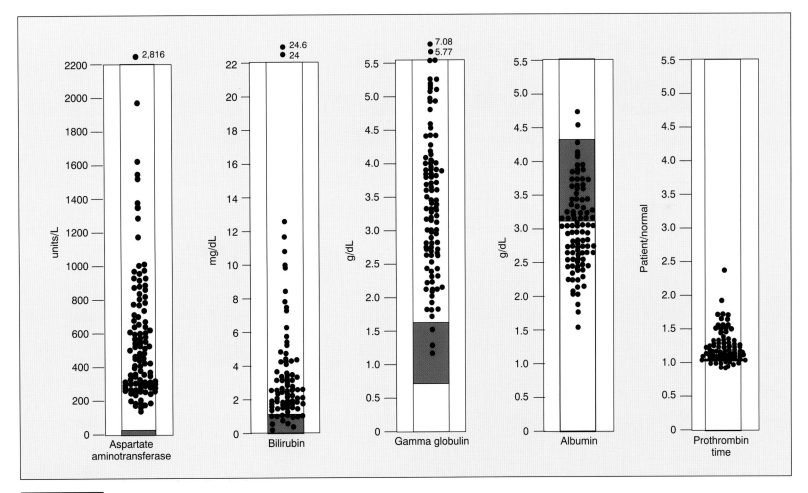

FIGURE 3-8.

Laboratory findings in severe type 1 autoimmune hepatitis. The range of serum aminotransferase, bilirubin, gamma globulin, and albumin levels at presentation may be wide [36,41]. Serum aminotransferase activity may resemble that of a severe acute hepatitis [37].

The serum gamma globulin level, however, is rarely normal, and the majority of patients have hypoalbuminemia [5]. The shaded areas in the figure indicate the normal range for each of the laboratory tests.

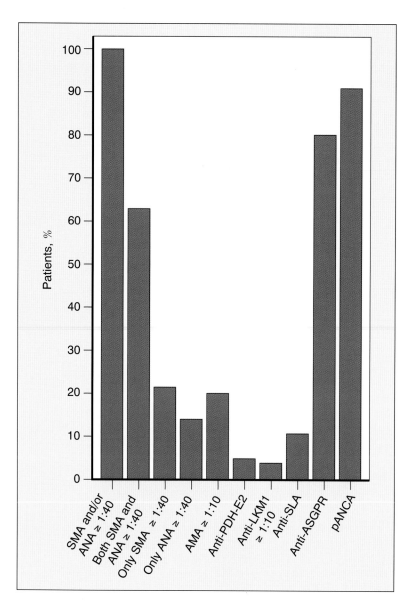

FIGURE 3-9.

Immunoserologic markers in type 1 autoimmune hepatitis. By definition, patients with type 1 autoimmune hepatitis are seropositive for smooth-muscle antibodies (SMA) or antinuclear antibodies (ANA) [1]. In 64% of patients, both markers are present concurrently [38]. Antimitochondrial antibodies (AMA) may be present in 20% of patients and are usually in low titer (≤1:40) [35]. In 27% of patients, the pattern of indirect immunofluorescence of antibodies to liver–kidney microsome type 1 (Anti-LKM1) has been confused with the AMA pattern, and the patients are diagnosed as falsely positive for AMA [34]. In 5% of patients, antibodies to the E2 subunits of the pyruvate dehydrogenase complex (Anti-PDH-E2) are present; these patients may in fact have primary biliary cirrhosis [35]. Antibodies to asialoglycoprotein receptor (Anti-ASGPR) are commonly present but do not distinguish specific subtypes of disease [23,42]. Perinuclear antineutrophil cytoplasmic antibodies (pANCA) are generally present in high titer, but the significance remains uncertain [43–45]. Anti-SLA—antibodies to soluble liver antigen.

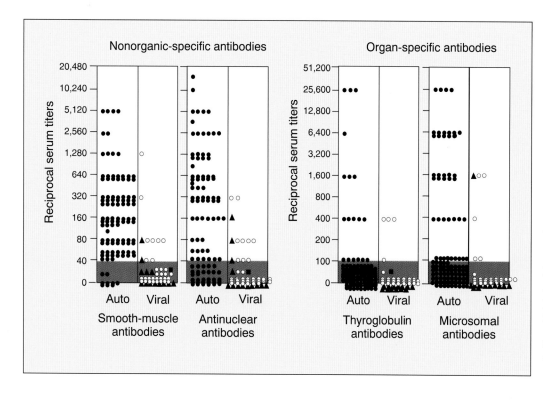

FIGURE 3-10.

Autoantibody titers in autoimmune hepatitis and chronic viral hepatitis. Patients with autoimmune hepatitis typically have titers of smooth-muscle antibodies (SMA) or antinuclear antibodies (ANA) that exceed 1:80 [20,21,38]. Patients with chronic hepatitis B (*triangles*), chronic hepatitis C (*open circles*), and posttransfusion hepatitis of unknown cause (*squares*) are seropositive for SMA (22% vs 90%, P < 0.0001) and ANA (22% vs 70%, P < 0.001) less commonly than those with autoimmune hepatitis, and they less frequently have autoantibody titers of greater than or equal to 1:80 (11% vs 84%, P < 0.0001) [20]. In contrast, organ-specific autoantibodies, such as thyroid antibodies, occur as commonly in chronic viral hepatitis as in autoimmune hepatitis, and the range of titer elevation for microsomal antibodies is similar in both groups [20]. The *shaded areas* in the figure indicate the range of seronegativity for each of the immunoserologic markers. (*From* Czaja *et al.* [20]; with permission.)

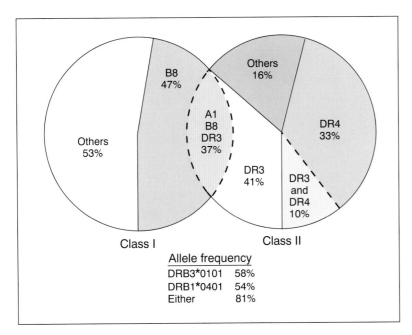

Allele frequency	
DRB3*0101	58%
DRB1*0401	54%
Either	81%

FIGURE 3-11.

Human leukocyte antigen phenotypes in type 1 autoimmune hepatitis. HLA-DR3 and HLA-DR4 are independent risk factors for autoimmune hepatitis in white patients of northern European background [46]. HLA-DR4 is the predominant phenotype in Japan [47]. The prevalence and behavior of autoimmune hepatitis in different regions of the world probably relate to HLA frequencies. HLA-B8 is in strong linkage dysequilibrium (94% concurrence) with HLA-DR3, and the phenotype A1-B8-DR3 characterizes type 1 autoimmune hepatitis [38]. The alleles DRB3*0101, which encodes for DR52a, and DRB1*0401 are present in 81% of patients [48]. These alleles encode the amino acid sequence of the DRB polypeptide, and they thereby determine the ability of each class II molecule to bind and present antigen to T cells [48]. This determination influences the specificity of the activated T-cell lymphocytes that are the effectors of the disease.

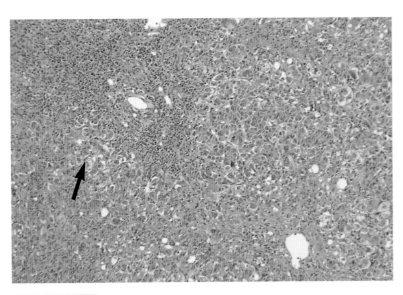

FIGURE 3-12.

Histologic findings of periportal hepatitis and bridging necrosis in severe type 1 autoimmune hepatitis (hematoxylin and eosin; original magnification, x100). The histologic hallmark of autoimmune hepatitis is periportal hepatitis (piecemeal necrosis), which is the *sine qua non* of the disease [1]. It is defined as disruption of the limiting plate of the portal tract by inflammatory infiltrate (*arrow*). Gamma globulin deposits were found in hepatic mesenchymal cells in association with lymphocytes, plasma cells, histocytes, and proliferated bile ductules, and the character of the lesion suggested an immunologically mediated cytodestructive process [3]. The specificity of piecemeal necrosis for autoimmune hepatitis is no longer recognized [4]. Extension of the inflammatory activity between portal tracts (portal–portal bridging necrosis) or between portal tracts and central vein (portal–central bridging necrosis) connotes a more severe lesion with a greater propensity for progression to cirrhosis [1]. Portal–central bridging has a higher predilection for cirrhosis than portal–portal bridging, but in most instances the lesions are of mixed character or indeterminate because of sampling variation [1].

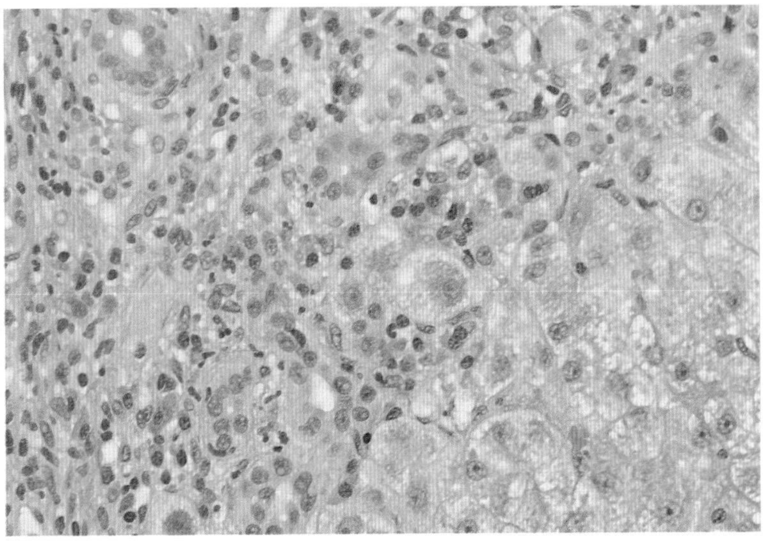

FIGURE 3-13.

Histologic findings of plasma cell infiltration of the portal tracts in type 1 autoimmune hepatitis (hematoxylin and eosin; original magnification, x400). Moderate-to-severe plasma cell infiltration of the portal tracts is found in 66% of tissue specimens [49]. Assessments using monoclonal antibodies have indicated that the major component of the inflammatory cell infiltrate in the portal tracts is the T lymphocyte [50]. Nevertheless, the recognition of plasma cells has diagnostic value [49]. In portal and periportal regions, the helper/inducer cells (CD4) are more numerous than the suppressor/cytotoxic T cells (CD8) [51]. In the lobule and in areas of piecemeal necrosis, the reverse is true [51].

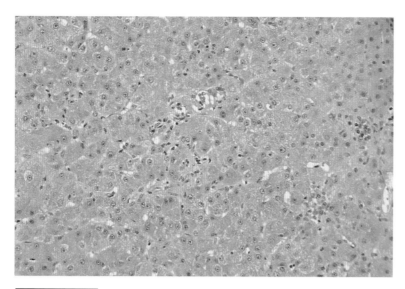

FIGURE 3-14.

Histologic findings of lobular hepatitis in severe type 1 autoimmune hepatitis (hematoxylin and eosin; original magnification, x100). Prominent cellular infiltrates that line sinusoidal spaces in association with liver cell degenerative or regenerative changes and Kupffer cell hyperplasia connote lobular hepatitis [49]. Moderate-to-severe lobular hepatitis can be found at presentation or during relapse of autoimmune hepatitis; its presence has diagnostic value in distinguishing autoimmune hepatitis from chronic hepatitis C [49,52]. The presence of lobular hepatitis is part of the histologic spectrum of autoimmune hepatitis [4].

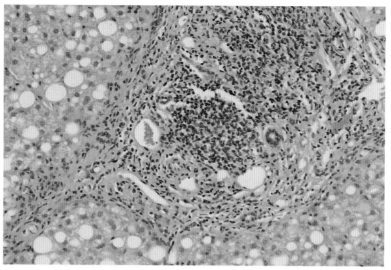

FIGURE 3-15.

Histologic findings that distinguish chronic hepatitis C from autoimmune hepatitis (hematoxylin and eosin; original magnification, x200). A germinal center with surrounding small lymphocytes or a densely packed collection of small lymphocytes within a portal tract connotes a portal lymphoid aggregate and suggests the diagnosis of chronic hepatitis C [49,52,53]. The presence of small, large, or mixed-size vacuoles of lipids within the cytoplasm of hepatocytes (steatosis) or bile duct damage or loss also suggests the diagnosis of chronic hepatitis C [49,52,53]. The absence of these changes and the presence of moderate-to-severe piecemeal necrosis, lobular inflammation, broad areas of parenchymal collapse, and multinucleated hepatocytes suggest the diagnosis of autoimmune hepatitis [49,52].

TABLE 3-1. IMPORTANT INDIVIDUAL HISTOLOGIC FEATURES THAT DISTINGUISH AUTOIMMUNE HEPATITIS FROM CHRONIC HEPATITIS C

	AUTOIMMUNE HEPATITIS, %	CHRONIC HEPATITIS C, %	P VALUE
Portal plasma cells	66	21	0.005
Piecemeal necrosis (moderate to severe)	23	0	0.02
Lobular hepatitis (moderate to severe)	47	16	0.04
Portal lymphoid aggregates	42	76	0.05
Steatosis	16	52	0.005

TABLE 3-1.

Careful histologic examination can have diagnostic value and can strengthen therapeutic decisions, especially in patients with clinical features of a mixed autoimmune and viral nature. Portal lymphoid aggregates, steatosis, or bile duct changes in the absence of moderate-to-severe piecemeal necrosis and lobular hepatitis support the diagnosis of chronic hepatitis C [49,52,53]. Unfortunately, there are no pathognomonic features. Immunohistochemical techniques using monoclonal antibodies against hepatitis C virus antigens identify sparse, focal changes that are limited by sampling variation and low sensitivity [54].

TABLE 3-2. PERFORMANCE PARAMETERS OF HISTOLOGIC INTERPRETATION IN AUTOIMMUNE HEPATITIS AND CHRONIC HEPATITIS C

	CLINICAL DIAGNOSES*, %	
PERFORMANCE PARAMETERS	AUTOIMMUNE HEPATITIS	CHRONIC HEPATITIS C
Sensitivity	40	57
Specificity	81	91
Positive predictability	68	67
Negative predictability	57	87
Overall predictability	62	82

*Gold standard for the diagnosis against which histologic assessments were measured

TABLE 3-2.

Histologic interpretation must be rendered on the basis of composite morphologic changes and the predominance of individual features previously identified as having diagnostic value [49]. Portal lymphoid aggregates or steatosis suggest the diagnosis of chronic hepatitis C with a sensitivity of 57% and specificity of 91% [49]. The absence of these changes and the presence of moderate-to-severe piecemeal necrosis or lobular inflammation suggest the diagnosis of autoimmune hepatitis with a sensitivity of 40% and specificity of 81% [49]. The high specificity and predictability of the histologic patterns are compromised by low sensitivity [49].

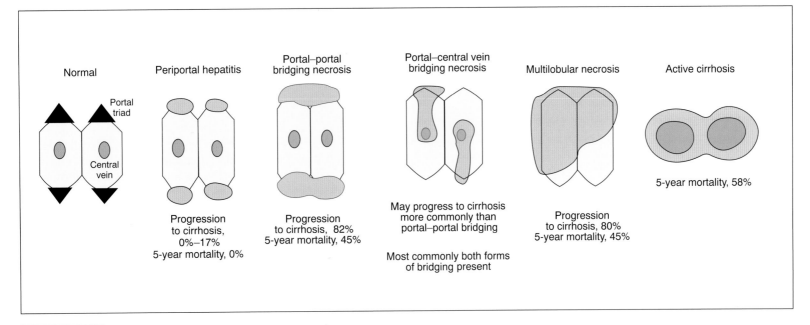

FIGURE 3-16.

Prognoses of initial histologic patterns in untreated type 1 autoimmune hepatitis. The severity and aggressiveness of the inflammatory process can be estimated by the histologic pattern at presentation [1,41]. The type and degree of hepatic inflammation can be assessed by needle biopsy with 90% accuracy [1]. Sampling variation and intraobserver interpretive error limit the ability of needle biopsy to evaluate cirrhosis [1]. Portal–portal and portal–central bridging necrosis are frequently mixed findings or are difficult to distinguish. Periportal hepatitis, which is the hallmark lesion of autoimmune hepatitis, typically has a benign prognosis and does not require therapy per se [1,25]. Transitions can occur between the various histologic patterns spontaneously or during therapy [1,25].

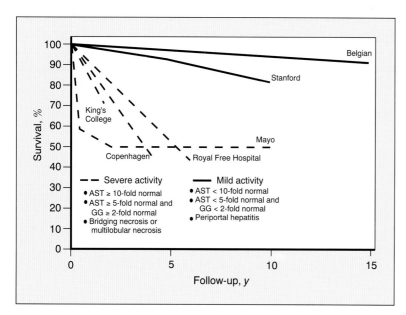

Figure 3-17.

Prognoses associated with different degrees of inflammatory activity in untreated type 1 autoimmune hepatitis. Sustained severe laboratory changes or histologic features of confluent necrosis have a poorer prognosis than laboratory and histologic changes of lesser magnitude [1]. Randomized treatment trials indicate that patients assigned to control or nonsteroidal therapies have a mortality as high as 40% within 6 months of presentation and a 5-year life expectancy of 45% to 50% [1]. AST—aspartate aminotransferase; GG—gamma globulin.

TYPE 2 AUTOIMMUNE HEPATITIS

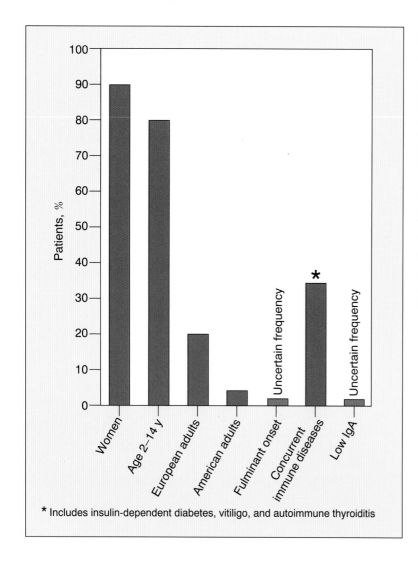

* Includes insulin-dependent diabetes, vitiligo, and autoimmune thyroiditis

Figure 3-18.

Clinical features of type 2 autoimmune hepatitis. The diagnosis requires the presence of antibodies to liver–kidney microsome type 1 (Anti-LKM1), but antibodies to hepatitis C virus and hepatitis C virus RNA may be present [28–30]. The disease has been described mainly in pediatric patients in Western Europe, but adults may also be afflicted [55]. In the United States, seropositivity for Anti-LKM1 has been found in only 4% of adults [34] and hepatitis C virus infection has not been a feature of the disease. Patients with type 2 autoimmune hepatitis typically have concurrent immunologic diseases, including autoimmune thyroiditis, insulin-dependent diabetes, vitiligo, and ulcerative colitis [55]. They have a high frequency of organ-specific autoantibodies, such as parietal cell antibodies, antibodies to the islets of Langerhans, and thyroid antibodies [55]. An acute, even fulminant, presentation may occur, and patients uncommonly have a pronounced hypergammaglobulinemia [55,56]. Interestingly, they may have a low serum immunoglobulin A (IgA) concentration [55].

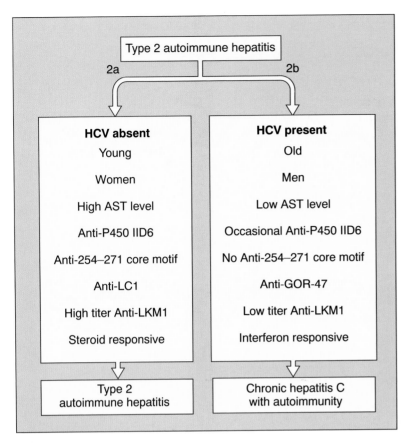

FIGURE 3-19.

Subtypes of type 2 autoimmune hepatitis. Patients with type 2a autoimmune hepatitis lack evidence of hepatitis C virus (HCV) infection [29,30]. These patients fit the profile typical of those with autoimmune hepatitis and they respond well to corticosteroid therapy. Patients with type 2b autoimmune hepatitis have HCV infection [29,30]. These individuals have the profile typical of patients with chronic viral hepatitis and may or may not respond to interferon therapy [27,57]. Patients with type 2a disease more commonly have antibodies to P450 IID6 than patients with type 2b disease [58,59]. Additionally, these patients have disease-specific immunoreactivity against synthetic peptides containing the amino acid sequence 254-271 of P450 IID6 [60]. In contrast, patients with type 2b disease and antibodies to P450 IID6 lack immunoreactivity against this core motif; they also have antibodies to GOR-47 (Anti-GOR-47) (common in chronic HCV infection) [29,60]. Antibodies to liver cytosol type 1 (Anti-LC1) characterize young patients with type 2a disease but are present in only 32% of such patients [61]. Anti-LKM1—antibodies to liver–kidney microsome type 1; AST—aspartate aminotransferase.

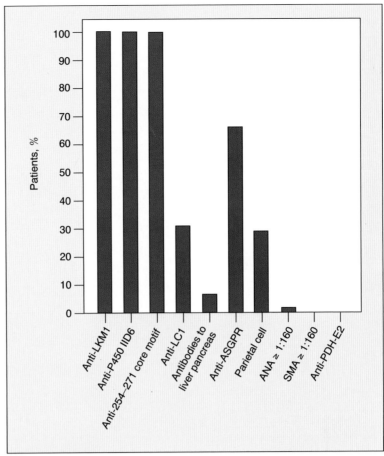

FIGURE 3-20.

Immunoserologic markers in nonviral type 2 autoimmune hepatitis. Antibodies to liver–kidney microsome type 1 (Anti-LKM1), P450 IID6 (Anti-P450 IID6), and the core motif 254-271 amino acid sequence (Anti-254-271) characterize these patients [58–60,62]. Antibodies to asialoglycoprotein receptor (Anti-ASGPR) are common, but they do not distinguish this subgroup [23,42]. Organ-specific autoantibodies, such as parietal cell antibodies, are frequently demonstrated [55]. Smooth-muscle antibodies (SMA) and antinuclear antibodies (ANA) rarely occur together with Anti-LKM1 [34,55]. Anti-LC1—antibodies to liver cytosol type 1; Anti-PDH-E2—antibodies to the E2 subunits of the pyruvate dehydrogenase complex.

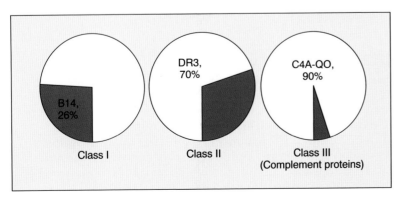

FIGURE 3-21.

Human leukocyte antigen phenotypes in nonviral type 2 autoimmune hepatitis. Preliminary studies indicate an association with B14, DR3, and C4A-QO [63]. The linkages among the class I, class II, and class III antigens are unknown, and it is unclear how significantly these phenotypes differ from those in ethnically matched patients with type 1 autoimmune hepatitis.

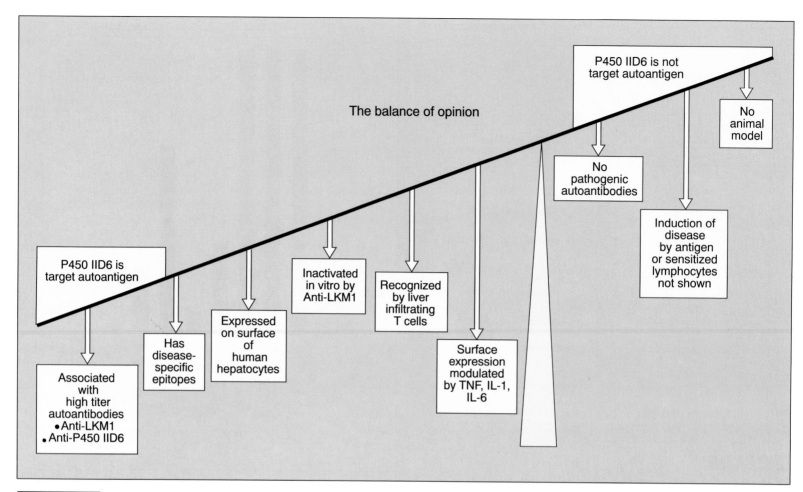

FIGURE 3-22.

Recognition of cytochrome monooxygenase P450 IID6 as the target autoantigen of type 2 autoimmune hepatitis. The balance of opinion favors the candidacy of P450 IID6 as the target autoantigen of type 2 autoimmune hepatitis because of its association with high titer autoantibodies and disease-specific epitopes, expression on hepa-tocyte membrane surfaces, inactivation in vitro by antibodies to liver–kidney microsome type 1 (Anti-LKM1), recognition by liver-infiltrating T cells, and modulation by cytokines [62,64–67]. Anti-P450 IID6—antibodies to P450 IID6; IL-1—interleukin 1; IL-6—interleukin 6; TNF—tumor necrosis factor.

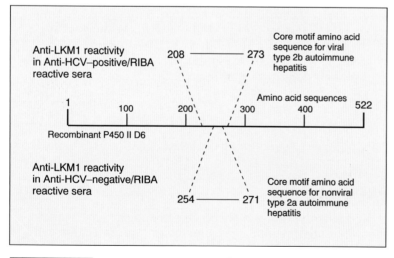

FIGURE 3-23.

Epitopes for antibodies to liver–kidney microsome type 1 (Anti-LKM1) on recombinant P450 IID6 in patients with and without hepatitis C virus (HCV) infection. The core amino acid sequence 254–271 is recognized only by sera from patients with Anti-LKM1 and no evidence of HCV infection [60]. The amino acid sequence 208-273 is recognized by the majority of sera obtained from patients with Anti-LKM1 and HCV infection [60]. The different immunoreactivities suggest that the Anti-LKM1 are different in patients with and without HCV infection. Anti-HCV—antibodies to HCV; RIBA—recombinant immunoblot assay.

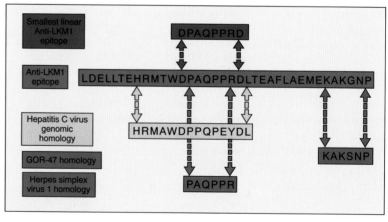

FIGURE 3-24.

Amino acid sequences within P450 IID6 that are recognized by antibodies to liver–kidney microsome type 1 (Anti-LKM1) and the presence of homologies with other epitopes. The smallest epitope of recombinant P450 IID6 recognized by Anti-LKM1 is eight amino acids [62]. The majority of antibodies will react against a 33–amino acid epitope. Amino acid sequences within the Anti-LKM1 epitope have homology with the hepatitis C virus genome, the genome of herpes simplex type 1, and GOR-47 [62]. These homologies suggest that cross-reacting antibodies may be gener-ated by any of these antigens.

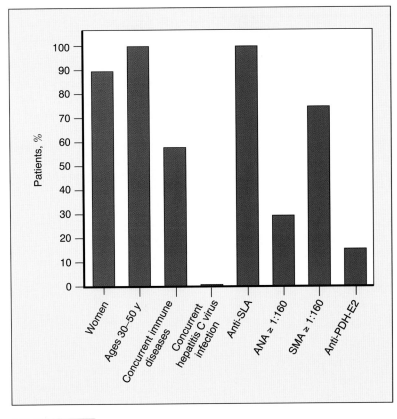

FIGURE 3-25.

Clinical and immunoserologic features of type 3 autoimmune hepatitis. This subtype is characterized by the presence of antibodies to soluble liver antigen (Anti-SLA) [31]. The clinical and immuno-serologic profiles resemble that of type 1 autoimmune hepatitis [31,35]. The validity of type 3 autoimmune hepatitis as a distinct subgroup remains uncertain. ANA—antinuclear antibodies; Anti-PDH-E2—antibodies to the E2 subunits of the pyruvate dehydro-genase complex; SMA—smooth muscle antibodies.

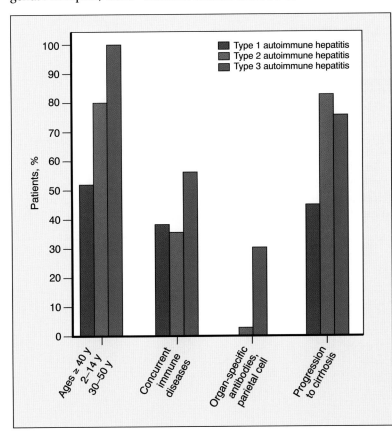

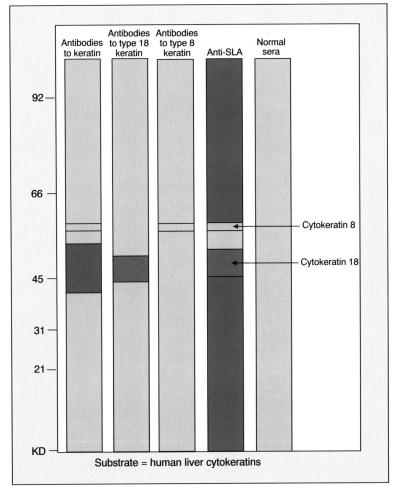

FIGURE 3-26.

Immunoblot analysis indicating reactivity of antibodies to soluble liver antigen (Anti-SLA) against liver cytokeratins. Reactivity against cytokeratins 8 and 18 can be demonstrated in Anti-SLA specimens by using human liver cytokeratins as substrate and applying anti-bodies to keratin and monoclonal antibodies to keratin type 1 through 8 and 18, normal sera, and sera from patients with Anti-SLA [68]. These findings indicate that cytokeratins 8 and 18 are the target antigens of Anti-SLA [68]. (*Adapted from* Wachter *et al.* [68]; with permission.)

FIGURE 3-27.

Pertinent differences among the three proposed subtypes of autoimmune hepatitis. The major differences are in age, frequency of organ-specific autoantibodies, and prognoses. Preliminary studies suggest that patients with type 2 autoimmune hepatitis more commonly progress to cirrhosis than patients with type 1 [55].

TABLE 3-3. PLETHORA OF AUTOANTIBODIES ASSOCIATED WITH AUTOIMMUNE HEPATITIS

Autoantibody species	Target antigen(s)	Implication(s)
Nuclear	Centromere 52K SSA/Ro Histones Ribonucleoproteins Complex subcellular particle (?)	Type 1 hepatitis Epiphenomenon Affects nuclear functions
Smooth muscle	Actin (F,G) Tubulin Intermediate filaments	Type 1 hepatitis Nonactin activity in viral disease
Actin	Polymerized F actin	High specificity in type 1 hepatitis May facilitate surface binding of antibody
Liver-kidney microsome type 1	P450 IID6	Type 2 hepatitis Inhibits P450 IID6 Present in hepatitis C virus
P450 IID6	Recombinant P450 IID6	Type 2 hepatitis
254–271 core motif	Synthetic peptides of P450 IID6	Nonviral type 2
Liver cytosol 1	Cytosolic protein	Nonviral hepatitis type 2a
Soluble liver antigen	Cytokeratins 8, 18	Type 3 hepatitis Cryptogenic marker
Liver-pancreas	Cytosolic noncytokeratins	Type 3 hepatitis Cryptogenic marker
Asialoglycoprotein receptor	Transmembrane glycoprotein	Autoimmune marker
Perinuclear antineutrophil cytoplasmic antibodies	Neutrophil granule components	High titer High frequency IgG1 isotype Unknown function

TABLE 3-3.

Antibodies to polymerized F-actin have been proposed as specific for type 1 autoimmune hepatitis and, in some regions, type 1 disease is already referred to as *antiactin hepatitis* [1,25,55]. Antibodies to liver–pancreas are present in 33% of patients with cryptogenic chronic hepatitis and have been proposed as a better marker for type 3 autoimmune hepatitis than antibodies to soluble liver antigen [32].

AUTOANTIBODY-NEGATIVE AUTOIMMUNE HEPATITIS

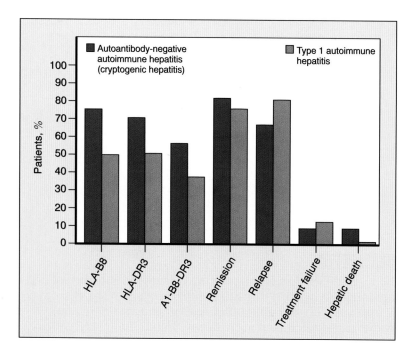

FIGURE 3-28.

Autoantibody-negative autoimmune hepatitis (*ie*, cryptogenic chronic hepatitis) is indistinguishable from type 1 autoimmune hepatitis by HLA and response to corticosteroids. These patients satisfy all criteria for autoimmune hepatitis, including histologic features [33]. However, they lack conventional immunoserologic markers. Such patients must be differentiated from those with cryptogenic chronic liver disease, which usually connotes nondescript end-stage inactive cirrhosis [2,33].

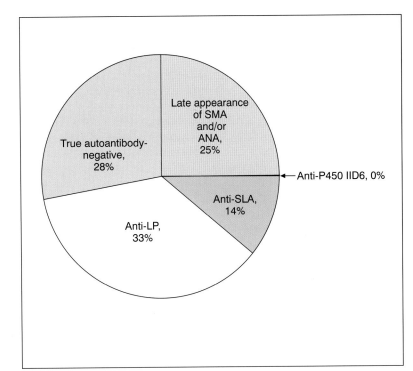

FIGURE 3-29.

Reclassification of autoantibody-negative autoimmune hepatitis by novel autoantibodies and serial testing for conventional immuno-serologic markers. The majority of marker-negative patients can be reclassified as having marker-positive autoimmune hepatitis by repeated testing or by assessments for antibodies to liver–pancreas (Anti-LP) or soluble liver antigen (Anti-SLA) [32,35]. Smooth-muscle antibodies (SMA) and antinuclear antibodies (ANA) may not be detected at initial screening because titers may fluctuate spontaneously [3]. Sequential testing may disclose their presence later in the course of the disease. Unfortunately, many patients still lack a diagnostic immunoserologic marker despite these measures [2].

PATHOGENESIS

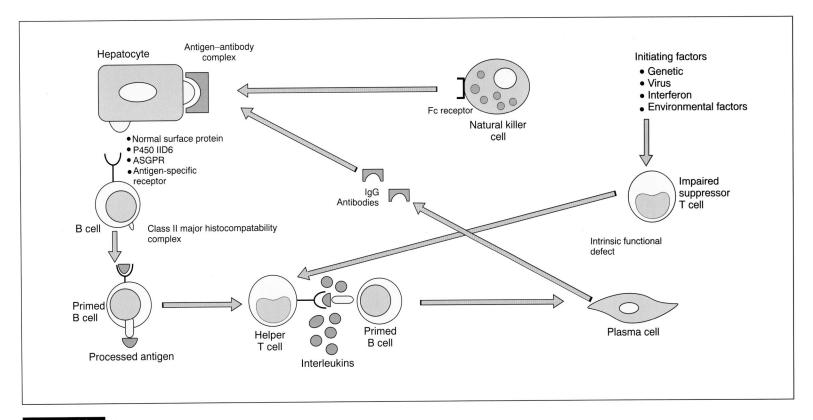

FIGURE 3-30.

Pathogenic hypothesis based on antibody-dependent, cell-mediated cytotoxicity. The principal defect is impairment of suppressor T-cell function [1,69]. Immunoglobulin G (IgG) production by plasma cells is inadequately modulated and antibodies complex with normal proteins on the hepatocyte surface. Candidate target antigens are asialoglycoprotein receptor (ASGPR) and P450 IID6. The antigen–antibody complex is the target for natural killer cells that have Fc receptors. The natural killer cells do not require prior sensitization to a specific antigen, but the antibody complex does provide some antigen specificity. Causes for suppressor cell dysfunction are unknown, but initiating factors may include genetic predisposition, viral infection, exogenous or endogenous interferon, and environmental factors. Corticosteroids improve nonantigen–specific suppressor T-cell dysfunction. Antigen-specific suppressor T-cell dysfunction is not affected by corticosteroid treatment and may perpetuate the disease. Unfortunately, this type of defect has not been consistently demonstrated in autoimmune hepatitis. (*Adapted from* Czaja [70]; with permission.)

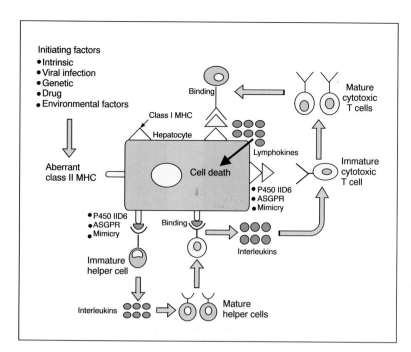

FIGURE 3-31.

Pathogenic hypothesis based on cell-mediated cytotoxicity. Aberrant expression of class II antigens on the antigen-presenting cell (shown here theoretically as the hepatocyte) may be induced by intrinsic factors associated with inflammatory activity, viral infection, genetic predisposition, drugs, or environmental factors. The presentation of target antigens, such as asialoglycoprotein receptor (ASGPR) and P450 IID6, to immature helper T cells may thereby be facilitated and a cascade of events initiated that results in the clonal expansion of cytotoxic T cells. Alternatively, the target antigen may be another protein that has homology with ASGPR or P450 IID6, initiating the sequence by molecular mimicry. Class I antigens, which are normally present on the hepatocyte membrane, may also facilitate direct expression of these same target antigens to immature cytotoxic T cells. Their activation and clonal expansion can then also lead to cytodestruction. MHC—major histocompatibility complex. (*Modified from* Czaja [70]; with permission.)

TREATMENT STRATEGIES

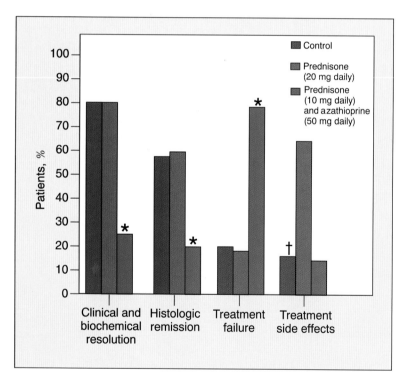

FIGURE 3-32.

Justifications for corticosteroid therapy in autoimmune hepatitis and the preference for administration of prednisone in combination with azathioprine. Several controlled clinical trials have demonstrated that corticosteroids ameliorate symptoms, improve laboratory abnormalities, induce histologic remission, and enhance immediate survival compared with untreated counterparts with disease of similar severity [1]. In the Mayo Clinic experience, prednisone alone or in a lower dose in combination with azathioprine induces clinical, biochemical, and histologic remission with frequencies comparable with each other and superior to that in a control population [1]. The combination regimen has significantly fewer side effects and is preferred over the regimen using a higher dose of prednisone alone [1]. The *asterisk* indicates significantly different results from prednisone alone or prednisone in combination with azathioprine. The *dagger* indicates significantly different results from prednisone alone.

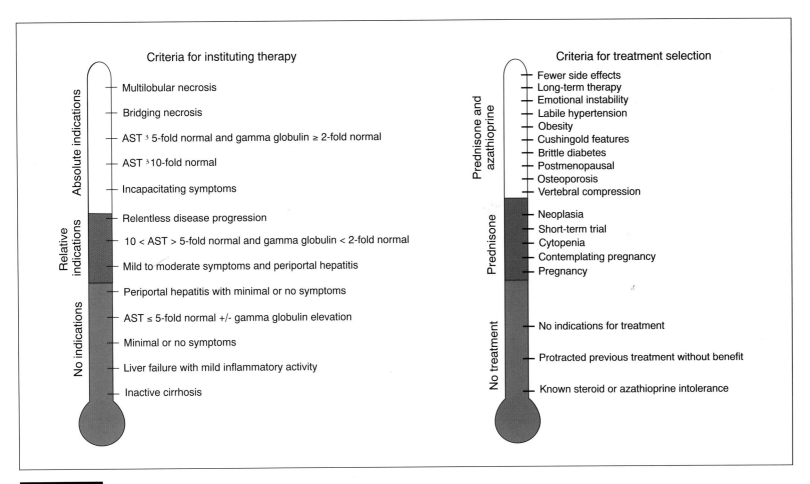

FIGURE 3-33.

Criteria for instituting therapy and selecting the appropriate treatment regimen. Disease severity, as assessed by symptoms, laboratory tests, and histologic examination, is the determinant for treatment [1]. Prednisone in combination with azathioprine is the preferred therapy, but it may not be indicated in all patients [1,25].

Previously untreated postmenopausal patients should be treated as vigorously as their premenopausal counterparts. Consequences such as vertebral compression develop mainly after multiple relapses and re-treatments [71]. AST—aspartate aminotransferase.

TREATMENT RESULTS

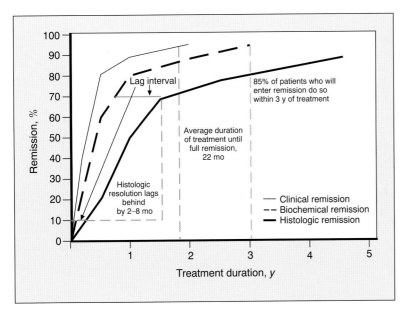

FIGURE 3-34.

Probabilities of clinical, biochemical, and histologic remission during corticosteroid therapy. The majority of patients (85%) who enter remission during therapy do so within 3 years [1]. The average duration of treatment to achieve remission is 22 months [1,25,36]. Because histologic remission lags behind clinical and biochemical remission by 3 to 6 months, treatment should be continued for at least this long following laboratory resolution. A liver biopsy assessment is necessary to establish a confident treatment endpoint [72].

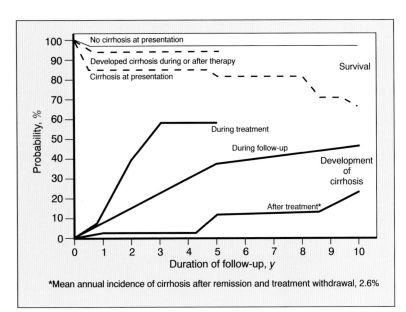

FIGURE 3-35.

Survival expectations and probability of developing cirrhosis
during and after corticosteroid treatment. Patients without
cirrhosis at presentation have better 5- and 10-year survival rates
than patients with cirrhosis at presentation [1]. Cirrhosis develops
in 47% of patients within 10 years after presentation despite corticosteroid treatment [1]. The highest probability of cirrhosis is
during initial therapy when the disease is most active. The mean
annual incidence of cirrhosis after initial remission is 2.6% [1].
Survival after the development of cirrhosis during or after treatment is similar to that of patients without cirrhosis [1,25]. These
findings suggest that the prognosis of cirrhosis after treatment is
related to the stage of the disease and the degree of inflammatory
activity accompanying the process.

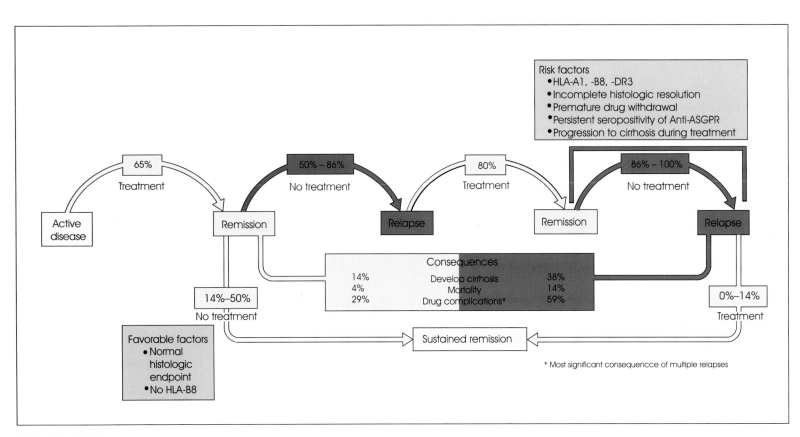

FIGURE 3-36.

Relapse after remission and drug withdrawal. Relapse after drug
withdrawal occurs in 50% to 86% of patients [73,74]. Reinstitution
of the original treatment regimen typically induces another remission, but the probability of another relapse after drug withdrawal
increases [73]. Premature drug withdrawal, incomplete histologic
resolution, persistence of antibodies to asialoglycoprotein receptor
(Anti-ASGPR), and the HLA-B8 or DRB3*0101 are factors that

augur relapse [1,25,42,48,72]. Progression to cirrhosis during
initial therapy is invariably associated with this outcome [72].
The principal consequences of relapse and re-treatment are drug-
induced side effects that diminish the net benefit–risk ratio of
therapy [75]. Treatment to a normal histologic endpoint reduces
the probability of relapse to 20% [72].

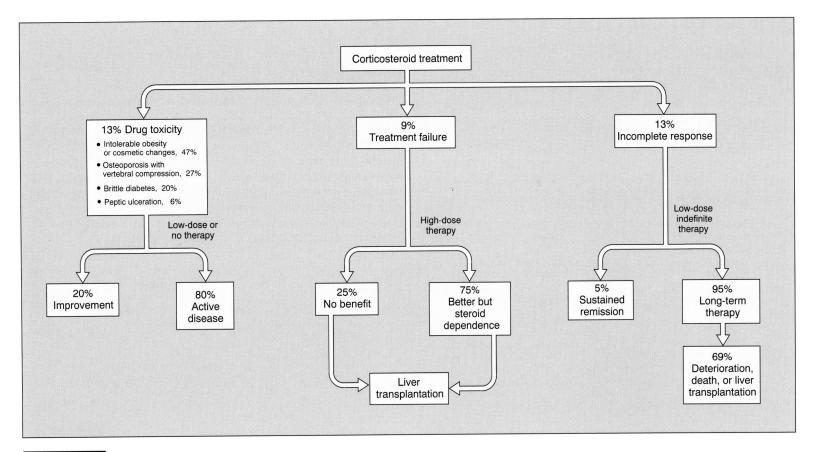

FIGURE 3-37.

Adverse responses to corticosteroid therapy and treatment strategies. Patients may develop serious drug toxicities, deteriorate despite compliance with the treatment regimen (*ie*, treatment failure), or fail to achieve remission after protracted therapy

(*ie*, incomplete response) [1]. These outcomes justify changes in the original treatment strategy. Liver transplantation is an option for the decompensated patient [76].

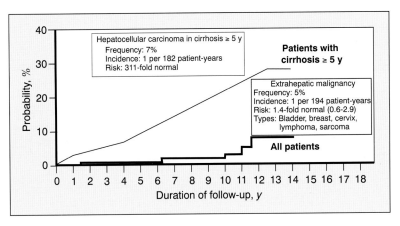

FIGURE 3-38.

Hepatocellular carcinoma and extrahepatic malignancy in corticosteroid-treated autoimmune hepatitis. As patients with cirrhosis live longer with effective therapy, the risk of hepatocellular carcinoma increases [77]. Surveillance programs using regular hepatic ultrasonography and serum α-fetoprotein determinations have not been assessed in this condition, and follow-up regimens must be determined on an individual basis [78]. The risk of extrahepatic malignancy is higher than normal in treated patients but does not contraindicate the use of potentially life-saving immunosuppressive drugs [79]. However, the risk of neoplasia does underscore the importance of carefully selecting patients for such treatment.

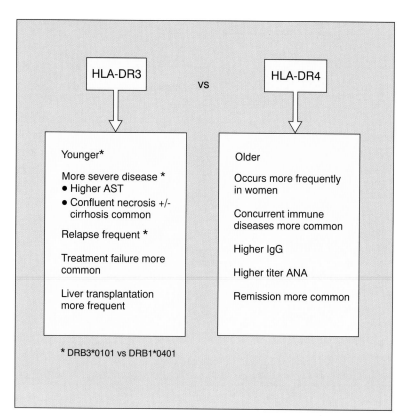

FIGURE 3-39.

Human leukocyte antigen phenotypes and disease behavior. The clinical expression of autoimmune hepatitis and its behavior during and after corticosteroid therapy are different in patients with HLA-DR3 and HLA-DR4 phenotypes [38,40,46,48,76]. In general, patients with HLA-DR3 have more severe and aggressive liver disease than patients with HLA-DR4 [40,48,76]. As yet, classification of patients by HLA phenotype has not been endorsed but may have a better rationale than classification schemes based on immunoserologic markers. ANA—antinuclear antibodies; AST—aspartate aminotransferase; IgG—immunoglobin G.

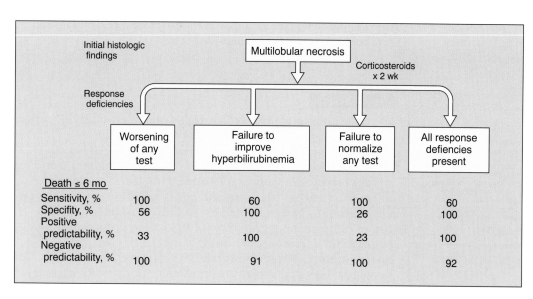

FIGURE 3-40.

Immediate treatment response as a prognostic index. There are no findings at presentation that confidently predict prognosis. Outcome can only be determined after assessment of response to corticosteroid therapy. Usually, this assessment can be done after 2 weeks of treatment. Prognosis is poorest in patients with multilobular necrosis at presentation [41]. If hyperbilirubinemia does not improve within 2 weeks, the patient invariably dies within 6 months. These patients should be evaluated expeditiously for liver transplantation [41]. Alternatively, improvement or normalization of any test during this interval predicts immediate survival in 92% of patients [41].

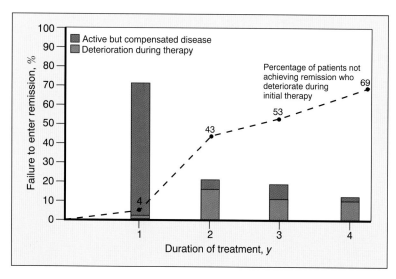

FIGURE 3-41.

Failure to enter remission after protracted treatment as a prognostic index. The majority of patients enter remission within 3 years after institution of treatment [76]. Failure to enter remission is associated with a risk of deterioration, and this risk increases with the duration of time that remission is not achieved [76]. Sixty-nine percent of patients who have not entered remission after 4 years of continuous therapy deteriorate and become candidates for liver transplantation [76]. The most common manifestation of decompensation is the development of ascites [76].

TREATMENT SCHEDULES

TABLE 3-4. RECOMMENDED PREDNISONE TREATMENT SCHEDULES FOR AUTOIMMUNE HEPATITIS

	DAILY DOSES ALONE, mG	DAILY DOSES WITH 50 mG AZATHIOPRINE
Week 1	60	30
Week 2	40	20
Week 3	30	15
Week 4	30	15
Until endpoint	20	10

TABLE 3-4.

Regimens are designed to control inflammatory activity rapidly with high initial doses. The dose of prednisone is then reduced systematically over a 4-week period until a fixed daily maintenance dose is achieved [1,25,80,81]. Laboratory tests are performed at the 2-week and 3-month intervals to document disease response [80].

Dose reduction does not have to be monitored by frequent laboratory tests. After 3 months, testing at 6-month intervals is appropriate [80]. The daily maintenance dose should not be reduced until histologic remission is achieved. Treatment failure or major drug toxicity are the only indications for interim dose adjustments [1,81].

MANAGEMENT OF SUBOPTIMAL RESPONSES

TABLE 3-5. PREDNISONE TREATMENT FAILURE REGIMENS

	DAILY DOSES ALONE, mG	DAILY DOSES (WITH AZATHIOPRINE), mG
Month 1	60	30 (150)
Month 2*	50	20 (100)
Month 3*	40	10 (50)
Month 4*	30	10 (50)
Month 5*	20	10 (50)

*Dose reductions each month only if clinical and laboratory improvement

TABLE 3-5.

Worsening of the serum aspartate aminotransferase level, increase in the serum bilirubin level by at least 67% of the pretreatment value, worsening of the histologic pattern of inflammatory activity, development of ascites, or emergence of endogenous encephalopathy during treatment connotes treatment failure [1]. Doses higher than conventional regimens are warranted [1]. Fixed doses must be administered for at least 1 month before attempting dose reduction. Dose reductions each month are justified by sustained

clinical and biochemical improvements [1,25]. When conventional maintenance doses are reached, no further dose reductions are necessary until remission is achieved. The high-dose regimens induce clinical and laboratory improvement in 75% of patients within 2 years, but histologic remission is achieved in only 25% of patients [1,25]. These patients commonly become dependent on indefinite corticosteroid therapy and are at risk for drug-related side effects and disease progression.

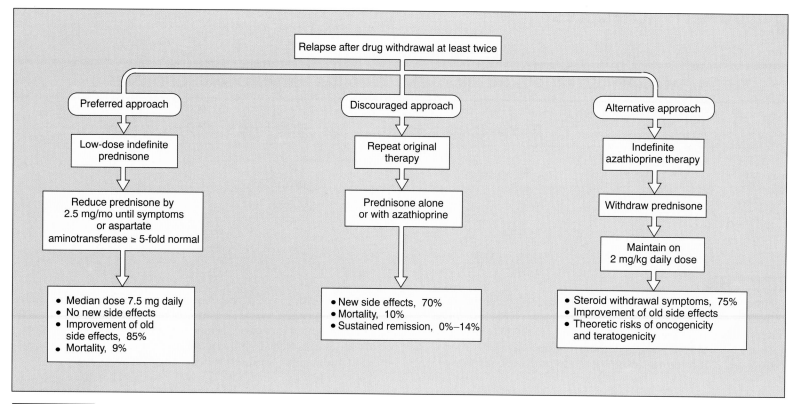

FIGURE 3-42.

Treatment strategies after multiple relapses. The benefit–risk ratio of re-treatment with conventional regimens after at least two relapses diminishes greatly [75]. Low-dose indefinite corticosteroid therapy adequately controls inflammatory activity and is well tolerated [82].

Indefinite azathioprine therapy is another approach, but it is usually associated with corticosteroid withdrawal symptoms and there are theoretic risks of oncogenicity and teratogenicity [83].

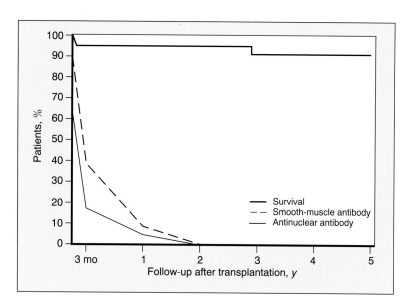

FIGURE 3-43.

Liver transplantation for autoimmune hepatitis. Decompensated patients should be considered for liver transplantation. The 5-year survival rate after transplantation is 92%. Recurrence of disease is rare but possible in inadequately immunosuppressed recipients and in HLA-DR3–positive recipients of HLA-DR3–negative grafts [76,84]. The immunoserologic markers and hypergammaglobulinemia resolve within 2 years [76].

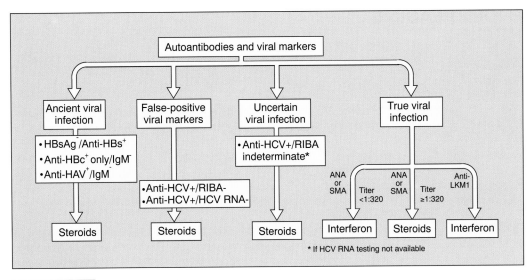

FIGURE 3-44.

Treatment strategies for patients with autoantibodies and viral markers. Interferon therapy in patients with predominant autoimmune features may exacerbate the liver disease [57,85–87]. Corticosteroid therapy in patients with predominant viral disease can increase the virus burden and not improve the inflammatory activity [88]. In patients with mixed features, the treatment strategy is dictated by the predominant manifestations [21]. Patients with ancient viral infection, false-positive viral markers, uncertain viral infection, and high titers ($\geq$ 1:320) of smooth-muscle antibodies (SMA) or antinuclear antibodies (ANA) are candidates for corticosteroid therapy [21]. In the latter instance, corticosteroids do not worsen the disease and 57% of patients enter remission [19]. Most importantly, a possible deterioration induced by interferon therapy is avoided. Patients with true viral infection and low titers (< 1:320) of SMA, ANA, or antibodies to liver–kidney microsome type 1 (Anti-LKM1) are candidates for interferon therapy [21,27,57]. Anti-HAV—antibodies to hepatitis A virus; Anti-HBc—antibodies to hepatitis B core antigen; Anti-HBs—antibodies to hepatitis B surface antigen; Anti-HCV—antibodies to HCV; HBsAg—hepatitis B surface antigen; HCV—hepatitis C virus; IgM—immunoglobin M; RIBA—recombinant immunoblot asssay.

TABLE 3-6. INVESTIGATIONAL TREATMENT CONSIDERATIONS FOR AUTOIMMUNE HEPATITIS

IMUNOSUPPRESSANTS		CYTOPROTECTIVE AGENTS	
Cyclosporine[†]	Inhibits lymphokine release	Phosphatidylcholine*	Modifies liver membrane
FK-506[‡]	Prevents clonal expansion of cytotoxic T cells; inhibits IL-2 receptor; impairs antibody production	Thiazolidine-carboxylate*	
		Ursodeoxycholic acid[†]	Alters class I HLA expression; reduces hydrophobic bile acids; protective physical barrier to liver membrane
Thymic extracts*	Stimulates suppressor cells; inhibits antibody production		
Intravenous immunoglobin[†]	Interferes with Fc receptors; induces suppressor cells; anti-idiotypic suppression of autoantibodies		
Brequinar[§]	Inhibits pyrimidine synthesis; prevents lymphocyte proliferation		
Rapamycin[§]	Blocks after IL-2 and receptor binding; prevents clonal expansion		

*Controlled trial
[†]Anecdotal experience
[‡]Open-label trial
[§]Untested hypothetical agents

TABLE 3-6.

Novel treatment possibilities include immunosuppressant agents that have emerged from the transplantation arena and cytoprotective agents [89–96]. Experiences have been limited and preliminary in most instances. Brequinar and rapamycin have hypothetic advantages that remain to be tested [94–97]. IL-2—interleukin 2.

REFERENCES AND RECOMMENDED READING

1. Czaja AJ: Diagnosis, prognosis, and treatment of classical autoimmune chronic active hepatitis. In *Autoimmune Liver Diseases*. Edited by Krawitt EL, Wiesner RH. New York: Raven Press; 1991:143–166.

2. Czaja AJ: Chronic active hepatitis: The challenge of a new nomenclature. *Ann Intern Med* 1993, 119:510–517.

3. Czaja AJ: Autoimmune chronic active hepatitis—a specific entity? *J Gastroenterol Hepatol* 1990, 5:343–351.

4. Johnson PJ, McFarlane IG, Alvarez F, *et al.*: Meeting report. International autoimmune hepatitis group. *Hepatology* 1993, 18:998–1005.

5. Nikias GA, Batts KP, Czaja AJ: The nature and prognostic implications of autoimmune hepatitis with an acute presentation. *J Hepatol* 1994, 21:866–871.

6. Lenzi M, Ballardini G, Fusconi M, *et al.*: Type 2 autoimmune hepatitis and hepatitis C virus infection. *Lancet* 1990, 335:258–259.

7. Magrin S, Craxi A, Fiorentino G, *et al.*: Is autoimmune hepatitis an HCV-related disease? *J Hepatol* 1991, 13:56–60.

8. Magrin S, Craxi A, Fabiano C, *et al.*: Hepatitis C virus replication in "autoimmune" chronic hepatitis. *J Hepatol* 1991, 13:364–367.

9. Vento S, Garofano T, DiPerri G, *et al.*: Identification of hepatitis A virus as a trigger for autoimmune chronic hepatitis type 1 in susceptible patients. *Lancet* 1991, 337:1183–1187.

10. Laskus T, Slusarczyk J: Autoimmune chronic active hepatitis developing after acute type B hepatitis. *Dig Dis Sci* 1989, 34:1294–1297.

11. Berk L, Schalm SW, Heijtink RA: Severe chronic active hepatitis (autoimmune type) mimicked by coinfection of hepatitis C and human immunodeficiency viruses. *Gut* 1991, 32:1198–1200.

12. Robertson DAF, Zhang SL, Guy EC, Wright R: Persistent measles virus genome in autoimmune chronic active hepatitis. *Lancet* 1987, 2:9–11.

13. Silva MO, Reddy KR, Jeffers LJ, *et al.*: Interferon-induced chronic active hepatitis? *Gastroenterology* 1991, 101:840–842.

14. Czaja AJ, Taswell HF, Rakela J, Schimek C: Frequency and significance of antibody to hepatitis C virus in severe corticosteroid-treated autoimmune chronic active hepatitis. *Mayo Clin Proc* 1991, 66:572–582.

15. Lenzi M, Johnson PJ, McFarlane IG, *et al.*: Antibodies to hepatitis C virus in autoimmune liver disease: Evidence for geographical heterogeneity. *Lancet* 1991, 338:277–280.

16. Silva E, Sallie R, Tibbs C, *et al.*: Absence of hepatitis C virus in British patients with type 1 autoimmune chronic active hepatitis—a polymerase chain reaction and serological study. *J Hepatol* 1993, 19:211–215.

17. Mitchel LS, Jeffers LJ, Reddy KR, *et al.*: Detection of hepatitis C virus antibody by first and second generation assays and polymerase chain reaction in patients with autoimmune chronic active hepatitis types I, II, and III. *Am J Gastroenterol* 1993, 88:1027–1034.

18. Czaja AJ, Magrin S, Fabiano C, *et al.*: Hepatitis C virus infection as a determinant of behavior in type 1 autoimmune hepatitis. *Dig Dis Sci* 1995, 40:33–40.

19. McFarlane IG, Smith HM, Johnson PJ, *et al.*: Hepatitis C virus antibodies in chronic active hepatitis: pathogenetic factor or false positive result? *Lancet* 1990, 335:754–757.

20. Czaja AJ, Carpenter HA, Santrach PJ, *et al.*: Evidence against hepatitis viruses as important causes of severe autoimmune hepatitis in the United States. *J Hepatol* 1993, 18:342–352.

21. Czaja AJ: Autoimmune hepatitis and viral infection. *Gastroenterol Clin North Am* 1994, 23:547–566.

22. Manns MP, Griffin KJ, Sullivan KF, Johnson EF: LKM-1 autoantibodies recognize a short linear sequence in P450 IID6, a cytochrome P-450 monooxygenase. *J Clin Invest* 1991, 8:1370–1378.

23. Poralla T, Treichel U, Lohr H, Fleischer B: The asialoglycoprotein receptor as target structure in autoimmune liver diseases. *Semin Liver Dis* 1991, 11:215–222.

24. Desmet VJ, Gerber M, Hoofnagle JH, *et al.*: Classification of chronic hepatitis: Diagnosis, grading and staging. *Hepatology* 1994, 19:1513–1520.

25. Czaja AJ: Autoimmune hepatitis: Current therapeutic concepts. *Clin Immunother* 1994, 1:413–429.

26. Choo Q-L, Kuo G, Weiner AJ, *et al.*: Isolation of a cDNA clone from a blood-borne non-A, non-B viral hepatitis genome. *Science* 1989, 244:359–361.

27. Todros L, Touscoz G, D'Urso N, *et al.*: Hepatitis C virus-related chronic liver disease with autoantibodies to liver-kidney microsomes (LKM). Clinical characterization from idiopathic LKM-positive disorders. *J Hepatol* 1991, 13:128–131.

28. Garson JA, Lenzi M, Ring C, *et al.*: Hepatitis C viraemia in adults with type 2 autoimmune hepatitis. *J Med Virol* 1991, 34:223–226.

29. Michel G, Ritter A, Gerken G, *et al.*: Anti-GOR and hepatitis C virus in autoimmune liver diseases. *Lancet* 1992, 339:267–269.

30. Lunel F, Abuaf N, Frangeul L, *et al.*: Liver/kidney microsome type 1 and hepatitis C virus infection. *Hepatology* 1992, 16:630–636.

31. Manns M, Gerken G, Kyriatsoulis A, *et al.*: Characterization of a new subgroup of autoimmune chronic active hepatitis by autoantibodies against a soluble liver antigen. *Lancet* 1987, 1:292–294.

32. Stechemesser E, Klein R, Berg PA: Characterization and clinical relevance of liver–pancreas antibodies in autoimmune hepatitis. *Hepatology* 1993,18:1–9.

33. Czaja AJ, Carpenter HA, Santrach PJ, *et al.*: The nature and prognosis of severe cryptogenic chronic active hepatitis. *Gastroenterology* 1993, 104:1755–1761.

34. Czaja AJ, Manns MP, Homburger HA: Frequency and significance of antibodies to liver–kidney microsome type 1 in adults with chronic active hepatitis. *Gastroenterology* 1992, 103:1290–1295.

35. Czaja AJ, Carpenter HA, Manns MP: Antibodies to soluble liver antigen, P450IID6, and mitochondrial complexes in chronic hepatitis. *Gastroenterology* 1993, 105:1522–1528.

36. Czaja AJ, Davis GL, Ludwig J, *et al.*: Autoimmune features as determinants of prognosis in steroid-treated chronic active hepatitis of uncertain etiology. *Gastroenterology* 1983, 85:713–717.

37. Amontree JS, Stuart TD, Bredfeldt JE: Autoimmune chronic active hepatitis masquerading as acute hepatitis. *J Clin Gastroenterol* 1989, 11:303–307.

38. Czaja AJ, Carpenter HA, Santrach PJ, Moore SB: Genetic predispositions for the immunological features of chronic active hepatitis. *Hepatology* 1993,18:816–822.

39. Perdigoto R, Carpenter HA, Czaja AJ: Frequency and significance of chronic ulcerative colitis in severe corticosteroid-treated autoimmune hepatitis. *J Hepatol* 1992, 14:325–331.

40. Czaja AJ, Carpenter HA, Santrach PJ, Moore SB: Significance of HLA DR4 in type 1 autoimmune hepatitis. *Gastroenterology* 1993, 105:1502–1507.

41. Czaja AJ, Rakela J, Ludwig J: Features reflective of early prognosis in corticosteroid-treated severe autoimmune chronic active hepatitis. *Gastroenterology* 1988, 95:448–453.

42. Treichel U, Poralla T, Hess G, *et al.*: Autoantibodies to human asialoglycoprotein receptor in autoimmune-type chronic hepatitis. *Hepatology* 1990, 11:606–612.

43. Warny M, Brenard R, Cornu C, *et al.*: Antineutrophil antibodies in chronic hepatitis and the effect of α-interferon therapy. *J Hepatol* 1993, 17:294–300.

44. Mulder AHL, Horst G, Haagsma EB, *et al.*: Prevalence and characterization of neutrophil cytoplasmic antibodies in autoimmune liver diseases. *Hepatology* 1993, 17:411–417.

45. Targan S, Landers C, Vidrich A, Czaja A: High level perinuclear antineutrophil cytoplasmic antibodies (P-ANCA) are present in almost all autoimmune hepatitis (AIH) type 1 patients. *Gastroenterology* 1994, 106:A997.

46. Donaldson PT, Doherty DG, Hayllar KM, *et al.*: Susceptibility to autoimmune chronic active hepatitis: Human leukocyte antigens DR4 and A1-B8-DR3 are independent risk factors. *Hepatology* 1990, 13:701–706.

47. Seki T, Kiyosawa K, Inoko H, Ota M: Association of autoimmune hepatitis with HLA-Bw54 and DR4 in Japanese patients. *Hepatology* 1990, 12:1300–1304.

48. Doherty DG, Donaldson PT, Underhill JA, *et al.*: Allelic sequence variation in the HLA class II genes and proteins in patients with autoimmune hepatitis. *Hepatology* 1994, 19:609–615.

49. Czaja AJ, Carpenter HA: Sensitivity, specificity and predictability of biopsy interpretations in chronic hepatitis. *Gastroenterology* 1993, 105:1824–1832.

50. Frazer IH, Mackay IR, Bell J, Becker G: The cellular infiltrate in the liver in auto-immune chronic active hepatitis: Analysis with monoclonal antibodies. *Liver* 1985, 5:162–172.

51. Hashimoto E, Lindor KD, Homburger HA, *et al.*: Immunohisto-chemical characterization of hepatic lymphocytes in primary biliary cirrhosis in comparison with primary sclerosing cholangitis and autoimmune chronic active hepatitis. *Mayo Clin Proc* 1993, 68:1049–1055.

52. Bach N, Thung SN, Schaffner F: The histological features of chronic hepatitis C and autoimmune chronic hepatitis: A comparative analysis. *Hepatology* 1992, 15:572–577.

53. Scheuer PJ, Ashrafzadeh P, Sherlock S, *et al.*: The pathology of hepatitis C. *Hepatology* 1992, 15:567–571.

54. Hiramatsu N, Hayashi N, Haruna Y, *et al.*: Immunohistochemical detection of hepatitis C virus-infected hepatocytes in chronic liver disease with monoclonal antibodies to core, envelope and NS3 regions of the hepatitis C virus genome. *Hepatology* 1992,16:306–311.

55. Homberg J-C, Abuaf N, Bernard O, *et al.*: Chronic active hepatitis associated with antiliver–kidney microsome antibody type 1: A second type of "autoimmune" hepatitis. *Hepatology* 1987, 7:1333–1339.

56. Porta G, Da Costa Gayotto LC, Alvarez F: Anti-liver-kidney microsome antibody-positive autoimmune hepatitis presenting as fulminant liver failure. *J Pediatr Gastroenterol Nutr* 1990, 11:138–140.

57. Muratori L, Lenzi M, Cataleta M, *et al.*: Interferon therapy in liver–kidney microsome antibody type 1-positive patients with chronic hepatitis C. *J Hepatol* 1994, 21:199–203.

58. Ma Y, Peakman M, Lenzi M, *et al.*: Case against subclassification of type II autoimmune chronic active hepatitis. *Lancet* 1993, 3411:60.

59. Vergani D, Mieli-Vergani G: Type II autoimmune hepatitis. What is the role of the hepatitis C virus? *Gastroenterology* 1993, 104:1870–1873.

60. Yamamoto AM, Cresteil D, Homberg JC, Alvarez F: Characterization of the anti-liver-kidney microsome antibody (anti-LKM1) from hepatitis C virus-positive and -negative sera. *Gastroenterology* 1993, 104:1762–1767.

61. Abuaf N, Johanet C, Chretien P, *et al.*: Characterization of the liver cytosol antigen type 1 reacting with autoantibodies in chronic active hepatitis. *Hepatology* 1992, 16:892–898.

62. Manns MP, Griffin KJ, Sullivan KF, Johnson EF: LKM-1 autoantibodies recognize a short linear sequence in P450IID6, a cytochrome P-450 monooxygenase. *J Clin Invest* 1991, 88:1370–1378.

63. Manns MP, Kruger M: Immunogenetics of chronic liver diseases. *Gastroenterology* 1994, 106:1676–1697.

64. Loeper J, Descatoire V, Maurice M, *et al.*: Cytochromes P-450 in human hepatocyte plasma membrane: recognition by several autoantibodies. *Gastroenterology* 1993, 104:203–216.

65. Manns M, Zanger U, Gerken G, *et al.*: Patients with type II autoimmune hepatitis express functionally intact cytochrome P-450 db1 that is inhibited by LKM-1 autoantibodies *in vitro* but not *in vivo*. *Hepatology* 1990, 12:127–132.

66. Lohr H, Manns M, Kyriatsoulis A, *et al.*: Clonal analysis of liver-infiltrating T cells in patients with LKM-1 antibody-positive autoimmune chronic active hepatitis. *Clin Exp Immunol* 1991, 84:297–302.

67. Trautwein C, Ramadori G, Gerken G, *et al.*: Regulation of cytochrome P450 IID6 by acute phase mediators in C3H/HeJ mice. *Biochem Biophys Res Commun* 1992, 182:617–623.

68. Wachter B, Kyriatsoulis A, Lohse AW, *et al.*: Characterization of liver cytokeratin as a major target antigen of anti-SLA antibodies. *J Hepatol* 1990, 11:232–239.

69. Krawitt EL, Kilby AE, Albertini RJ, *et al.*: An immunogenetic study of suppressor cell activity in autoimmune chronic active hepatitis. *Clin Immunol Immunopathol* 1988, 46:249–257.

70. Czaja AJ: Autoimmune hepatitis; evolving concepts and treatment strategies. *Dig Dis Sci* 1995, 40:435–456.

71. Wang KK, Czaja AJ: Prognosis of corticosteroid-treated hepatitis B surface antigen-negative chronic active hepatitis in postmenopausal women: A retrospective analysis. *Gastroenterology* 1989, 97:1288–1293.

72. Czaja AJ, Davis GL, Ludwig J, Taswell HF: Complete resolution of inflammatory activity following corticosteroid treatment of HBsAg-negative chronic active hepatitis. *Hepatology* 1984, 4:622–627.

73. Czaja AJ, Ammon HV, Summerskill WHJ: Clinical features and prognosis of severe chronic active liver disease (CALD) after corticosteroid-induced remission. *Gastroenterology* 1980, 78:518–523.

74. Hegarty JE, Nouri-Aria KT, Portmann B, *et al.*: Relapse following treatment withdrawal in patients with autoimmune chronic active hepatitis. *Hepatology* 1983, 3:685–689.

75. Czaja AJ, Beaver SJ, Shiels MT: Sustained remission following corticosteroid therapy of severe HBsAg-negative chronic active hepatitis. *Gastroenterology* 1987, 92:215–219.

76. Sanchez-Urdazpal L, Czaja AJ, van Hoek B, *et al.*: Prognostic features and role of liver transplantation in severe corticosteroid-treated autoimmune chronic active hepatitis. *Hepatology* 1992, 15:215–221.

77. Wang KK, Czaja AJ: Hepatocellular cancer in corticosteroid-treated severe autoimmune chronic active hepatitis. *Hepatology* 1988, 8:1679–1683.

78. Colombo M, De Franchis R, Del Ninno E, *et al.*: Hepatocellular carcinoma in Italian patients with cirrhosis. *N Engl J Med* 1991, 325:675–680.

79. Wang KK, Czaja AJ, Beaver SJ, Go VLW: Extrahepatic malignancy following long-term immunosuppressive therapy of severe hepatitis B surface antigen-negative chronic active hepatitis. *Hepatology* 1989, 10:39–43.

80. Czaja AJ: Chronic active hepatitis. In *Current Therapy in Allergy, Immunology, and Rheumatology.* Edited by Lichtenstein LM, Fauci AS. St. Louis: Mosby-Year Book; 1992:273–278.

81. Czaja AJ: Treatment of autoimmune hepatitis. In *Autoimmune Hepatitis.* Edited by Nishioka M, Toda G, Zeniya M. Amsterdam: Elsevier Science B.V.; 1994:283–304.

82. Czaja AJ: Low dose corticosteroid therapy after multiple relapse of severe HBsAg-negative chronic active hepatitis. *Hepatology* 1990, 11:1044–1049.

83. Stellon AJ, Keating JJ, Johnson PJ, *et al.*: Maintenance of remission in autoimmune chronic active hepatitis with azathioprine after corticosteroid withdrawal. *Hepatology* 1988, 8:781–784.

84. Wright HL, Bou-Abboud CF, Hassanein T, *et al.*: Disease recurrence and rejection following liver transplantation for autoimmune chronic active liver disease. *Transplantation* 1992, 53:136–139.

85. Vento S, DiPerri G, Garofano T, *et al.*: Hazards of interferon therapy for HBV-seronegative chronic hepatitis. *Lancet* 1989, 2:926.

86. Papo T, Marcellin P, Bernuau J, *et al.*: Autoimmune chronic hepatitis exacerbated by α-interferon. *Ann Intern Med* 1992, 116:51–53.

87. Shindo M, DiBisceglie AM, Hoofnagle JH: Acute exacerbation of liver disease during interferon alfa therapy for chronic hepatitis C. *Gastroenterology* 1992, 102:1406–1408.

88. Magrin S, Craxi A, Fabiano C, *et al.*: Hepatitis C viremia in chronic liver disease: Relationship to interferon-alpha or corticosteroid therapy. *Hepatology* 1994, 19:273–279.

89. Faulds D, Goa KL, Benfield P: Cyclosporin: A review of its pharmacodynamic and pharmacokinetic properties, and therapeutic use in immunoregulatory disorders. *Drugs* 1993, 45:953–1040.

90. Peters DH, Fitton A, Plosker GL, Faulds D: Tacrolimus: A review of its pharmacology,and therapeutic potential in hepatic and renal transplantation. *Drugs* 1993, 46:746–794.

91. Thomson AW, Carroll PB, McCauley J, *et al.*: FK-506: A novel immunosuppressant for treatment of autoimmune disease. Rationale and preliminary clinical experience at the University of Pittsburgh. *Springer Semin Immunopathol* 1993, 14:323–344.

92. Van Thiel DH, Wright H, Carroll P, *et al.*: FK 506 in the treatment of autoimmune chronic active hepatitis: Preliminary results. *Am J Gastroenterol* 1992, 87:1309.

93. Carmassi F, Morale M, Puccetti R, *et al.*: Efficacy of intravenous immunoglobulin therapy in a case of autoimmune-mediated chronic active hepatitis. *Clin Exper Rheumatol* 1992, 10:13–17.

94. Schwartsmann G, Peters GJ, Laurensse E, *et al.*: DUP 785 (NSC 368390): Schedule-dependency of growth inhibitory and antipyrimidine effects. *Biochem Pharmacol* 1988, 37:3257–3266.

95. Cramer DV, Chapman FA, Jaffee BD, *et al.*: The effect of a new immunosuppressive drug, brequinar sodium, on heart, liver, and kidney allograft rejection in the rat. *Transplantation* 1992, 53:303–308.

96. Bierer BE, Jin YJ, Fruman DA, *et al.*: FK 506 and rapamycin: Molecular probes of T-lymphocyte activation. *Transplant Proc* 1991, 23:2850–2855.

97. Crosignani A, Battezzati PM, Setchell KDR, *et al.*: Effects of ursodeoxycholic acid on serum liver enzymes and bile acid metabolism in chronic active hepatitis: A dose-response study. *Hepatology* 1991, 13:339–344.

Chapter 4

Acute and Chronic Hepatitis B

MILTON G. MUTCHNICK

Hepatitis B virus (HBV) infection is a serious worldwide public health problem with an estimated 300 million people exhibiting evidence of chronic infection [1]. Over 250,000 of these individuals die annually from acute or chronic liver disease [1]. Newly acquired HBV infection in the United States occurs in 200,000 to 300,000 individuals annually, accounting for 43% of the acute viral hepatitis cases reported [2]. Approximately 4.8% of the US population has been infected with HBV, and there are an estimated 1 to 1.25 million carriers [2,3]. This viral pathogen produces both acute and chronic infection with polymorphic clinical presentations that range from an asymptomatic carrier state to fulminant disease.

Hepatitis B virus is an enveloped, partially double-stranded DNA virus, showing both nucleotide and protein sequence similarity to the retroviruses, suggesting a common ancestry [4]. HBV is the only hepadnavirus afflicting humans; other members of this family of hepatotropic viruses infect other species [4]. These viral pathogens are not believed to be cytopathic for hepatocytes under most conditions. Rather, host-mediated immune response to HBV and to HBV peptides on hepatocyte membranes results in lysis of the hepatocyte [5].

In the acute form, HBV–induced hepatitis is a predominantly nonicteric illness with approximately 25% of patients presenting with jaundice. The vast majority of patients with acute HBV will proceed to recovery, but a very small proportion (1% to 12%) will progress to a chronic carrier state not necessarily associated with inflammatory changes in the liver. The risk of developing chronic HBV infection is increased if the patient is immune suppressed or if the virus is acquired by the patient at a young age [6–11].

The consequences of a chronic HBV infection, with concomitant evidence of active viral replication, include progressive liver disease, hepatic failure, and hepatocellular carcinoma

[12,13]. These potential sequelae provide ample motivation to engage in therapeutic efforts to decrease both the morbidity and mortality promoted by the virus in patients with chronic HBV. At present interferon-α_{2b} is the only licensed drug in the United States approved for use in chronic HBV. This antiviral and immune-modulating protein has been shown effective in promoting disease remission in 30% to 40% of patients with chronic HBV [14–16]. The impact of successful interferon therapy on the natural history of the disease remains to be determined. For example, it is not known if progression to cirrhosis or development of hepato-cellular carcinoma is prevented or delayed.

Investigational drugs used alone or in combination are currently undergoing the scrutiny of clinical trials. The role of orthotopic liver transplantation in the treatment of the failing liver in chronic HBV remains problematic as well as contro-versial. A requirement also exists to develop treatment strate-gies for patients with chronic HBV deemed unsuitable for standard interferon therapy. Furthermore, treatment regimens in the future will likely reflect a patient-specific orientation, *ie*, selecting from a menu of therapeutic agents that will be used alone, in combination, or perhaps sequentially with the timing of drug intervention dependent on the status of host-HBV interaction.

■ THE HEPATITIS B VIRUS

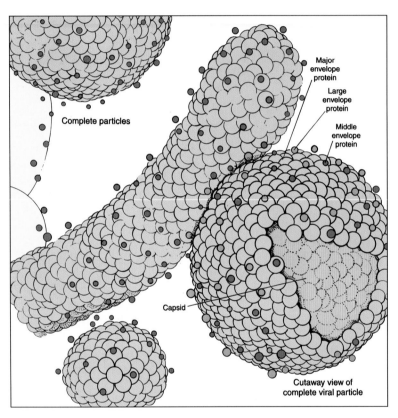

Major envelope protein

Large envelope protein

Middle envelope protein

Complete particles

Capsid

Cutaway view of complete viral particle

FIGURE 4-1.

The hepatitis B virus (HBV) is a member of the smallest known group of animal DNA viruses called *hepadnaviridae* [17]. The virus consists of two concentric protein coats. The inner coat, or capsid, is a single core protein that envelops and interacts with the HBV DNA. Note that in contrast to the complete viral particle where the outer coat contains the large, middle, and major surface proteins, only the middle and major proteins are found in incomplete and noninfectious viral particles [18]. These small 22-nm particles are produced in much greater abundance than the larger 42-nm complete viral particle [19]. (*Adapted from* Tiollais and Buendia [19]; with permission.)

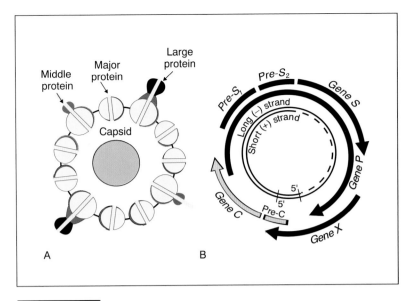

FIGURE 4-2.

The hepatitis B virus (HBV) genome and protein products. The HBV genome is a small, circular, and partly double-stranded DNA molecule of about 3200 nucleotide subunits. An asymmetry exists in the length of the strands. The full length strand that is complementary to the viral messenger RNAs is designated to have minus polarity, the L(-) strand. The other strand, S(+), is 50% to 80% the length of the L(-) strand [19,20]. The HBV genome contains only four potential genes (S, C, P, and X), which overlap as shown in **panel B** [21]. The strategic placement of open reading frames permits encoding for the synthesis of different specific proteins from the same genetic material. The surface (S) gene encodes for the major envelope protein (hepatitis B surface antigen [HBsAg]) as shown in **panel A**. The color code of the genes in *panel B* correspond to the proteins in *panel A*. The middle protein is encoded by Pre-S$_2$ and S genes whereas the large protein is encoded by a combination of Pre-S$_1$, Pre-S$_2$, and S. All three proteins contain HBsAg. The C (core) gene encodes the protein of the nucleocapsid (hepatitis B core antigen) and is preceded by a short Pre-C region that with the core region forms a large protein that is eventually degraded and secreted into the serum (hepatitis B e antigen). The P gene encodes enzymes (DNA polymerase) required for viral replication. P, shown in *panel B*, is the longest gene incorporating parts of all the other genes. Finally, the X gene protein product regulates the transcription of all viral genes by interacting with a DNA sequence in the genome. The X protein may participate in hepatocyte injury leading to hepatocellular carcinoma. (*Adapted from* Tiollas and Buendia [19]; with permission.)

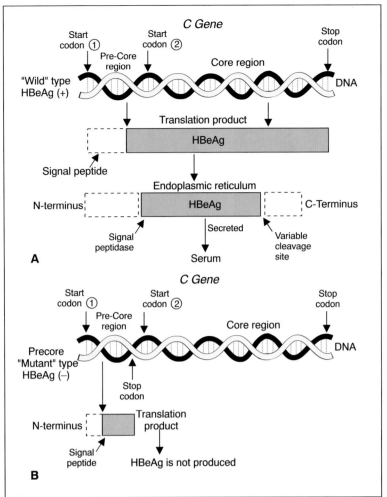

FIGURE 4-3.

Wild type and mutant forms of the hepatitis B virus (HBV). Identification of mutant HBV DNA genomes unable to synthesize hepatitis B e antigen (HBeAg) has resulted in efforts to associate these mutants with clinical outcomes. Several studies have reported on an apparent linkage between the mutant HBV and fulminant HBV in the acute setting [22] or more severe liver injury in the setting of a chronic hepatitis [23]. Absence of HBeAg production was initially viewed to portend an ominous development. Emergence of the mutant type HBV, however, may suggest that these viral variants are a consequence of, rather than the cause for, the severe clinical outcomes reported [24,25]. Mixed wild and mutant HBV populations are found frequently in HBeAg–positive patients with evidence to suggest eventual displacement of the wild type by the mutant virus in some patients [26]. In **panel A**, hepatitis B core antigen (HBcAg) is synthesized by the core region of C gene beginning at start codon 2 (not shown). A codon is a genetic sequence that initiates the translation and production of protein. HBeAg is synthesized by the C gene beginning at start codon 1. The precore region encodes a signal peptide for transport of the large protein to the endoplasmic reticulum where a signal peptidase cleaves the signal peptide from the N-terminus. A protease cleaves a variable length peptide from the C-terminus [20]. The HBeAg is then secreted from the cell into the serum. **Panel B** depicts the precore "mutant" type, which is unable to synthesize HBeAg. Note the presence of a translational stop codon that is located in the precore region as a consequence of a mutation in one of 10 possible sites [25,27]. Although this precludes the synthesis of HBeAg which requires the encoding of the entire C gene, encoding for HBcAg is not affected because its synthesis is initiated at start codon 2 (not shown).

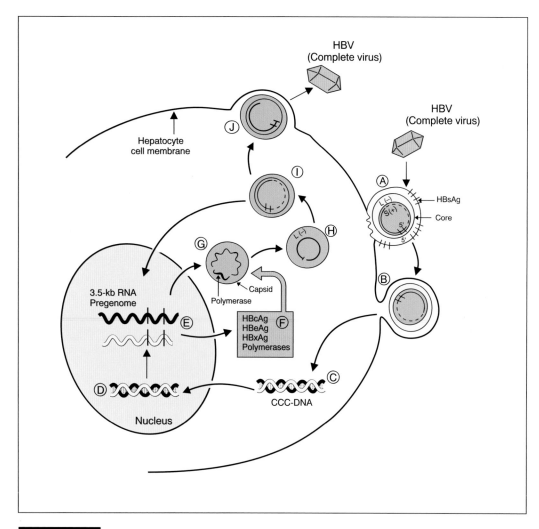

protein sequences bind with pHSA, which in turn form a link between the HBV and the liver cell pHSA receptor [29]), 2) a Pre-S1 receptor on the liver cell [28,29], and 3) annexin V protein (a Ca^{++}–dependent phospholipid binding protein) present in liver which combines with the hepatitis B surface antigen (HBsAg) [30]. Other potential receptors for HBV that bind to HBsAg include interleukin-6 [31], the receptor for transferrin [32], and apolipoprotein H [33]. As the virus is taken up by the cell (B), the envelope is removed and enzymes extend the S(+) strand to form a covalently closed circular double-stranded DNA (CCC-DNA) (C). The HBV genome in its core migrates to the nucleus (D), where cellular polymerases transcribe it into a long RNA. The 3.5-kb strand constitutes the pregenome containing all viral DNA sequence information. Additional viral structural protein messenger RNAs (E) pass into the cytoplasm and are translated (F). The pregenome and viral DNA polymerase are packaged into new capsids (G). The polymerase reverse transcribes the RNA pregenome into a new L(-) DNA strand. The pregenome is then destroyed. The L(-) strand (H) is then used as a template for formation of the S(+) strand (I). Some capsids containing double-stranded DNA return to the nucleus to amplify the pool of CCC-DNA. Subsequently, the mature cores (I) are packaged into HBsAg particles, which accumulate in the endoplasmic reticulum and exit the cell (J). When the virus leaves the cell, elongation of the S(+) strand stops immediately. HBcAg—hepatitis B core antigen; HBeAg—hepatitis B e antigen; HBxAg—hepatitis B x antigen.

FIGURE 4-4.

Hepatitis B virus (HBV) replication in hepatocytes [19,20]. The HBV invades the cell by binding to surface receptors (A). Although the specific receptor for HBV has not been defined, a candidate receptor binding site would likely be located on the sinusoidal border of the hepatocyte [28]. Target receptors proposed include 1) a polymerized human serum albumin (pHSA) receptor on the membrane (according to this hypothesis Pre-S2

PATHOGENESIS

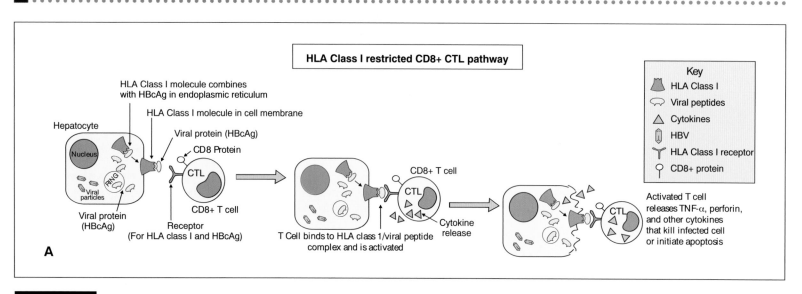

FIGURE 4-5.

The mechanism of hepatocyte injury in acute hepatitis B virus (HBV) infection mainly results from cellular immune response. It is generally believed that the HBV is not directly cytopathic and that the host immune response to the presence of infected hepatocytes results in elimination of these cells, most likely by CD8+ cytotoxic T

(Continued on next page)

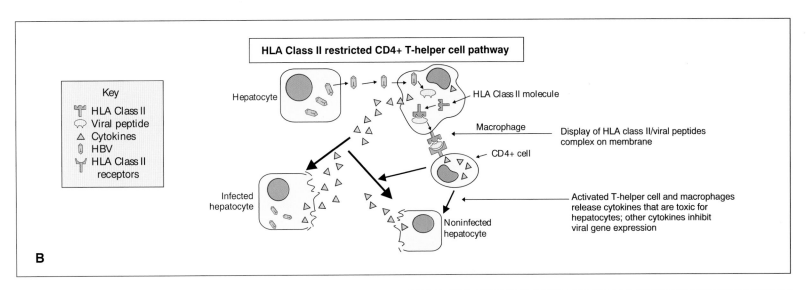

HLA Class II restricted CD4+ T-helper cell pathway

Key
- HLA Class II
- Viral peptide
- Cytokines
- HBV
- HLA Class II receptors

Hepatocyte

HLA Class II molecule

Macrophage — Display of HLA class II/viral peptides complex on membrane

CD4+ cell

Infected hepatocyte

Noninfected hepatocyte

Activated T-helper cell and macrophages release cytokines that are toxic for hepatocytes; other cytokines inhibit viral gene expression

B

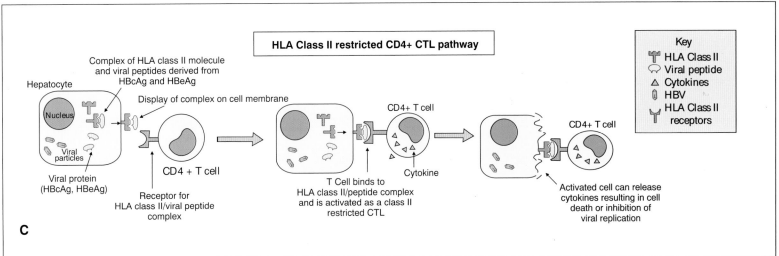

HLA Class II restricted CD4+ CTL pathway

Complex of HLA class II molecule and viral peptides derived from HBcAg and HBeAg

Hepatocyte

Nucleus

Display of complex on cell membrane

CD4+ T cell

CD4+ T cell

Key
- HLA Class II
- Viral peptide
- Cytokines
- HBV
- HLA Class II receptors

Viral particles

Viral protein (HBcAg, HBeAg)

CD4 + T cell

Receptor for HLA class II/viral peptide complex

Cytokine

T Cell binds to HLA class II/peptide complex and is activated as a class II restricted CTL

Activated cell can release cytokines resulting in cell death or inhibition of viral replication

C

FIGURE 4-5. (CONTINUED)

lymphocytes (CTL) [34,35]. CTLs and natural killer cells are found in large numbers in the liver of patients with acute hepatitis [36]. In acute HBV, interferon is produced in large quantities leading to increased expression of HLA antigens classes I and II [37]. Interferon also promotes the production of a group of enzymes (*RING* genes) that process HBV antigens for presentation on the cell membrane by HLA class I molecules.

A, The HLA antigen and viral protein complex on the hepatocyte membrane provokes a vigorous immune response with activation of CTLs that release cytotoxins, which can eventuate in cell death or trigger cell suicide through a process called *apoptosis*. CTL directed towards HBV envelope and nucleocapsid proteins have been described in patients with acute or chronic HBV with the core protein believed to serve as the primary target antigen [37,38]. Other alternative pathways involving CD4+ T cells may play a role in the necroinflammatory response acting individually or in concert with CTL lysis. **B**, Viral particles secreted by hepatocytes are taken up by macrophages, processed, and the derived viral peptides presented to CD4+ T cells in an HLA class II restricted manner. These T cells respond to several epitopes within the hepatitis B core antigen

(HBcAg) and hepatitis B e antigen (HBeAg). A number of these epitopes are immunodominant and recognized in patients with diverse HLA backgrounds [39]. These activated macrophages and T cells that enter a proliferative phase then release a series of cytokines that are cytotoxic for HBV–infected, as well as noninfected, hepatocytes [40]. Evidence to support this mechanism for cytolysis was provided by studies in a patient receiving a completely HLA class I mismatched liver allograft, who then redeveloped active HBV disease. Because HLA class I restricted CTL could not account for the hepatocyte injury, the HLA class I independent pathway described emerges as the most likely explanation [41]. **C**, The final potential mechanism to account for destruction of HBV–infected hepatocytes involves the presentation of HBV antigens, which are processed in hepatocytes, fragmented, and then combined with HLA class II molecules in the endoplasmic reticulum. The HLA class II molecule and viral peptide complex is displayed on the cell membrane for presentation to CD4+ T cells. The activated cell is an HLA class II restricted CD4+ CTL, which secretes cytokines leading to liver cell injury. This pathway is considered least efficient and may not constitute a major pathway for cell injury [41].

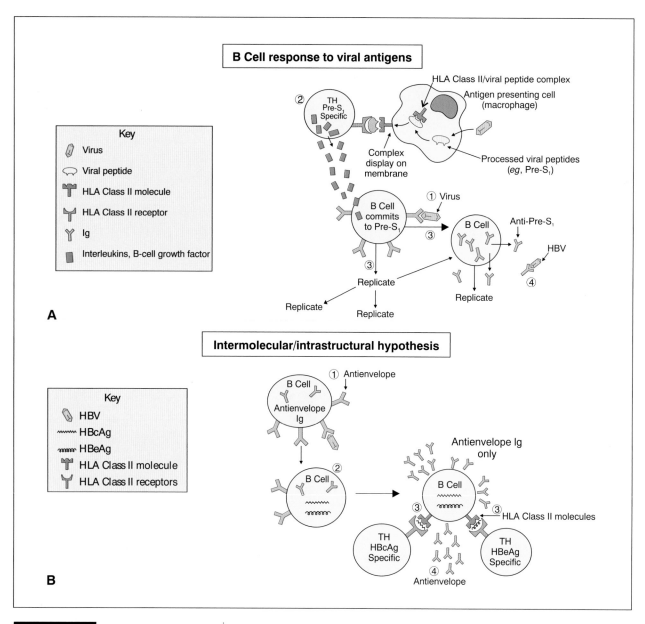

B Cell response to viral antigens

Key
- Virus
- Viral peptide
- HLA Class II molecule
- HLA Class II receptor
- Ig
- Interleukins, B-cell growth factor

② TH Pre-S₁ Specific

HLA Class II/viral peptide complex

Antigen presenting cell (macrophage)

Complex display on membrane

Processed viral peptides (eg, Pre-S₁)

① Virus

B Cell commits to Pre-S₁

③

B Cell

Anti-Pre-S₁

HBV

③

④

Replicate

Replicate

Replicate

Replicate

A

Intermolecular/intrastructural hypothesis

Key
- HBV
- HBcAg
- HBeAg
- HLA Class II molecule
- HLA Class II receptors

① Antienvelope

B Cell

Antienvelope Ig

② B Cell

Antienvelope Ig only

B Cell

③ ③ HLA Class II molecules

TH HBcAg Specific

TH HBeAg Specific

④ Antienvelope

B

FIGURE 4-6.

The humoral immune role in acute hepatitis B. B lymphocytes respond to the presence of HBV antigens producing multiple antibodies. The antibody to hepatitis B core antigen (HBcAg) is not viral neutralizing, whereas antibodies to hepatitis B surface antigen (HBsAg) are. Antibodies to hepatitis B e antigen (HBeAg) correlate with loss of viral replication and are not protective after emerging at long intervals following resolution of an acute infection. HLA class II restricted CD4+ T helper cells (TH) that specifically recognize envelope (HBsAg, Pre-S₁, and Pre-S₂) peptides can promote the production by B cells of antibodies against components of the envelope. These neutralizing antibodies bind extracellular free viruses and help prevent cell-to-cell spread. **A,** Uncommitted B lymphocytes (*1*) recognizing a viral antigen bind the antigen (in this example, Pre-S₁ envelope peptide) to an immunoglobulin (Ig) receptor. TH cells specific for Pre-S₁ (*2*), but recognizing a different epitope, proliferate and release various B-cell growth factors. These interleukins stimulate clonal expansion of the now committed B cell (*3*) with production of a specific

antibody to Pre-S₁. Released antibody binds to the Pre-S₁ site on the HBV preventing cell-to-cell spread and viral clearance (*4*). **B,** HBcAg (or HBeAg)–specific TH cells can also provide "help" for production of antienvelope antibodies by a process termed *intermolecular-intrastructural T-cell help* [42]. According to this hypothesis, a B cell primed to produce antibody to an envelope peptide binds through its Ig receptor to that epitope located on the HBV (*1*). The entire viral particle (*2*) is internalized and processed into a variety of viral peptides, some of which (*3*) are expressed on the B-cell membrane in a complex with HLA class II molecules. HBcAg– or HBeAg–specific TH cells that recognize epitopes in HBcAg– or HBeAg–derived viral peptides in the complex bind to the B cell and help increase production of specific antienvelope Ig by cell-specific but not Ig-specific cytokines (*4*). Thus, the increased production of antienvelope Ig by the B cell "helped" by an HBcAg TH did not require the presence of both HBcAg and HBsAg on the same molecule at the B-cell surface (intermolecular) but did necessitate that both antigens be in the same particle, the internalized HBV (intrastructural).

TABLE 4-1. POTENTIAL MECHANISMS PROMOTING DEVELOPMENT OF CHRONIC HBV INFECTION IN ADULTS

MECHANISM	ACUTE HEPATITIS	CHRONIC INFECTION
Interferon production [37]	Large quantities	Impaired
Response to interferon [37]	Increased expression of HLA class antigens	Inhibited
Cellular immune response	Not inhibited	Blocked or interfered with
		Immunocytes infected with HBV
		Altered production of cytokines
		State of tolerance created by high levels of HBsAg, HBeAg, or HBcAg
HLA Class I restricted [43] CD8+ T cell	CD8+ T Cells efficiently lyse hepatocytes displaying HLA class I/core protein complex	Possible defect in HLA antigen conformation precluding effective complex with viral protein; results in defective CD8+ T cell response
HLA Class II restricted CD4+ T cell response	Effective and dynamic; directed against HBcAg and HBeAg epitopes Associated with clearance of HBsAg	Weak, less effective, no HBsAg clearance
HBV Mutations [37]	Elimination of infection is efficient, disallowing emergence of mutant forms	Spontaneous mutation occurs and dominant HBV strain changes–with a survival advantage, eg, HBeAg–negative mutant form; immune system does not "recognize" viral antigens

TABLE 4-1.

The propensity for development of a chronic hepatitis B virus (HBV) infection is related to age at the time of exposure, immunologic status, and factors promoting viral persistence. HBcAg—hepatitis B core antigen; HBeAg—hepatitis B e antigen; HBsAg—hepatitis B surface antigen.

HEPATITIS B INFECTION

Epidemiology

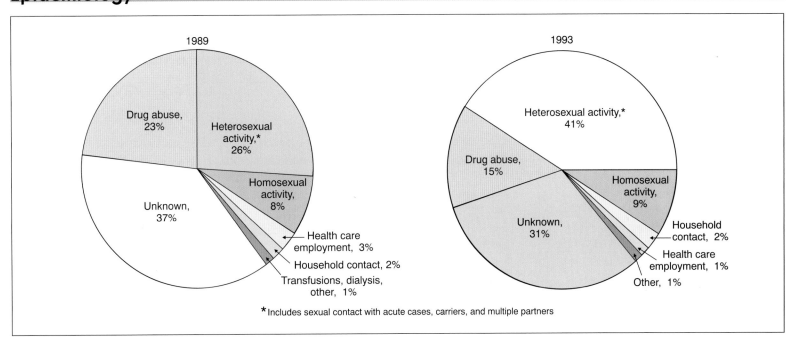

*Includes sexual contact with acute cases, carriers, and multiple partners

FIGURE 4-7.

Risk factors associated with reported cases of acute hepatitis B (HBV) in the United States. Shifts have developed in the frequency of some risk factors between the 1980s and 1990s. Heterosexual activity as a risk factor increased from 26% in 1989 to 41% in 1993, whereas cases involving drug abuse, health care employment, and unknown risk associations have decreased. Interestingly, cases associated with homosexual activity have increased slightly. Over the past decade the number of cases reported annually has been decreased by half. This lowered frequency of acute HBV probably reflects changes in behavior as a consequence of the AIDS epidemic as well as the impact of previous vaccination programs. It is anticipated that emphasizing HBV immunization for infants, children, and adolescents will serve to limit the population at risk for acquiring HBV and should gradually result in disappearance of the disease in the United States. (*Adapted from* McQuillan *et al.* [2] and Centers for Disease Control Sentinel Counties; with permission.)

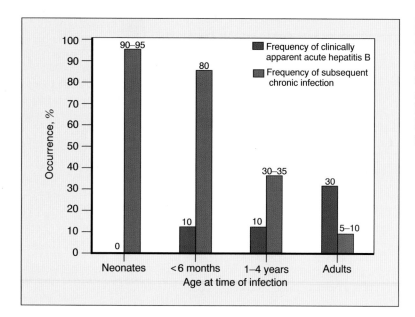

FIGURE 4-8.

Detection of acute hepatitis B. Most patients with acute hepatitis B go undetected unless they present with obvious clinical symptoms such as jaundice or they undergo biochemical tests that disclose aminotransferase elevations. The younger the individual, the less likely the diagnosis of acute hepatitis will be made. Paradoxically, however, the younger the patient is at the time of initial infection, the more likely the development of a chronic infection [7].

TABLE 4-2. DIAGNOSTIC INTERPRETATIONS OF HBV MARKERS

HBV MARKER	DESCRIPTION	IMPLICATIONS
HBsAg	Noninfectious component of viral coat	Considered the *sine qua non* for acute and chronic infection; it may, however, also be present in the absence of HBV replication, produced by cells with integrated HBV DNA coding for HBsAg; loss of HBsAg accepted as hallmark of recovery
Anti-HBs	Antibody response to HBsAg	Usually indicates recovery and immunity to HBV; it is the protective antibody resulting from vaccination with HBsAg material; also may be present in acute disease or as an inconstant finding in nearly a third of patients with chronic infection [45]
HBeAg	Soluble antigen that correlates with HBV replication and infectivity	Presence in serum signals high level of infectivity because it parallels viral replication; may disappear before or after loss of serum HBV DNA with disease remission; sustained loss of HBeAg in the presence or absence of Anti-HBe with continuing viral replication (HBV DNA) may presage emergence of an HBeAg–negative "mutant" virus
Anti-HBe	Antibody response to HBeAg; not considered protective	Presence suggests decreasing levels of viral replication and HBV DNA and also indicates move towards disease remission or resolution
HBcAg	Found in core of virus	No practical purpose for detecting in serum; HBeAg and HBV DNA are surrogate markers
Anti-HBc IgM	Nonprotective antibody to the HBcAg	Present in recent HBV infection; may recur in reactivation of a chronic hepatitis
Anti-HBc IgG	As above	Presence indicative of acute, chronic, or remote HBV infection; however, titers can decline over many years to undetectable levels; not present in individuals immunized to HBV
HBV DNA	Replicative genetic material of HBV; infectious agent	Presence in serum (by non-PCR methodologies) correlates to viral replication and continued infection; disappears with complete resolution of disease; may become undetectable in disease remission only to emerge once again with disease activation; the significance of its presence in serum as detected only by PCR is unclear

TABLE 4-2.

A detailed medical history and complete physical examination are key for interpreting the significance of test results for hepatitis B virus (HBV) components (HBV DNA, hepatitis B surface antigen [HBsAg], hepatitis B e antigen [HBeAg], hepatitis B core antigen [HBcAg]) or host immune responses to the virus (antibodies to HBsAg [Anti-HBs], antibodies to HBeAg [Anti-HBe], antibodies to HBcAg [Anti-HBc]) in patients suspected to be infected with HBV. Positive test results for one or several HBV markers may indicate an acute process or raise suspicion of a chronic infection [44]. For example, very recent vaccination for HBV might yield a positive test for HBsAg, suggesting acute disease or a carrier state. Discovery of a HBsAg–negative and Anti-HBs–positive status does not confirm a previous HBV infection but could indicate past HBV vaccination. Clarification of this issue would be achieved by taking an immunization history and a negative test for Anti-HBc immunoglobulin G (IgG). The potential implications associated with the identification of specific HBV markers are shown. IgM—immunoglobulin M; PCR—polymerase chain reaction.

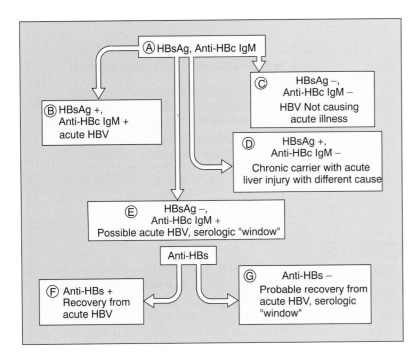

FIGURE 4-9.

Algorithm for the serologic approach to the diagnosis of acute hepatitis B. When a patient presents with suspected acute hepatitis, other etiologies must be considered. With respect to ascertaining the potential role for HBV, specific tests should be requested in a cost-effective and methodical manner. The hepatitis B surface antigen (HBsAg) and antibodies to hepatitis B core antigen (Anti-HBc) immunoglobulin M (IgM) class provide critical information on the candidacy of the HBV as the etiologic factor in acute liver injury (A). The results shown in B indicate acute HBV or, in the event the patient has an established chronic HBV infection, disease reactivation. The latter determination can be surmised only with preexisting evidence of HBV disease. The findings shown in C and D are consistent with non-HBV origin of the acute process. The positive HBsAg in D suggests an acute process of non-HBV cause superimposed on an HBV carrier. Patients who are recovering from an acute HBV infection may test HBsAg negative (E), although the Anti-HBc IgM will remain positive. Recovery is confirmed when antibody to HBsAg (Anti-HBs) is positive (F). In the event the Anti-HBs (G) is negative, the patient may be in the serologic "window" (characterized by absence of both HBsAg and Anti-HBs) before forming Anti-HBs.

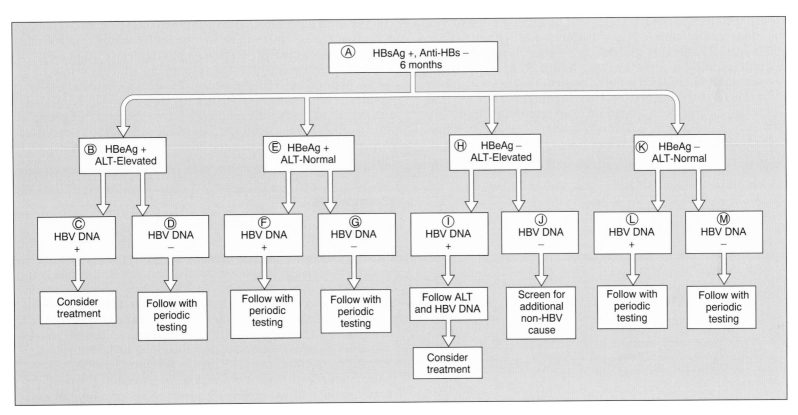

FIGURE 4-10.

Use of hepatitis B e antigen (HBeAg), antibodies to HBeAg (Anti-HBe), and hepatitis B virus (HBV) DNA testing in acute HBV. Little benefit is gained from routine assay for HBeAg, Anti-HBe, or HBV DNA in the setting of uncomplicated acute HBV. These markers should be reserved for situations where fulminant disease is a concern, when recovery appears delayed, or if there is progression to chronic disease. By general agreement, indication of chronic hepatitis occurs following 6 months of continuing necroinflammation [46]. If the illness appears protracted, *eg*, beyond 3 months, determination of the presence of HBeAg is warranted. Such presence suggests the likelihood for chronicity [47]. Following an acute hepatitis B, if hepatitis B surface antigen (HBsAg) persists for longer than 6 months, viral replicative activity should be assessed. Given the profile in A, viral replication may be determined with HBeAg and HBV DNA. Where the HBeAg is present with an elevated alanine aminotransferase level (ALT) (B), the presence of HBV DNA (C) indicates continuing active disease and candidacy for therapeutic intervention. Absence of HBV DNA (D) suggests possible clearance of virus-infected hepatocytes. When the HBeAg is positive with normal or near normal ALT (E), a positive HBV DNA (F) may represent an asymptomatic carrier status, whereas the absence of HBV DNA (G) could also reflect an asymptomatic carrier state or impending clearance of the HBV. The absence of HBeAg with elevated ALT (H) and a positive HBV DNA (I) could signal emergence of the HBeAg–negative "mutant" HBV with continuing disease or, less likely, that the original infection was with a mutant type HBV. It is also possible that clearance of the virus is occurring. Absence of HBV DNA (J) may signal resolution of the disease with delayed normalization of the ALT level or an additional undisclosed non-HBV etiology. When the HBeAg is negative with a normal ALT (K), a positive HBV DNA (L) indicates either clearing of the HBV infection or, again, infection with HBeAg–negative mutant HBV. Absence of HBeAg and HBV DNA with normal ALT levels (M) is consistent with a nonreplicative HBV status with continuing HBsAg antigenemia. Anti-HBs—antibodies to HBsAg.

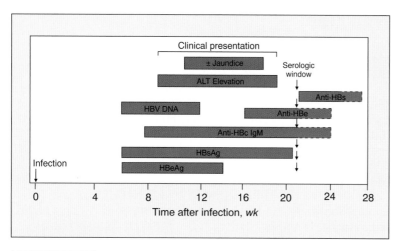

FIGURE 4-11.

Relationship between the appearance of hepatitis B virus (HBV) markers and the clinical presentation in uncomplicated acute HBV. Hepatitis B e antigen (HBeAg) and hepatitis B surface antigen (HBsAg) are detectable 4 to 8 weeks following infection and before onset of clinical illness. Symptoms of illness may be mild and go undetected, which is often the case, because a minority of patients present with jaundice [45,47]. The alanine aminotransferase (ALT) elevations usually subside before disappearance of the HBsAg and appearance of antibodies to HBsAg (Anti-HBs). Note the existence of a potential time gap, the serologic "window," when the HBsAg is not detected and Anti-HBs is not identified. Testing for antibodies to hepatitis B core antigen (Anti-HBc) immunoglobulin M (IgM) will bridge the gap, providing proof of an acute HBV illness. The HBV DNA is detected for a relatively short interval disappearing before normalization of the ALT or loss of HBeAg and HBsAg. Anti-HBe—antibodies to hepatitis B e antigen.

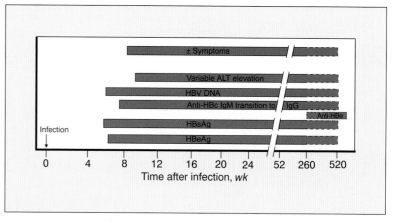

FIGURE 4-12.

Relationship between hepatitis B virus (HBV) markers, clinical presentation, and development of chronic infection. Symptoms may be mild and the illness may go undetected. Unlike a self-limited acute infection, the hepatitis B surface antigen (HBsAg) will persist along with the hepatitis B e antigen (HBeAg). The latter may not be detectable at times because its presence correlates with viral replication. The antibodies to hepatitis B core antigen (Anti-HBc) immunoglobulin M (IgM) class will disappear except during periods of disease reactivation, but the Anti-HBc immunoglobulin G (IgG) class will persist. Alanine aminotransferase (ALT) elevations will vary considerably and at times can achieve normal values. Antibodies to HBsAg are usually not detected but may be identified periodically [45]. Finally, the HBV DNA will be present and may show fluctuating serum levels over the course of years. After a variable period of time, the patient will usually seroconvert to an HBeAg–negative status and antibodies to HBeAg (Anti-HBe)–positive status.

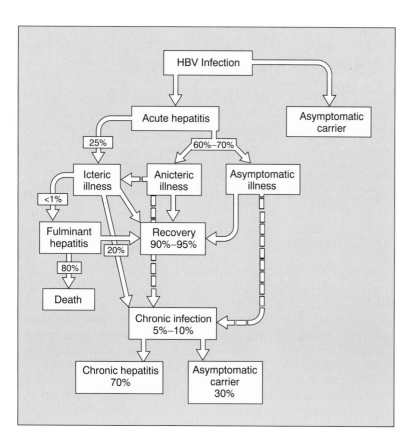

FIGURE 4-13.

Consequences of infection with hepatitis B virus (HBV). Most individuals who are exposed to the HBV will develop acute hepatitis. Those who become icteric are readily diagnosed; many who are anicteric but still display symptoms of illness may be identified. An additional asymptomatic group of patients exists who have abnormalities of one or several biochemical tests but do not exhibit symptoms and thus escape initial detection. The proportion of asymptomatic cases of acute HBV is problematic. Although patients with anicteric or asymptomatic hepatitis bear increased risk for progressing to chronicity [48], the overwhelming majority of patients with acute hepatitis recover without sequelae. A small proportion of patients experience a particularly effective immune clearance of infected hepatocytes that can result in fulminant disease. Although the survival rate is dismal in the absence of orthotopic liver transplantation, survival rates are highest when patients are less than 45 years of age [49]. Most patients with chronic infection have a chronic hepatitis, whereas a smaller proportion of chronically infected individuals manifest an asymptomatic carrier state.

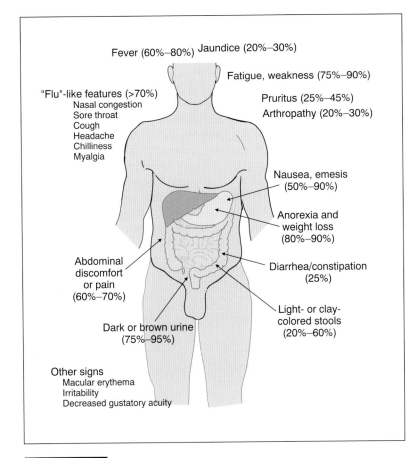

Fever (60%–80%)   Jaundice (20%–30%)

Fatigue, weakness (75%–90%)

"Flu"-like features (>70%)
Nasal congestion
Sore throat
Cough
Headache
Chilliness
Myalgia

Pruritus (25%–45%)
Arthropathy (20%–30%)

Nausea, emesis
(50%–90%)

Anorexia and
weight loss
(80%–90%)

Abdominal
discomfort
or pain
(60%–70%)

Diarrhea/constipation
(25%)

Light- or clay-
colored stools
(20%–60%)

Dark or brown urine
(75%–95%)

Other signs
Macular erythema
Irritability
Decreased gustatory acuity

FIGURE 4-14.

Constellation of symptoms reported by patients with acute hepatitis B. Most patients experiencing an acute HBV infection will have a nonicteric or asymptomatic illness [49]. The frequency of recognized acute hepatitis B is correlated to age at the time of infection as shown in Figure 4-8. Adults are more likely to manifest evidence of illness, whereas infants and children rarely do. Patients who do not have icterus in the presence or absence of symptoms are at higher risk for developing chronic disease [48]. Although only a quarter of patients will become clinically jaundiced [45], a larger proportion will report evidence consistent with a cholestatic process by describing changes in color of urine and stool. Most symptoms experienced by patients are protean and frequently attributed to a nonspecific "viral" syndrome.

TABLE 4-3. LABORATORY ASSESSMENT– POTENTIAL FINDINGS

BIOCHEMICAL	HEMATOLOGIC
Common	*Common*
Total bilirubin ↑	Lymphopenia, neutropenia
Direct > indirect	Elevated ESR
Alkaline phosphatase ↑	
ALT ↑	*Infrequent/rare*
AST ↑	Prolongation of prothrombin
LDH ↑	time
Serum IgG and IgM increased in a third of patients	Hemolytic anemic
Inconstant	**URINE/STOOLS**
Albumin–unchanged or ↓	Urobilinogen (bilirubinuria)
Globulin–unchanged or ↑	Clay-, gray-, or light-colored stools
Infrequent/rare	
Cholesterol, triglycerides ↑	Rarely proteinuria
α-Fetoprotein ↑	

TABLE 4-3.

Laboratory assessment in acute hepatitis B. Laboratory findings in acute hepatitis B resemble that seen for virtually all forms of acute viral hepatitis and cannot be used to distinguish between viral etiologies. Elevations seen in the total bilirubin, alkaline phosphatase (hepatic isoenzyme), alanine aminotransferase (ALT), and aspartate aminotransferase (AST) levels are quite variable in the magnitude, as well as duration, of these elevations [47,49]. Clearly, requests for multiple, daily laboratory assessments in uncomplicated acute hepatitis are not warranted, particularly when peak elevations are attained and resolution of illness is under way. The peak bilirubin level is usually seen approximately 2 weeks following onset of jaundice, and normalization of the bilirubin may take an additional month. Typically, the bilirubin level does not exceed 10 mg/dL but can reach 20 mg/dL [49]. ALT and AST elevations, peaking, and resolution occur over a longer period and display fluctuations in values. Hematologic changes are infrequent and of less moment. Lymphopenia, leukopenia, and neutropenia may occur early in the illness. Lymphocytosis with atypical lymphocytes can develop. ESR—erythrocyte sedimentation rate; IgG—immunoglobulin G; IgM—immunoglobulin M; LDH—lactic dehydrogenase.

TABLE 4-4. INFREQUENT OR RARE SEQUELAE OF ACUTE HEPATITIS B

Prolonged acute hepatitis (6%–15%)

Time duration: Weeks to months

Symptoms: Fatigue, anxiety, anorexia, right upper abdominal tenderness

Laboratory findings: Elevated ALT/AST, usually mild

Conclusion/response: Observation

Persistence beyond 6 months may herald progression to chronic hepatitis

Hematologic

Pancytopenia

Thrombocytopenia

Aplastic anemia

Immune complex disease (10%–25%)

Vasculitis

    Necrotizing vasculitis (polyarteritis)

    Glomerulonephritis (membranous or membranoproliferative)

Neurologic

    Guillain-Barré syndrome

    Polyneuritis

Unusual sequelae of acute hepatitis B. A small proportion of patients who seem to recover from an acute hepatitis will then experience a prolonged illness and more rarely, a relapse [47,50]. These entities represent a protracted acute hepatitis characterized by a milder clinical course and less striking changes in biochemical tests than the initial illness. Almost all patients go on to complete recovery within a year [50]. Monitoring such patients is important to identify individuals progressing towards an authentic chronic hepatitis. Immune complex disease may occur in the preicteric stage, during illness, or following apparent recovery [49,51]. Immune complexes consisting of hepatitis B surface antigen (HBsAg)–antibodies to HBsAg, hepatitis B e antigen (HBeAg)–antibodies to HBeAg, or hepatitis B core antigen (HBcAg)–antibodies to HBcAg have been described. Often, liver disease is minimal, whereas the consequence of vasculitis can prove severe and life threatening. ALT—alanine aminotransferase; AST—aspartate aminotransferase.

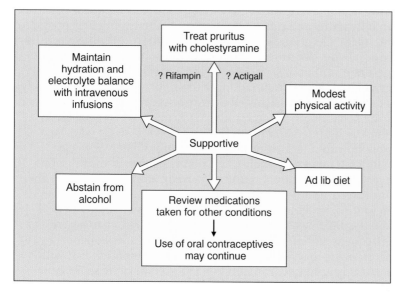

FIGURE 4-15.

Treatment modalities in acute hepatitis B. The provision of supportive care forms the basis of treatment in acute hepatitis B. Patients should not be advised to remain in bed, but rather that the level of physical activity should be commensurate with the state of well being. Dietary restrictions are no longer recommended. If, however, significant nausea or emesis accompany the illness, prudence would dictate avoidance of food likely to promote nausea. Avoidance of alcohol is sensible given its potential hepatotoxic effect. Nonetheless, alcohol ingestion (moderate, of course) is not contraindicated following complete recovery. Patients with significant emesis, dehydration, or electrolyte imbalance will require correction with the appropriate intravenous solutions. Individuals experiencing considerable discomfort associated with pruritus may be given cholestyramine. The use of ursodiol or rifampin should be considered, however, no conclusive evidence of benefit yet exists in acute viral hepatitis. Finally, patients who develop acute viral hepatitis may also have other conditions requiring medication. A review of such agents is necessary to forestall untoward reactions that develop consequent to compromised hepatic function.

CHRONIC HEPATITIS B

TABLE 4-5. DIFFERENTIAL DIAGNOSIS OF CHRONIC HEPATITIS

Viral hepatitis
    Hepatitis B
    Hepatitis C
    Hepatitis D
    Hepatitis non-A, non-B, non-C?
Autoimmune liver disease
Drug induced
    Wilson's disease
Cryptogenic
Chronic liver disease–not considered chronic hepatitis
    Primary biliary cirrhosis
    Primary sclerosing cholangitis
    Hemochromatosis
    α_1-Antitrypsin deficiency

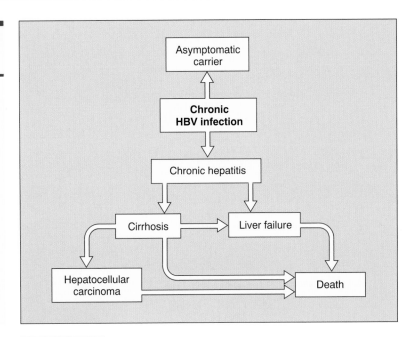

TABLE 4-5.

Patients displaying serologic evidence suggestive of hepatitis B virus (HBV) infection are at a comparable risk for developing other forms of acute or chronic liver disease to that seen in HBV–negative individuals. Admittedly, an index of suspicion is necessary to justify additional evaluation of patients who satisfactorily fulfill the diagnostic criteria for chronic HBV. The etiology to account for chronic hepatitis remains undetermined in 10% to 25% of patients and is referred to as "cryptogenic" [52,53]. Nonetheless, consideration must be given to concomitant extant diseases and, where indicated, appropriate assessment must be undertaken. A group of hepatic disorders such as primary biliary cirrhosis and primary sclerosing cholangitis exist, which may share features with the syndrome of chronic hepatitis but are not considered examples of that syndrome.

FIGURE 4-16.

Consequences of chronic hepatitis B. Chronic infection with HBV can result in the development of a chronic carrier state with little or no evidence of liver injury or progression to a chronic necroinflammatory condition. Chronic hepatitis may lead to hepatic failure over a relatively short time interval in the presence or absence of cirrhosis [54]. Alternatively, cirrhosis may result with subsequent development of hepatocellular carcinoma or hepatic failure [48].

TABLE 4-6. HISTOLOGICAL CLASSIFICATION OF CHRONIC HEPATITIS B

ETIOLOGY-CHRONIC HEPATITIS B

GRADING	(A) MINIMAL	(B) MILD	(C) MODERATE	(D) SEVERE
HAI Numerical equivalent	1–3	4–8	9–12	13–18

STAGE (FIBROSIS)	I. NONE	II. MILD	III. MODERATE	IV. SEVERE	V. CIRRHOSIS
HAI Numerical equivalent	0	1	(2)*	3	4

Examples of histologic classification	(1)	(2)
Etiology	Chronic hepatitis B	Chronic hepatitis B
Grade	Mild activity	Severe activity
Stage	Mild fibrosis	Severe fibrosis

*The original Knodell HAI did not include a "2" in scoring fibrosis; mild and moderate fibrosis were considered equivalent [57]

TABLE 4-6.

Histologic classification of chronic hepatitis B. Liver biopsy is an important component of patient care in chronic hepatitis B. Chronic hepatitis is a histologic diagnosis and examination of a tissue specimen provides information on the extent of damage and in predicting outcome [55]. Assessment of the pattern and extent of necroinflammation correlates with the distribution of replicating HBV in the liver [56]. Past attempts to define the histologic features observed in chronic hepatitis did not incorporate disease etiology or clinical status in the interpretive analysis. Several semiquantitative grading systems have, however, provided useful approaches for gauging disease severity, for providing short-term prognosis, and for monitoring response to therapeutic interventions [57,58]. Although the Knodell histologic activity index (HAI) and Scheuer scoring systems have been used extensively, they incorporate numeric scores for grading the severity of the necroinflammatory changes. They combine them with scores for the stage of disease (eg, fibrosis). A recently proposed classification takes into consideration clinical, etiologic, and histologic information in arriving at the final diagnosis of chronic hepatitis [46]. The aforementioned system characterizes disease etiology, grade, and stage as separate parameters. Application of this classification system to chronic hepatitis B is demonstrated in this table.

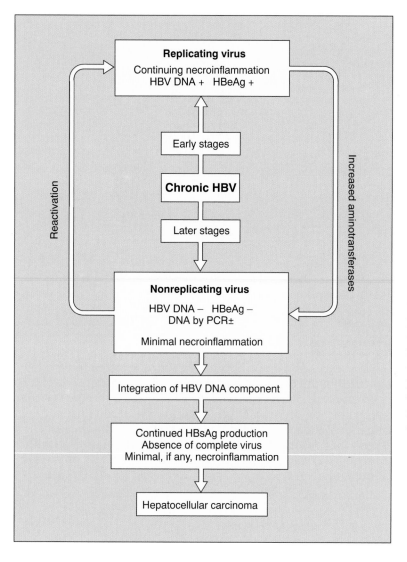

FIGURE 4-17.

Natural history of chronic hepatitis. With the advent of effective therapy, changes in the natural history of chronic hepatitis can be predicted, and although indications exist that such alterations have taken place in patients responding to treatment, accurate information on the nature and extent of disease modification will require many years of follow-up. Review of data from the preinterferon era has provided information on the long-term consequences of chronic hepatitis B virus (HBV) infection (*see* Fig. 4-18). In the early stages of disease characterized by viral replication and necroinflammation, continuing injury to the liver may result in irreversible damage in the presence, or absence, of cirrhosis. In time, the virus may lose the ability to replicate, usually signalled by loss of hepatitis B e antigen (HBeAg) and HBV DNA and accompanied by a transient increase in necroinflammation [59]. Some of these patients will harbor small quantities of HBV DNA detectable only by polymerase chain reaction (PCR) technology. Such individuals will, after variable time intervals and for undetermined reasons, reactivate their disease once again, thus producing HBeAg and larger amounts of HBV DNA. This relapse can result in additional liver damage which can lead to hepatic failure [59–61]. Other patients in the nonreplicating phase of disease may integrate part of the HBV genome resulting in the production of hepatitis B surface antigen (HBsAg) only, with no concomitant viral replication [62]. In such a setting there is little inflammation, however, the risks of developing hepatocellular carcinoma are increased [62,63].

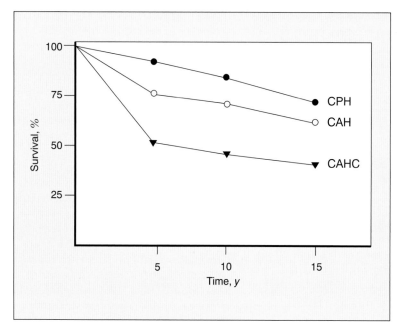

FIGURE 4-18.

An analysis of the mortality rate observed in 379 patients in the pre-interferon era [55]. Patients were categorized upon the basis of an initial liver biopsy. Those with mild disease (*n*=121), classified as having chronic persistent hepatitis (CPH), had minimal mortality. Patients with more severe disease (*n*=128), classified as having chronic active hepatitis (CAH), exhibited a higher mortality rate that was exceeded by patients with active cirrhosis (*n*=130). The differences between each of the groups were significant (*P*<0.001). The 5-year mortality rate with active cirrhosis is similar to that observed in other studies of hepatitis B–related cirrhosis [64,65]. The outcome analyses were based on the initial histologic classifications and did not take into account subsequent changes in histopathology. Thus, for example, progression of disease may not have occurred in some patients with CAH and indeed, regression of the histologic lesions may have taken place. In a study of 105 noncirrhotic patients with chronic hepatitis B who were studied for a mean of 3.7 years, initial histologic findings of moderate CAH were more likely to regress to findings of CPH on follow-up biopsy than to progress to cirrhosis [66]. CAHC—chronic active hepatitis with cirrhosis; HBsAg—hepatitis B surface antigen. (*Adapted from* Weissberg *et al.* [55] and Ladenheim *et al.* [67]; with permission.)

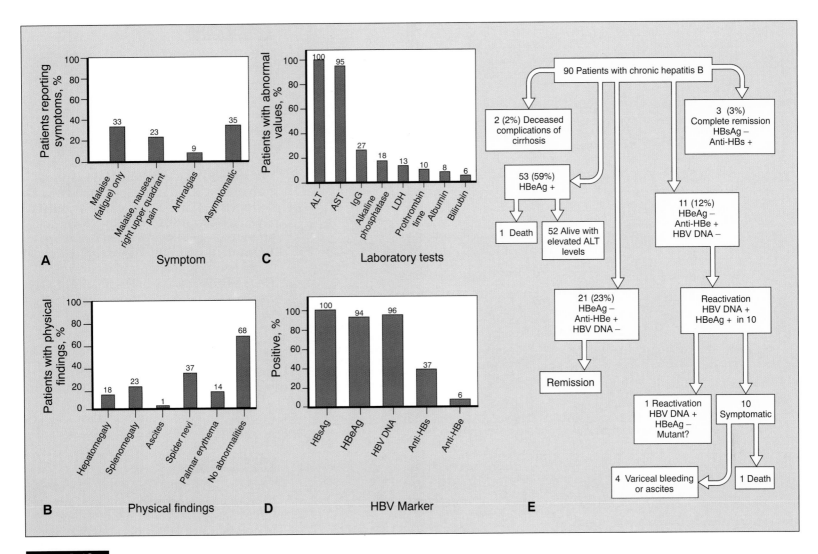

FIGURE 4-19.

Clinical, biochemical, and serologic profiles of patients with chronic hepatitis B. Data are presented at the outset of a long-term follow-up for 90 patients known to have chronic hepatitis B for a mean of 5.1 years and who were subsequently watched for 2.4 years (range 1 to 9 years; 59). **A**, Nearly two-thirds of the patients reported mild symptoms that were frequently self-limited or improved over time. Thirty-five percent of patients were asymptomatic. **B**, Physical findings were sparse with most patients displaying minimal (*eg*, spider nevi) or no abnormal features. Only 25% of the patients had hepatomegaly or splenomegaly. **C**, Virtually all patients had increased aminotransferases, with 6% showing elevations in the bilirubin. Of the 78 patients for whom liver histology was available, 27 (35%) had chronic persistent hepatitis, 32 (41%) had chronic active

hepatitis, and 19 (24%) had cirrhosis. **D**, The serologic findings are shown. All patients had hepatitis B surface antigen (HBsAg); more than a third of the patients had antibodies to HBsAg (Anti-HBs). **E**, Patient outcomes. Clearance of the hepatitis B e antigen (HBeAg) and hepatitis B virus (HBV) DNA was usually associated with disease remission in a majority of patients [59], although a small group redeveloped disease, often with severe episodes of reactivation resulting in disease progress and in one instance, death. One patient undergoing reactivation, but remaining HBeAg negative, may have experienced emergence of a mutant HBV form. ALT—alanine transaminase; AST—aspartate transaminase; Anti-HBe—antibodies to HBeAg; IgG—immunoglobulin G; LDH—lactic dehydrogenase.

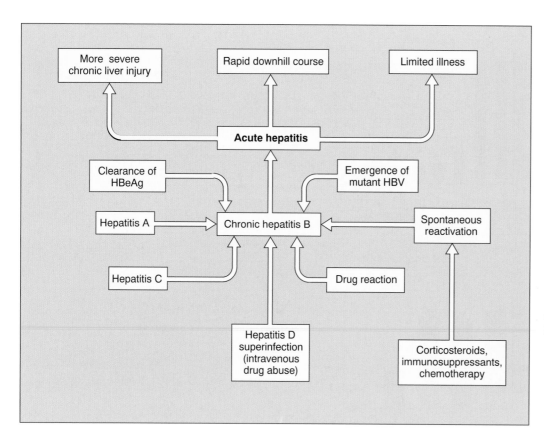

FIGURE 4-20.

Acute hepatitis superimposed on chronic hepatitis B. The sudden onset of acute hepatitis in an asymptomatic hepatitis B virus (HBV) carrier or in a patient with chronic hepatitis cannot be construed alone as resulting from entrance into a more active phase of HBV disease. Although reactivation of disease or emergence of a mutant HBV could account for exacerbation of illness, other etiologies must be considered. A carefully taken history might reveal risk factors such as intravenous drug abuse and exposure to a hepatitis D virus superinfection or HIV. Use of corticosteroids, other immunosuppressives, or chemotherapeutic agents could unwittingly result in reactivation of disease with grave consequences [9,10,68,69]. HBeAg—hepatitis B e antigen.

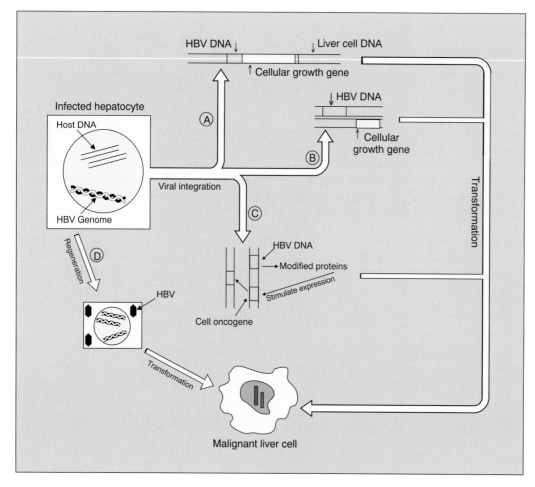

FIGURE 4-21.

The hepatitis B virus (HBV) is not believed to carry oncogenes that can transform infected hepatocytes. The long latency period between HBV infection and the development of hepatocellular carcinoma provides additional evidence for the absence of an HBV oncogene [19,70]. Although the mechanisms to account for the tumorigenic process have not been delineated, a number of possibilities have been proposed. Integration of viral DNA adjacent to cellular growth genes may transform hepatocytes into tumor cells by deregulating their expression and result in uncontrolled growth (A). On the other hand (B), insertion of the viral genome can occur at multiple sites in human chromosomes and result in considerable genetic rearrangements (deletions, translocations, or amplifications), features common in human tumors [19,70–72]. Integrated viral DNA may alone or with cellular DNA produce altered proteins which in turn activate expression of HBV and cellular genes, such as oncogenes (C). Another possibility is that the increased chronic necroinflammation increases cell turnover and regeneration leading to activation of cellular growth genes (D).

Treatment of chronic hepatitis B

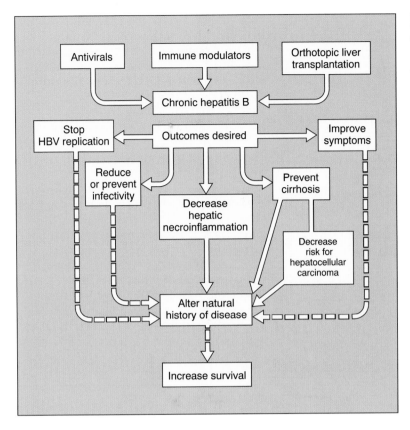

FIGURE 4-22.

The therapeutic objective in chronic hepatitis B is, in the final analysis, to rid the body of a viral infection. A variety of medications have been used, almost all of which have proven either ineffective or too toxic and will not be enumerated. The current approaches include therapy with antivirals, immune modulators, and when all else fails, orthotopic liver transplantation. The goal is to change the natural history of chronic hepatitis B and abrogate the consequences of hepatitis B virus (HBV) infection. Most patients who acquire HBV infection do quite well on their own and should not be interfered with. What characteristics would the ideal candidate for intervention have? The prospective patient should exhibit evidence of chronic infection associated with evidence of viral replication (hepatitis B e antigen [HBeAg], HBV DNA) and inflammation (elevated aminotransferases). Symptoms, such as they may be, and histologic findings are of less import in the decision to treat [73].

TABLE 4-7. ENDPOINTS DEFINING EFFICACY OF TREATMENT

Termination of HBV replication

Loss of HBeAg, seroconversion to Anti-HBe

Loss of HBV DNA by hybridization assay

Cessation of chronic liver injury

Normalization of aminotransferases

Decreased symptomatology, if any

Disease-free state

Seroconversion to HBsAg–negative and Anti-HBs–positive status

Absence of HBV DNA from serum and liver tissue by PCR

TABLE 4-7.

Absence of viral replication and cessation of the hepatic inflammatory reaction with normalization of the alanine and aspartate transaminase levels are the immediate goals of therapy. A quantitative hepatitis B e antigen (HBeAg) microparticle capture enzyme immunoassay (IMx; Abbott Laboratories; Abbott Park, IL) currently undergoing review may serve as a surrogate test for serum hepatitis B virus (HBV) DNA in future studies determining response to antiviral therapy [74]. Long-term objectives include eradication of all vestiges of HBV infection. Although achieving hepatitis B surface antigen (HBsAg)–negative status is clearly desired, by no means does it signal eradication of the HBV [75,76]. Anti-HBe—antibodies to HBeAg; Anti-HBs—antibodies to HBsAg; PCR—polymerase chain reaction.

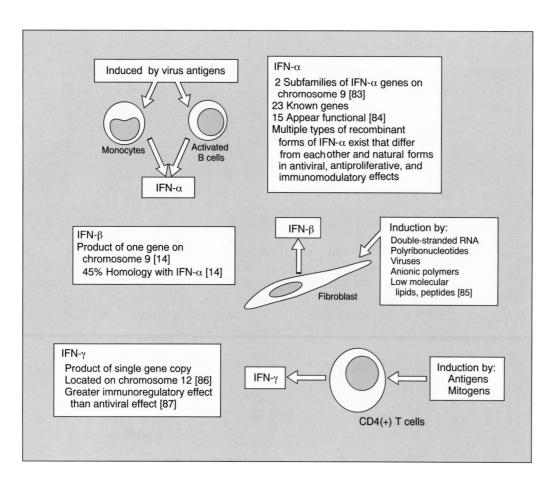

FIGURE 4-23.

Rationale for interferon (IFN) treatment in chronic hepatitis B. Patients with chronic hepatitis B have a deficiency of endogenous IFN in response to the chronic viral infection. Mononuclear cells isolated from patients with chronic hepatitis B show suboptimal production of IFN-α [77,78]. Evidence suggests that the core region of the hepatitis B virus (HBV) genome may suppress IFN production by host cells [79]. The ability of patients with chronic hepatitis B to respond to IFN nonetheless remains intact [43,80,81]. Although the precise mechanism of IFN action is not known, this family of polypeptides (α, β, and γ classes) was originally identified by their induction of an antiviral state [82]. In addition, IFNs also exert antiproliferative as well as immunomodulatory effects [14,82]. IFN-α and -β (type I IFN), which bind to the same receptor, exert a mainly antiviral effect. IFN-γ (type II IFN), which binds to a different receptor, has a predominantly immune modulatory effect.

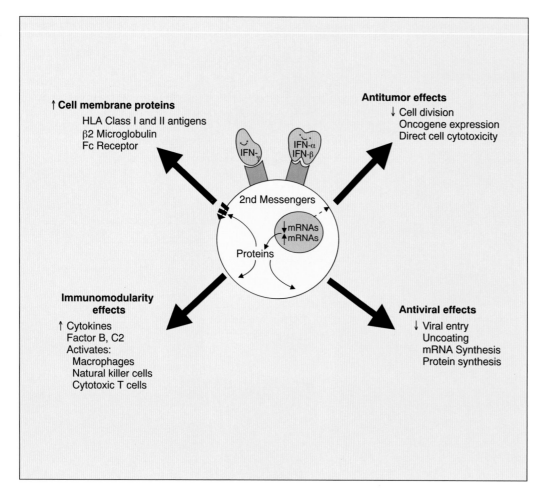

FIGURE 4-24.

Action of the interferons (IFNs). IFN-α and IFN-β share a common receptor that is encoded by a gene on chromosome 21. These receptors are found on a variety of human cells. IFN-γ binds to a receptor encoded by a gene on chromosome 6 [88], however, chromosome 21 may be required for activation of the gene on chromosome 6 [89]. Receptors for IFN-γ are located on many cell types including lymphocytes, fibroblasts, platelets, and tumor cell lines [14]. Internalization of the IFNs may not be critical for the subsequent actions, which are possibly mediated by second messengers. Recent studies on the IFN signal transduction pathway have characterized protein tyrosine kinases that in turn phosphorylate signal transducers that bind to DNA promoter sequences and activate gene transcription [90]. The IFNs induce a variety of known, as well as unidentified, proteins. The immunomodulatory, antiviral, and antiproliferative effects of the IFNs are shown. (*Adapted from* Peters [14]; with permission.)

TABLE 4-8. POSSIBLE IFN EFFECTS IN CHRONIC HEPATITIS B

Induction of HLA class I antigen	IFN-α, -β, -γ
Induction of HLA class II antigen	IFN-γ
Induction of 2' 5' oligoadenylate synthetase	IFN-α, -β, -γ
Inhibition of viral entry into cells	IFN-α, -β, -γ
Prevention of viral uncoating	IFN-α, -β, -γ
Inhibition of messenger RNA translation	IFN-α, -β, -γ
inhibition of viral assembly	IFN-α, -β, -γ
Induction of protein kinase	IFN-α and IFN-β more than IFN-γ

TABLE 4-8.

The ability of interferons (IFNs) to exert antiviral effects depend on their interactions with cell receptors and the subsequent induction of cellular proteins. In addition, ample evidence exists to suggest that their immunomodulatory and antiproliferative properties may also play a significant role in the therapeutic response in chronic hepatitis B [91]. The induction of HLA class I and II proteins may enhance immune recognition of viral proteins permitting clearance of the virus as illustrated previously (*see* Figs. 4-5 and 4-6). The 2' 5' oligoadenylate synthetase induction activates RNase L, which in turn preferentially cleaves viral RNA (and to a lesser extent, host RNA) [14]. Protein kinase promotes phosphorylation of several proteins that enhance the antiviral state of the cell [92].

Clinical trials with interferon

TABLE 4-9. CONSENSUS FINDINGS OF THERAPEUTIC TRIALS [95–100]

Loss of serum HBV DNA and HBeAg in approximately one-third of patients

Response associated with improvement in liver histology

Response associated with improvement in aminotransferases

Successful response requires treatment for a minimum of 3 months

Dosages of 5 to 10 MU are sufficient to suppress viral replication

Dosages of 1 or 2 MU are inadequate

Three times weekly administration of IFN is effective for suppressing viral replication and is better tolerated than daily administration

TABLE 4-9.

Interferon (IFN) treatment of chronic hepatitis B. IFN-α is at present the most effective treatment for chronic hepatitis B. It is the only drug approved for use in the United States, based in part on the landmark randomized controlled trial wherein IFN-α_{2b} was proven of benefit in the treatment of chronic hepatitis B [93]. A recent meta-analysis [16], which reviewed treatment outcomes in 16 prospective, randomized, controlled studies (including that of Perillo and coworkers [93]), showed that IFN-α was beneficial with loss of hepatitis B surface antigen observed 6% more often in treated patients than in controls. Loss of hepatitis B virus (HBV) replication (hepatitis B e antigen [HBeAg], HBV DNA) occurred 20% more often and normalization of alanine transaminase values was seen at a significantly higher frequency in IFN-treated patients [16]. Numerous therapeutic trials conducted between 1985 and 1990 permit a consensus of findings [94]. The overall treatment response rates were remarkably similar among the listed studies. Various types of IFN-α were used— recombinant as well as natural forms.

TABLE 4-10. PREDICTIVE FACTORS OF IFN RESPONSE

Low viral load (HBV DNA < 100 pg/mL) [92]

Elevated ALT levels (> 100 IU/ml)

Active necroinflammation in the liver

Horizontal acquisition of HBV infection (as an adult)

Female gender

HIV Negative

TABLE 4-10.

Predictive factors of response to interferon (IFN)-α. Low pretreatment serum hepatitis B virus (HBV) DNA levels and elevated alanine transaminase (ALT) values are the most useful factors for predicting a favorable response to treatment [93,94]. A low level of HBV DNA in association with an elevated ALT level appear indicative of an enhanced immune response with increased destruction of infected hepatocytes. The presence of concurrent viral infections (HIV, perhaps hepatitis D virus) and other disorders of the immune system comprise negative predictors for treatment response [94].

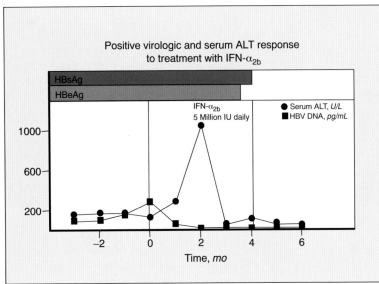

Positive virologic and serum ALT response to treatment with IFN-α$_{2b}$

HBsAg
HBeAg

IFN-α$_{2b}$
5 Million IU daily

● Serum ALT, *U/L*
■ HBV DNA, *pg/mL*

1000

600

200

−2   0   2   4   6

Time, *mo*

FIGURE 4-25.

FIGURE 4-25.

Typical successful response to interferon (IFN) treatment. Most patients responding to IFN will experience an alanine transaminase (ALT) flare several fold higher than the pretreatment value during the 16-week treatment course. This flare may signal activation of the host immune response to hepatitis B virus (HBV)–infected cells. Approximately 60% to 70% of responders and 25% to 30% of nonresponders will display ALT flares [101]. Patients usually tolerate the flare unless hepatic synthetic function is poor. Emergence from the flare is associated with clearance of HBV DNA and normalization of the ALT. The hepatitis B e antigen (HBeAg) may disappear shortly thereafter or some months later [93,94,101]. At times the flare may reach alarming proportions and be accompanied by jaundice and clinical symptomatology dictating dose reduction or treatment discontinuation. The phase of aggressive inflammatory reaction under certain conditions may end in hepatic failure and death. Identification of patients liable to experience this potentially lethal complication is addressed in Figure 4-27. HBsAg—hepatitis B surface antigen.

FIGURE 4-26.

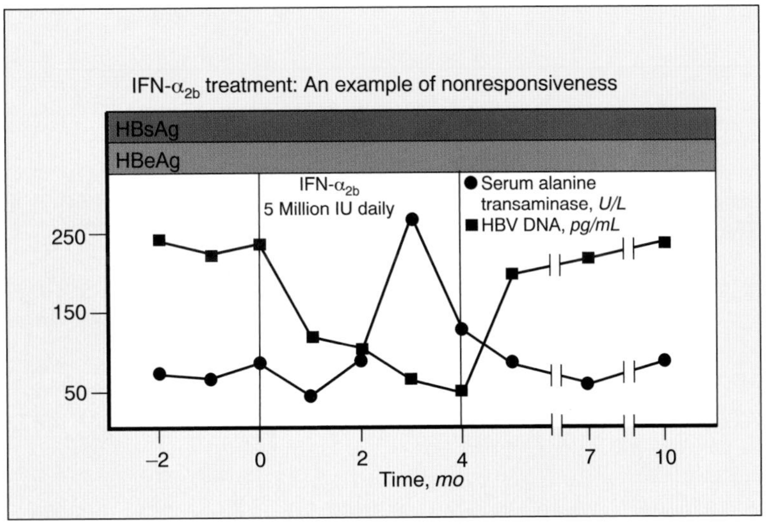

IFN-α$_{2b}$ treatment: An example of nonresponsiveness

HBsAg
HBeAg

IFN-α$_{2b}$
5 Million IU daily

● Serum alanine transaminase, *U/L*
■ HBV DNA, *pg/mL*

250

150

50

−2   0   2   4   7   10

Time, *mo*

Unsuccessful response to interferon (IFN). In this instance the hepatitis B virus (HBV) DNA load was high and correspondingly, the alanine transaminase elevation was modest. Although a flare occurred, it was apparently insufficient to adequately lyse infected hepatocytes. With cessation of treatment, values for HBV DNA and alanine transaminase returned to pretreatment levels. HBeAg—hepatitis B e antigen; HBsAg—hepatitis B surface antigen.

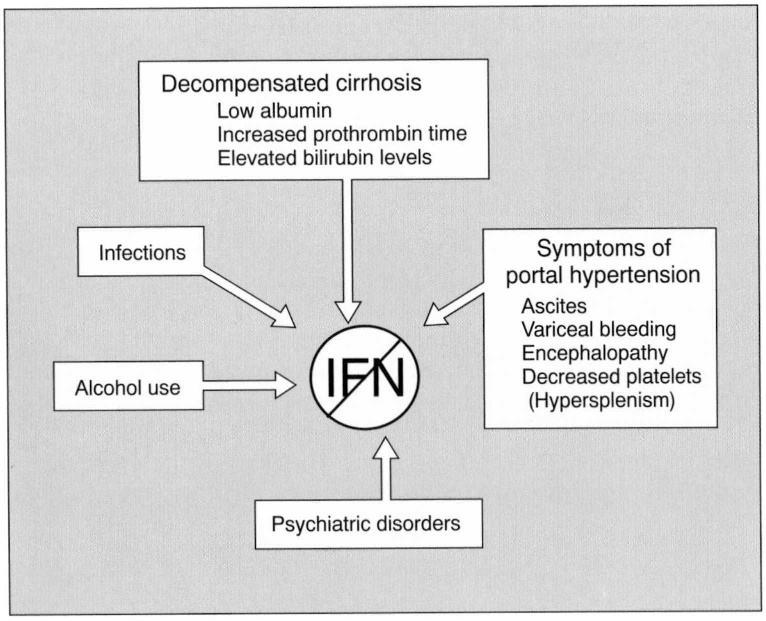

FIGURE 4-27.

Decompensated cirrhosis
Low albumin
Increased prothrombin time
Elevated bilirubin levels

Infections

Symptoms of portal hypertension
Ascites
Variceal bleeding
Encephalopathy
Decreased platelets
(Hypersplenism)

Alcohol use

IFN

Psychiatric disorders

Contraindications for engaging in interferon (IFN) therapy. As noted in Figure 4-25, there are patients at increased risk of suffering a calamitous experience when undergoing standard IFN therapy for chronic hepatitis B. Patients with decompensated cirrhosis [102] have little hepatic reserve to sustain what may represent a major inflammatory process that is instrumental in clearance of the virus. Evidence of a predisposition towards liver failure include findings of low albumin levels, increased prothrombin time, and elevated bilirubin. Signs of portal hypertension portend danger when ascites, encephalopathy, episodes of esophageal or gastric variceal bleeding, and hematologic abnormalities are present. Use of IFN in such patients may also promote severe infections particularly if leukocyte counts are low. Continued consumption of alcohol is also a contraindication either when starting treatment or for continuing therapy when informed of the alcohol intake. Finally, clinically relevant psychiatric dysfunction may be aggravated by IFN.

FIGURE 4-28.

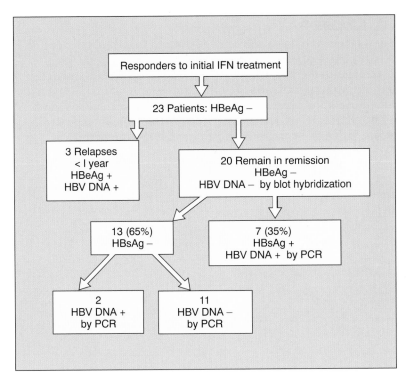

Long-term outcomes for responders to interferon (IFN). Most of the clinical trials to assess IFN efficacy have evaluated patients over the course of 1 to 2 years. Recurrence of hepatitis B virus (HBV) replication has been reported in 5% to 50% of responders within the 1st year and in 10% to 20% of patients during the 2nd year of follow-up [94,101]. Furthermore, despite seroconversion to a hepatitis B surface antigen (HBsAg)–negative and antibodies to HBsAg–positive condition in patients, low levels of HBV DNA can be identified indefinitely in liver tissue [103]. Although traces of the HBV DNA can be retained for long periods in the liver, the significance of this observation remains unknown. What is clear is that patients responding to IFN are not likely to reactivate nor to demonstrate findings of chronic inflammation in the liver. Clearly, the disease in such responders has entered a stage of remission (forever, it is hoped) and such people behave as if they are free of disease. Twenty three (36%) of 64 patients responding to IFN and followed for a mean of 4.3 years at the National Institutes of Health (NIH) are presented [104]. As shown, 65% of patients with sustained loss of hepatitis B e antigen (HBeAg) lost HBsAg. Other studies from Spain report a 24% seroconversion to HBsAg–negative status and in a study of Chinese patients, no patients lost HBsAg during a follow-up period similar to that of the NIH study [105,106]. PCR—polymerase chain reaction.

TABLE 4-11. ADVERSE EFFECTS OF INTERFERON

Fatigue, malaise, chills

Alopecia

Anorexia, nausea

Significant depression, difficulty sleeping

Emotional lability

Suppression of bone marrow elements

Autoantibodies

Interferon neutralizing antibodies

Infections

Decreased libido

TABLE 4-11.

Almost all patients receiving interferon will experience some type of adverse effect. Most of these individuals will tolerate these difficulties, motivated by the desire to be rid of the disease. Modification in dose may be necessary, particularly if symptoms become debilitating or if compliance with treatment is threatened. Some patients must discontinue therapy when hematologic problems arise [94,107].

TABLE 4-12. PROBLEM PATIENT GROUPS REQUIRING EVALUATION

Nonresponders to standard IFN treatment

Perinatally infected patients

Children

Transplant recipients

HBeAg–Negative precore mutant HBV–Infected patients

Decompensated cirrhosis

HBV Carriers

Hemodialysis patients

HBV–Related immune complex disease

HIV–Positive patients

TABLE 4-12.

Additional studies are required in select groups of patients who are not considered candidates for standard interferon (IFN) therapy. Nonresponders to standard IFN therapy may be candidates for a short course of prednisone followed by standard IFN treatment. Of five large scale randomized controlled studies [94], four failed to show any benefit of prednisone priming followed by IFN as compared to IFN alone. However, patients with low alanine transaminase (ALT) values are likely to undergo an ALT flare 4 to 6 weeks after a short course of prednisone treatment and then respond to IFN [93,108]. Prednisone may induce increased production of viral peptides that bind to HLA class I molecules, which are expressed on the membrane. As shown in Figure 4-5A, the viral peptides are exposed to the immune system (cytotoxic T lymphocytes), which then lyse the infected cell [101]. Although IFN treatment of patients with decompensated cirrhosis is fraught with anxiety, not to speak of danger, such patients have responded to standard, tapered, or low dose IFN with sustained clearance of HBV DNA [101,109]. Side effects were frequent. Treatment of patients with decompensated cirrhosis should be accomplished with great care because the risk of infection and liver failure is considerable. HBeAg—hepatitis B e antigen; HBV—hepatitis B virus.

TABLE 4-13. CURRENT EXPERIMENTAL THERAPIES FOR CHRONIC HBV

THERAPEUTIC AGENT	INITIAL BENEFIT OBSERVED	CLINICAL TRIALS UNDER WAY
IFNs		
IFN-β	[110]	?
Nucleoside analogs		
Lamivudine	[111] [112]	+
Immunomodulators		
HBV Vaccine	[113]	?
Vaccine containing HBcAg epitopes	[94]	+
Combination therapy		
IFN-α + thymosin-α$_1$	[114]	−

TABLE 4-13.

Many agents have been subjected to clinical trials and have either failed the test of efficacy or were found to be too toxic [94]. Combination therapy using one or several antivirals or antivirals with immunomodulators are undergoing, and will continue to undergo, clinical testing. As insight is gained on hepatitis B virus (HBV)–host interactions, more precise therapeutic strategies will evolve. HBcAg—hepatitis B core antigen; IFN—interferon.

REFERENCES AND RECOMMENDED READING

1. Maynard JE: Hepatitis B: Global importance and need for control. *Vaccine* 1990, 8(suppl):18–20.

2. McQuillan GM, Alter MJ, Everhart JE: Viral hepatitis. In *Digestive Diseases in the United States: Epidemiology and Impact*. Edited by Everhart JE. Washington, DC: US Department of Health and Human Services, Public Health Service, National Institutes of Health, US Government Printing Office; 1994:125–156.

3. Margolis HS, Alter MJ, Hadler SC: Hepatitis B: Evolving epidemiology and implications for control. *Semin Liver Dis* 1991, 11:84–92.

4. Miller RH: Comparative molecular biology of the hepatitis viruses. *Semin Liver Dis* 1991, 11:113–120.

5. Alberti A, Trevisan A, Fattovich G, Realdi G: The role of hepatitis B virus replication and hepatocyte membrane expression in the pathogenesis of HBV-related hepatic damage. In *Advances in Hepatitis Research*. Edited by Chisari FV. New York: Masson, 1984:134–143.

6. Beasley RP, Hwang L-Y: Postnatal infectivity of hepatitis B surface antigen-carrier mothers. *J Infect Dis* 1983, 147:185–190.

7. McMahon BJ, Alward WLM, Hall DB, *et al.*: Acute hepatitis B virus infection: Relation of age to the clinical expression of disease and subsequent development of the carrier state. *J Infect Dis* 1985, 151:599–603.

8. Lok ASF: Natural history and control of perinatally acquired hepatitis B virus infection. *Dig Dis* 1992, 10:46–52.

9. Hoofnagle JH, Dusheiko GM, Schafer DF, *et al.*: Reactivation of chronic hepatitis B virus infection by cancer chemotherapy. *Ann Intern Med* 1982, 96:447–449.

10. Lau JYN, Lai CL, Lin HJ, *et al.*: Fatal reactivation of chronic hepatitis B virus infection following withdrawal of chemotherapy in lymphoma patients. *Q J Med* 1989, 73:911–917.

11. Davis G: Interferon treatment of viral hepatitis in immunocompromised patients. *Semin Liver Dis* 1989, 9:267–272.

12. Hoofnagle JH, Alter HJ: Chronic viral hepatitis. In *Viral Hepatitis and Liver Disease*. Edited by Vyas GN, Dienstag JL, Hoofnagle JH. Orlando: Grune & Stratton, 1984:97–113.

13. Liaw YF, Tai D-I, Chu C-M, *et al.*: The development of cirrhosis in patients with chronic type B hepatitis: A prospective study. *Hepatology* 1988, 8:493–496.

14. Peters M: Mechanisms of action of interferons. *Semin Liver Dis* 1989, 9:235–239.

15. Peters M: Immunological aspects of antiviral therapy. *Springer Semin Immunopathol* 1990, 12:47–56.

16. Wong DKH, Cheung AM, O'Rourke K, *et al.*: Effect of α-interferon treatment in patients with hepatitis B e antigen-positive chronic hepatitis B: A meta-analysis. *Ann Intern Med* 1993, 119:312–323.

17. Robinson WS, Marion P, Feitelson M, Siddiqui A: The hepadna virus group: Hepatitis B and related viruses. In *Viral Hepatitis*. Edited by Szmuness W, Alter HJ, Maynard JE. Philadelphia: Franklin Institute Press, 1982: 57–68.

18. Heerman KH, Goldman U, Schwartz W, *et al.*: Large surface proteins of hepatitis B virus containing the pre-S sequence. *J Virol* 1984, 52:396–402.

19. Tiollais P, Buendia MA: Hepatitis B virus. *Sci Am* 1991, 264:116–123.

20. Pugh JC, Bassendine MF: Molecular biology of hepadnavirus replication. *BMJ* 1990, 46:329–353.

21. Miller R, Kaneko S, Chung C, *et al.*: Compact organization of the hepatitis B virus genome. *Hepatology* 1989, 9:322–327.

22. Omata M, Ehata T, Yokosuka O, *et al.*: Mutations in the precore region of hepatitis B virus DNA in patients with fulminant and severe hepatitis. *N Engl J Med* 1991, 324:1699–1704.

23. Brunetto M, Stemler M, Bonino F, *et al.*: A new hepatitis B virus strain in patients with severe anti-HBe positive chronic hepatitis B. *J Hepatol* 1990, 10:258–261.

24. Okamato H, Yotsumoto S, Akahane Y, *et al.*: Hepatitis B virus with precore region defects prevail in persistently infected hosts always with seroconversion to the antibody against e antigen. *J Virol* 1990, 64:1298–1303.

25. Brown JL, Carman WF, Thomas HC: The clinical significance of molecular variation within the hepatitis B virus genome. *Hepatology* 1992, 15:144–148.

26. Hamasaki K, Nakata K, Nagayama Y, *et al.*: Changes in the prevalence of HBeAg negative mutant hepatitis B virus during the course of chronic hepatitis B. *Hepatology* 1994, 20:8–14.

27. Foster GR, Carman WF, Thomas HC: Replication of hepatitis B and delta viruses: Appearance of viral mutants. *Semin Liver Dis* 1991, 11:121–127.

28. Theilmann L, Goeser T: Interactions of hepatitis B virus with hepatocytes: Mechanism and clinical relevance. *Hepatogastroenterology* 1991, 38:10–13.

29. Pontisso P, Petit M-A, Bankowski MJ, *et al.*: Human liver plasma membranes contain receptors for the hepatitis B virus pre-S1 region and via polymerized human serum albumin for the pre-S2 region. *J Virol* 1989, 63:1981–1988.

30. Hertogs K, Depla E, Crabbe T, *et al.*: Spontaneous development of anti-hepatitis B virus envelop (anti-idiotypic) antibodies in animals immunized with human liver endonexin II or with the F (ab^1)$_2$ fragment of anti-human liver endonexin II immunoglobulin G: Evidence for a receptor-ligand–like relationship between small hepatitis B surface antigen and endonexin II. *J Virol* 1994, 68:1516–1521.

31. Neurath AR, Strick N, Li Y-Y: Cells transfected with human interleukin 6 cDNA acquire binding sites for the hepatitis B virus envelope protein. *J Exp Med* 1992, 176:1561–1569.

32. Franco A, Paroli M, Testa U, *et al.*: Transferrin receptor mediates uptake and presentation of hepatitis B envelope antigen by T lymphocytes. *J Exp Med* 1992, 175:1195–1205.

33. Mehdi H, Kaplan MJ, Anlar FY, *et al.*: Hepatitis B virus surface antigen binds to apolipoprotein H. *J Virol* 1994, 68:2415–2424.

34. Carman WF, Thomas HC: Genetic variation in hepatitis B virus. *Gastroenterology* 1992, 102:711–719.

35. Mills CT, Lee E, Perrillo R: Relationship between histology, aminotransferase levels, and viral replication in chronic hepatitis B. *Gastroenterology* 1990, 99:519–524.

36. Thomas HC, Jacyna M, Waters J, *et al.*: Virus-host interaction in chronic hepatitis B virus infection. *Semin Liver Dis* 1988, 8:342–349.

37. Foster GR, Thomas HC: Recent advances in the molecular biology of hepatitis B virus: Mutant virus and the host response. *Gut* 1993, 34:1–3.

38. Van Hecke E, Paradijs J, Molitor C, *et al.*: Hepatitis B virus—specific cytotoxic T lymphocyte responses in patients with acute and chronic hepatitis B virus infection. *J Hepatol* 1994, 20:514–523.

39. Ferrari C, Bertoletti A, Penna A, *et al.*: Identification of immunodominant T cell epitopes of the hepatitis B virus nucleocapsid antigen. *J Clin Invest* 1991, 88:214–222.

40. Moriyama T, Guilhot S, Klopchin K, *et al.*: Immunobiology and pathogenesis of hepatocellular injury in hepatitis B virus transgenic mice. *Science* 1990, 248:361–364.

41. Missale G, Brems JJ, Takiff H, *et al.*: Human leukocyte antigen class I—Independent pathways may contribute to hepatitis B virus-induced liver disease after liver transplantation. *Hepatology* 1993, 18:491–496.

42. Milich DR, McLachlan A, Thornton GB, *et al.*: Antibody production to the nucleocapsid and envelope of the hepatitis B virus primed by a single synthetic T cell site. *Nature* 1987, 329:547–549.

43. Pignatelli M, Waters J, Brown D, *et al.*: MHC Class I antigens on the hepatocyte membrane during recovery from acute hepatitis B virus infection and during interferon therapy in chronic hepatitis B virus infection. *Hepatology* 1986, 6:349–353.

44. Peters M, Vierling J, Gershwin ME, *et al.*: Immunology and the liver. *Hepatology* 1991, 13:977–994.

45. Hoofnagle JH, Schafer DF: Serologic markers of hepatitis B virus infection. *Semin Liver Dis* 1986, 6:1–10.

46. Desmet VJ, Gerber M, Hoofnagle JH, *et al.*: Classification of chronic hepatitis: Diagnosis, grading and staging. *Hepatology* 1994, 19:1513–1520.

47. Sherlock S: *Diseases of the Liver and Biliary System*. Oxford: Blackwell Scientific Publications; 1989.

48. Seeff LB, Koff RS: Evolving concepts of the clinical and serologic consequences of hepatitis B infection. *Semin Liver Dis* 1986, 6:11–22.

49. Koff RS: Viral hepatitis. In *Diseases of the Liver*. Edited by Schiff L, Schiff ER. Philadelphia: JB Lippincott Company, 1993: 492–577.

50. Chalmers TC, Eckhardt RD, Reynolds WE, *et al.*: The treatment of acute infectious hepatitis: Controlled studies of the effects of diet, rest, and physical reconditioning on the acute course of the disease and on the incidence of relapses and residual abnormalities. *J Clin Invest* 1955, 34:1163–1235.

51. Gocke DJ: Extrahepatic manifestations of viral hepatitis. *Am J Med Sci* 1975, 270:49–52.

52. Jeffers J, Hasan F, deMedina M, *et al.*: Prevalence of antibodies to hepatitis C virus among patients with cryptogenic chronic hepatitis and cirrhossis. *Hepatology* 1992, 15:187–190.

53. Czaja AJ, Carpenter HA, Santrach PJ, *et al.*: The nature and prognosis of severe cryptogenic chronic active hepatitis. *Gastroenterology* 1993, 104:1755–1761.

54. Hoofnagle JH, Seeff LB: Natural history of chronic type B hepatitis. In *Progress in Liver Diseases*. Edited by Popper H, Schaffner F. New York: Grune & Stratton, 1982:469–479.

55. Weissberg JL, Andres LL, Smith CI, *et al.*: Survival in chronic hepatitis B. An analysis of 379 patients. *Ann Intern Med* 1984, 101:613–616.

56. Chu C-M, Liaw Y-F: Intrahepatic distribution of hepatitis B surface and core antigens in chronic hepatitis B virus infection. *Gastroenterology* 1987, 92:220–225.

57. Knodell RG, Ishak KG, Black WC, *et al.*: Formulation and application of a numerical scoring system for assessing histological activity in asymptomatic chronic active hepatitis. *Hepatology* 1981, 1:431–435.

58. Scheuer PJ: Classification of chronic viral hepatitis: A need for reassessment. *J Hepatol* 1991, 13:372–374.

59. Hoofnagle JH, Davis GL, Hanson RG: Chronic type B hepatitis: Clinical course. In *Viral Hepatitis and Delta Infection*. Edited by Verme G, Bonino F, Rizzetto M. New York: Alan R. Liss, 1983:41–53.

60. Davis GL, Hoofnagle JH, Waggoner JG: Spontaneous reactivation of chronic hepatitis B infection. *Gastroenterology* 1984, 86:230–235.

61. Davis GL, Hoofnagle JH: Reactivation of chronic type B hepatitis presenting as acute viral hepatitis. *Ann Intern Med* 1985, 102:762–765.

62. Shafritz DA, Shouval D, Sherman HI, *et al.*: Integration of hepatitis B virus DNA into the genome of liver cells in chronic liver disease and hepatocellular carcinoma: Studies in percutaneous liver biopsies and postmortem tissue specimens. *N Engl J Med* 1981, 305:1067–1073.

63. Brechot C, Nalpas B, Courouce A-M, *et al.*: Evidence that hepatitis B virus has a role in liver-cell carcinoma in alcoholic liver disease. *N Engl J Med* 1982, 306:1384–1387.

64. Tanaka R, Itoshima T, Nagashima H: Follow-up study of 582 liver cirrhosis patients for 26 years in Japan. *Liver* 1987, 7:316–324.

65. Liaw YF, Lin DY, Chen TJ, *et al.*: Natural course after the development of cirrhosis in patients with chronic type B hepatitis: A prospective study. *Liver* 1989, 9:235–241.

66. Fattovich G, Brollo L, Giustina G, *et al.*: Natural history and prognostic factors for chronic hepatitis type B. *Gut* 1991, 32:294–298.

67. Ladenheim J, Yao F, Martin MC, *et al.*: Survival in chronic hepatitis B: A 15-year follow-up [Abstract]. *Hepatology* 1993, 18:119A.

68. Scullard GH, Smith CI, Merigan TC, *et al.*: Effects of immunosuppressive therapy on viral markers in chronic active hepatitis B. *Gastroenterology* 1981, 81:987–991.

69. Rakela J, Redecker AG, Weliky B: Effect of short-term prednisone in chronic type B hepatitis. *Gastroenterology* 1983, 84:956–960.

70. Dusheiko GM: Hepatocellular carcinoma associated with chronic viral hepatitis. *Br Med Bull* 1990, 46:492–511.

71. Rogler CE, Sherman M, Su CY, *et al.*: Deletion in chromosome 11P associated with a hepatitis B integration site in hepatocellular carcinoma. *Science* 1985, 230:319–322.

72. Yang DY, Schirmacher P, Held W, *et al.*: Growth factors, oncogenes, tumor suppressor genes, and carcinogenic mechanisms in the liver. In *Viral Hepatitis and Liver Disease*. Edited by Hollinger FB, Lemon SM, Margolis HS. Baltimore: Williams & Wilkins, 1991:547–556.

73. Hoofnagle JH: Chronic hepatitis B. *N Engl J Med* 1990, 323:337–339.

74. Perrillo R, Mimms L, Schectman K, *et al.*: Monitoring of antiviral therapy with quantitative evaluation of HBeAg: A comparison with HBV DNA testing. *Hepatology* 1993, 18:1306–1312.

75. Fong T-L, DiBisceglie AM, Gerber MA, *et al*: Persistence of hepatitis B virus DNA in the liver after loss of HBsAg in chronic hepatitis B. *Hepatology* 1993, 18:1313–1318.

76. Kuhns M, McNamara A, Mason A, *et al.*: Serum and liver hepatitis B virus DNA in chronic hepatitis B after sustained loss of surface antigen. *Gastroenterology* 1992, 103:1649–1656.

77. Alexander GJM: Immunology of hepatitis B virus infection. *Br Med Bull* 1990, 46:354–367.

78. Abb J, Zachoval R, Eisenburg J, *et al.*: Production of interferon α and interferon γ by peripheral blood leukocytes from patients with chronic hepatitis B virus infection. *J Med Virol* 1985, 16:171–176.

79. Twu JS, Lee CH, Liu PM, *et al.*: Hepatitis B virus suppresses expression of human β-interferon. *Proc Natl Acad Sci U S A* 1988, 85:252–256.

80. Shindo M, Okuno T, Matsumoto M, *et al.*: Serum 2′,5′-oligoadenylate synthetase activity during interferon treatment of chronic hepatitis B. *Hepatology* 1988, 8:366–370.

81. Nishiguchi S, Kuroki T, Otani S, *et al.*: Relationship of the effects of interferon on chronic hepatitis B and the induction of 2′,5′-oligoadenylate synthetase. *Hepatology* 1989, 10:29–33.

82. Samuel CE: Antiviral actions of interferon. Interferon-regulated cellular proteins and their surprisingly selective antiviral activities. *Virology* 1991, 183:1–11.

83. Pestka S, Langer JA, Zoon KC, *et al.*: Interferons and their actions. *Annu Rev Biochem* 1987, 56:727–777.

84. Henco K, Brosius J, Fujisawa A, *et al.*: Structural relationships of human interferon α genes and pseudogenes. *J Mol Biol* 1985, 185:227–260.

85. Stewart WE: *The Interferon System*, edn 2. New York: Springer-Verlag, 1979.

86. Taniguchi T: Regulation of cytokine gene expression. *Annu Rev Immunol* 1988, 6:439–464.

87. Kirchner H: Interferons, a group of multiple lymphokines. *Springer Semin Immunopathol* 1984, 7:347–374.

88. Rashidbaigi A, Langer JA, Jung V, *et al.*: The gene for the human immune interferon receptor is located on chromosome 6. *Proc Natl Acad Sci U S A* 1986, 83:384–388.

89. Jung V, Rashidbaigi A, Jones C, *et al.*: Human chromosomes 6 and 21 are required for sensitivity to human interferon γ. *Proc Natl Acad Sci U S A* 1987, 84:4151–4155.

90. Muller M, Ibelgaufts H, Kerr IM: Interferon response pathways—A paradigm for cytokine signalling? *J Viral Hepatitis* 1994, 1:87–103.

91. Peters M, Walling DM, Kelly K, *et al.*: Immunologic effects of α interferon in man: Treatment with human recombinant α interferon suppresses in vitro immunoglobulin production in patients with chronic type B hepatitis. *J Immunol* 1986, 137:3147–3152.

92. Samuel CE: The interferon-induced protein P1/eIF-2 α kinase. In *The Interferon System: A Current Review to 1987*. Edited by Baron S, Stanton GJ, Fleischmann WR. Austin: Univ Texas Pr, 1987: 373–381.

93. Perrillo RP, Schiff ER, Davis GL, *et al.*: A randomized controlled trial of interferon alfa-2b alone and after prednisone withdrawal for the treatment of chronic hepatitis B. *N Engl J Med* 1990, 323:295–301.

94. Lok ASF: Treatment of chronic hepatitis B. *J Viral Hepatitis* 1994, 1:105–124.

95. Alexander GJM, Brahm J, Fagan E, *et al.*: Loss of HBsAg with interferon therapy in chronic hepatitis B virus infection. *Lancet* 1987, 2:66–69.

96. McDonald JA, Caruso L, Karayiannis P, *et al*: Diminished responsiveness of male homosexual chronic hepatitis B virus carriers with HILV-III antibodies to recombinant α-interferon. *Hepatology* 1987, 7:719–723.

97. Fattovich G, Brollo L, Boscaro S, *et al*: Long-term effect of low dose recombinant interferon therapy in patients with chronic hepatitis B. *J Hepatol* 1989, 9:331–337.

98. Hoofnagle JH, Peters M, Mullen KD, *et al.*: Randomized, controlled trial of recombinant human α-interferon in patients with chronic hepatitis B. *Gastroenterology* 1988, 95:1318–1325.

99. Brook MG, Chan G, Yap I, *et al.*: Randomized controlled trial of lymphoblastoid interferon alfa in europid men with chronic hepatitis B virus infection. *BMJ* 1989, 299:652–656.

100. Saracco G, Mazzella G, Rosina F, *et al.*: A controlled trial of human lymphoblastoid interferon in chronic hepatitis B in Italy. *Hepatology* 1989, 10:336–341.

101. Perrillo RP: The management of chronic hepatitis B. *Am J Med* 1994, 96:34S–40S.

102. Kassianides C, DiBisceglie AM, Hoofnagle JH, *et al.*: α-Interferon therapy in patients with decompensated chronic type B hepatitis. In *Viral Hepatitis and Liver Disease*. Edited by Zuckerman A. New York: Alan R. Liss, 1988: 840–843.

103. Kuhns M, McNamara A, Mason A, *et al.*: Serum and liver hepatitis B virus DNA in chronic hepatitis B after sustained loss of surface antigen. *Gastroenterology* 1992, 103:1649–1656.

104. Korenman J, Baker B, Waggoner J, *et al.*: Long-term remission of chronic hepatitis B after α-interferon therapy. *Ann Intern Med* 1991, 114:629–634.

105. Carreno V, Castillo I, Molina J, *et al.*: Long-term follow-up of hepatitis B chronic carriers who responded to interferon therapy. *J Hepatol* 1992, 15:102–106.

106. Lok ASF, Chung HT, Liu VWS, *et al.*: Long-term follow-up of chronic hepatitis B patients treated with interferon alfa. *Gastroenterology* 1993, 105:1833–1838.

107. Renault PF, Hoofnagle JH: Side effects of α interferon. *Semin Liver Dis* 1989, 9:273–277.

108. Fevery J, Elewaut A, Michielsen P, *et al.*: Efficacy of interferon alfa-2b with or without prednisone withdrawal in the treatment of chronic viral hepatitis B. A prospective double-blind Belgian-Dutch study. *J Hepatol* 1990, 11:S108–S112.

109. Hoofnagle JH, DiBisceglie AM, Waggoner JG, *et al.*: Interferon alfa for patients with clinically apparent cirrhosis due to chronic hepatitis B. *Gastroenterology* 1993, 104:1116–1121.

110. Kagawa T, Morizane T, Saito H, *et al.*: A pilot study of long-term weekly interferon-β administration for chronic hepatitis B. *Am J Gastroenterol* 1993, 88:212–216.

111. Tyrrel DLJ, Mitchell MC, DeMan RA, *et al.*: Phase II trial of lamivudine for chronic hepatitis B. *Hepatology* 1993, 18:112A.

112. Dienstag JL, Perrillo RP, Schiff ER, *et al.*: Double-blind, randomized, three-month, dose-ranging trial of Lamivudine for chronic hepatitis B. *Hepatology* 1994, 20:199A.

113. Pol S, Driss F, Carnot F, *et al.*: Vaccination against hepatitis B virus: An efficient immunotherapy against hepatitis B multiplication. *CR Acad Sci III* 1993, 316:688–691.

114. Rasi G, Mutchnick MG, DiVirgilio D, *et al.*: Combination low-dose lymphoblastoid interferon (L-IFN α) and thymosin α₁(T α₁) therapy in the treatment of chronic hepatitis B. *Hepatology* 1994, 20:299A.

Chapter 5

Hepatitis C

DAVID BERNSTEIN
EUGENE R. SCHIFF

Hepatitis C virus (HCV) was identified in 1989. In the few years since its discovery, a remarkable amount of information has been amassed regarding HCV–induced disease. HCV is an RNA virus transmitted in large measure by exposure to blood and blood products. Individuals who use illicit drugs and share needles are likely to acquire HCV. It appears HCV can be transmitted by close (sexual) contact, although such transmission appears to be much less common than is the case with hepatitis B. HCV is occasionally transmitted from mother to child; such transmission is facilitated if the mother is also infected with HIV. Fully 40% of patients with HCV infection have no history of exposure, which might explain the methods of transmission.

Introduction of serologic markers for HCV infection has led to a better understanding of the virus itself, the epidemiology of the disease, and the natural history of chronic HCV. Soon after its discovery, HCV was established to cause most posttransfusion non-A, non-B hepatitis. Subsequently, it has been established that transfusion accounted for approximately 15% of cases of HCV infection. Current available serologic tests (enzyme-linked immunosorbent assay and recombinant immunoblot assay) are quite sensitive and specific incorporating epitopes from several parts of the virus.

Approximately 70%, and maybe even more, of the patients who acquire acute hepatitis will progress to chronic HCV. Furthermore, development of methods to determine the presence of HCV-RNA has enhanced the diagnosis of acute viral infection within weeks of exposure and has facilitated the ability to determine infectivity among patients who have antibodies to HCV (Anti-HCV). Quantitation of HCV-RNA can be useful in adjusting dose and duration of antiviral therapy among patients with chronic HCV.

It has become apparent that HCV is the most common cause of chronic liver disease, cirrhosis, and hepatocellular carcinoma in·the United States. HCV has also been established to cause a variety of disorders whose predominant manifestations are extrahepatic. These disorders include cryoglobulinemia, membranous glomerulonephritis, polyarteritis, and porphyria cutanea tarda. There is a type of autoimmune hepatitis (Type II) that is characterized by the presence of liver-kidney-microsomal antibodies, the absence of antinuclear antibodies, and evidence of HCV, suggesting this disorder is caused by the virus.

It has further been established that several quasispecies of HCV exist. These quasispecies result from relatively minor changes in the HCV genome. There are considerable geographic variations in the frequency of the various quasispecies, which differ in their natural history and response to antiviral therapy.

The diagnosis of chronic HCV is most often established following identification of Anti-HCV in a patient who is evaluated following identification of an elevated alanine aminotransferase (ALT) level. Scant correlation exists among clinical symptoms, degree of elevation of ALT increases, or histologic evidence of liver disease. Liver biopsy is useful in evaluation in allowing determination of the extent of disease and presence of other liver disorders. The usual natural history of chronic HCV is that of a smoldering illness that slowly progresses over years to cause cirrhosis and subsequent liver decompensation. Unfortunately, a protective antibody has not been identified, and no means of passive nor active immunization is available. Interferon therapy has been established to be useful in attenuating or eradicating HCV in 10% to 30% of patients. Factors that seem to be important in determining the likelihood of response to interferon therapy include young age (<45 years), low levels of HCV-RNA, absence of cirrhosis, and the identified quasispecies. A selection of figures that illustrate pertinent features of HCV infection is provided.

ACUTE VIRAL HEPATITIS

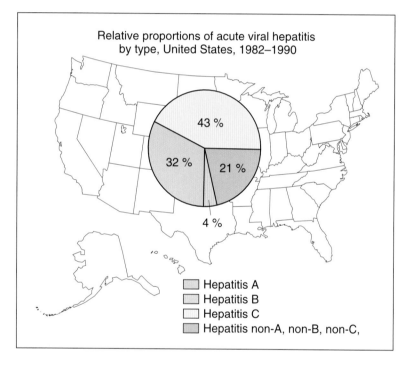

Relative proportions of acute viral hepatitis by type, United States, 1982–1990

43 %
32 %
21 %
4 %

- Hepatitis A
- Hepatitis B
- Hepatitis C
- Hepatitis non-A, non-B, non-C,

FIGURE 5-1.

Relative proportions of acute viral hepatitis. Hepatitis C represents 21% of all cases of acute hepatitis seen in the United States from 1982 to 1990. The most prevalent types of viral hepatitis infections reported to occur during that time period were hepatitis B and A, respectively. Hepatitis C testing has been commercially available since 1989. More sensitive assays are likely to increase the detection of both acute and chronic hepatitis caused by hepatitis C virus [1].

HEPATITIS C VIRUS

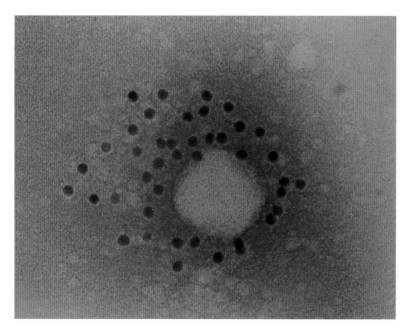

FIGURE 5-2.

Hepatitis C virus (HCV). This figure depicts the HCV coated with radiogold-labeled antibodies to HCV. HCV is an enveloped virus with an average diameter of 30 to 70 nm. It is a single-stranded RNA virus. The classification of HCV has been difficult. The virus shares similar features with both *Pestiviruses* and *Flaviviruses* [2,3]. (*Courtesy of* X. Li, Miami, FL)

Modes of transmission

TABLE 5-1. HCV

MODES OF TRANSMISSION

PARENTERAL	SEXUAL	PERINATAL
Transfusion	Uncommon	Rare
Intravenous drug abuse	Heterosexual	Coinfection with HIV
Needle stick	Homosexual?	

TABLE 5-1.

Modes of transmission. Hepatitis C virus (HCV) accounted for at least 90% of posttransfusion hepatitis before the initiation of the screening of blood donors in 1989. Recent reports have shown sexual transmission to occur, although the frequency is uncertain and likely low. There are data to suggest an increased risk of HCV in heterosexual patients with large numbers of sexual partners and also in those who engage in sexual relations with prostitutes. Less risk of HCV has been shown in the homosexual community. Perinatal transmission has been shown to occur in newborns of mothers with high levels of HCV-RNA and is especially likely if the mother is coinfected with HIV [4–6].

Risk factors

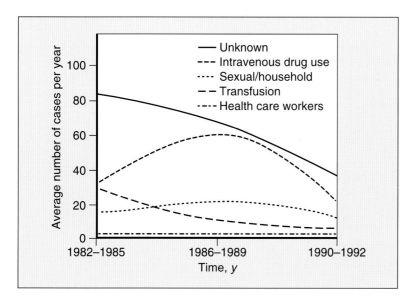

FIGURE 5-3.

Risk factors of non-A, non-B hepatitis C. The average number of cases per year of hepatitis C reported appears to be decreasing from that of the period 1982 to 1992. The "unknown" category is made up largely of individuals from lower socioeconomic levels, who have a higher prevalence of parenteral drug abuse and sexually transmitted disease as noted in the past but not immediately before the development of the acute episode [7,8].

TABLE 5-2. RISK FACTORS FOR HCV

HEALTH CARE SETTING

Transfusion of blood products before 1989
Needle stick injuries
Use of nondisposable syringes or needles
Hemodialysis
Transplantation of infected organs

TABLE 5-2.

Health care workers are at increased risk for the development of hepatitis C virus (HCV). Recent evidence in the United States estimated a 10% chance of acquiring HCV infection by needle stick. Blood products have been routinely screened for HCV since 1989 so that the risk of acquiring it from blood transfusions in the United States is negligible. Hemodialysis patients have been shown to be at increased risk of acquiring HCV infection [9–11].

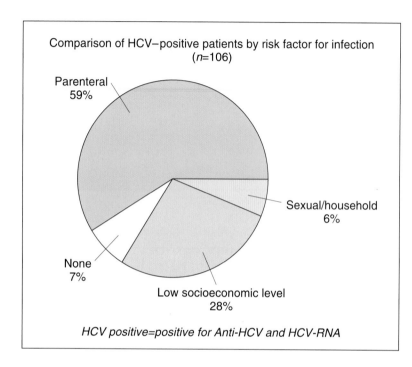

Comparison of HCV–positive patients by risk factor for infection (*n*=106)

Parenteral 59%

Sexual/household 6%

None 7%

Low socioeconomic level 28%

HCV positive=positive for Anti-HCV and HCV-RNA

FIGURE 5-4.

Risk factors among reported cases of acute hepatitis C virus (HCV). HCV is commonly seen in lower socioeconomic settings. Approximately 10% to 40% of patients have no identifiable risk factor for HCV. Sporadic infections of HCV have been attributed to close contact with patients with acute HCV or with chronic carriers. A thorough history of household events can increase the possibility of identifying risk factors for HCV [7]. Anti-HCV—antibodies to HCV. (*Adapted from* Alter *et al.* [7]; with permission.)

Evolution

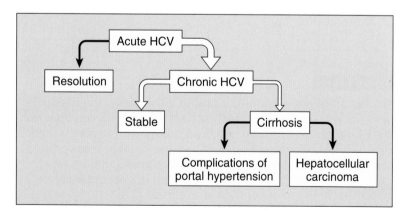

Acute HCV

Resolution

Chronic HCV

Stable

Cirrhosis

Complications of portal hypertension

Hepatocellular carcinoma

FIGURE 5-5.

Evolution of acute hepatitis. The natural history of hepatitis C virus (HCV) is not fully known. At least 80% of infected patients will develop chronic disease. Cirrhosis occurs in 20% to 40% of chronic HCV patients and in 16% to 32% of all patients infected with HCV. Complications of cirrhosis and hepatocellular carcinoma develop in 4% to 8% of infected patients. The time course to the development of cirrhosis and its complications is highly variable [12–15].

Geographic distribution

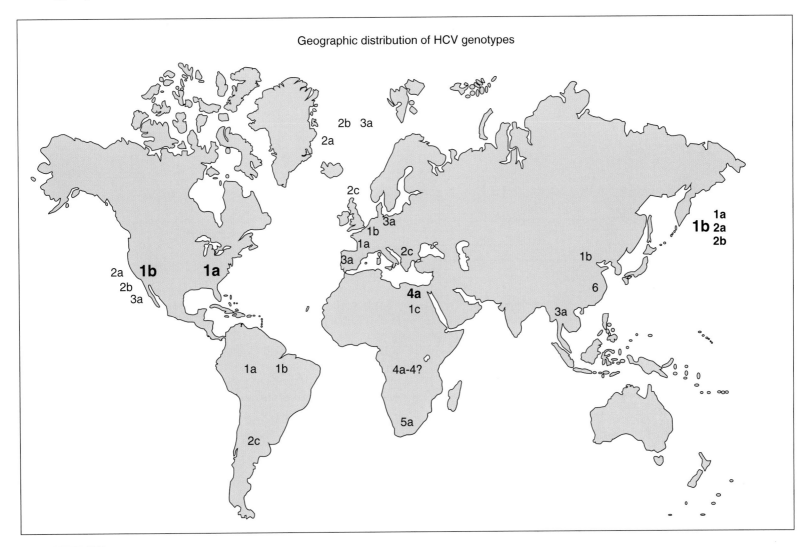

Geographic distribution of HCV genotypes

FIGURE 5-6.

Geographic distribution of hepatitis C virus (HCV) genotypes. There are six major genotypes. The most common genotype seen in the United States and Canada is type 1. Type 1b is associated with a more aggressive clinical course and appears to be more resistant to inter- feron therapy [16–18]. Several studies have associated genotype 1b with a higher risk for the development of hepatocellular carcinoma. Type 2 is commonly seen in Japan and Europe and appears to respond better to interferon therapy. (*Courtesy of* M. Urdea, Emeryville, CA)

Diagnosis

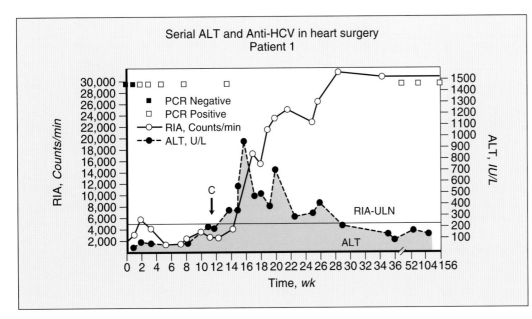

Serial ALT and Anti-HCV in heart surgery
Patient 1

- ■ PCR Negative
- □ PCR Positive
- —○— RIA, Counts/min
- –●– ALT, U/L

FIGURE 5-7.

This figure illustrates the development of hepatitis C after blood transfusions received at cardiac surgery. The first marker to appear is a positive hepatitis C virus (HCV)-RNA. Several weeks after the appearance of HCV-RNA, the alanine aminotransferase (ALT) will peak. Antibody to HCV (Anti-HCV) appears several months after the appearance of HCV-RNA and as illustrated, peaks approximately 4 to 6 months after exposure [19–21]. C signifies the onset of clinical symptoms. PCR—polymerase chain reac- tion; RIA—radioimmunoassay; ULN— upper limit of normal.

TABLE 5-3. DIFFERENTIAL DIAGNOSIS OF HISTOLOGICALLY DOCUMENTED CHRONIC HEPATITIS

Chronic viral hepatitis (B, C, D)

Autoimmune hepatitis

Drug-induced chronic hepatitis

Wilson's disease

TABLE 5-3.

Differential diagnosis of chronic hepatitis. The diagnosis of chronic hepatitis is considered in patients with persistent alanine aminotransferase elevation of at least 6 months' duration. Liver biopsy will document the presence of chronic hepatitis; the differential diagnosis includes both viral and nonviral etiologies. Nonalcoholic steatohepatitis also may mimic chronic hepatitis.

Serologic sequence

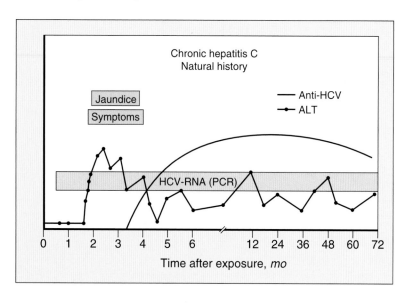

FIGURE 5-8.

Serologic sequence in chronic hepatitis C virus (HCV). HCV-RNA appears approximately 2 to 4 weeks after exposure. Symptoms and jaundice may appear 6 to 24 weeks after exposure. Antibody to HCV (Anti-HCV) appears 12 to 14 weeks after exposure and its presence is lifelong. Anti-HCV does not denote chronicity or active infection. HCV-RNA denotes active disease. Nevertheless, most patients do not present during the acute phase of the illness but instead are diagnosed years later with chronic HCV [22,23]. ALT—alanine aminotransferase; PCR—polymerase chain reaction. (*Adapted from* Hoofnagle [24]; with permission.)

Histologic features

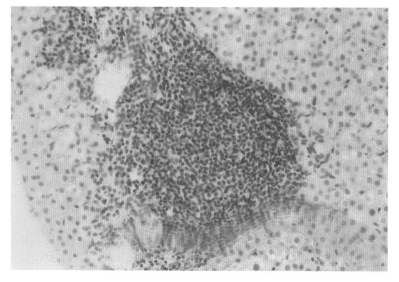

FIGURE 5-9.

Although the histologic features of chronic hepatitis C are not diagnostic, there are certain characteristic findings that are frequently found. Lymphoid follicular-like aggregates in the portal areas, fatty infiltration, bile ductular changes, and sinusoidal inflammation are common. Furthermore, there may be secondary iron deposition, evidence of coinfection with hepatitis B, or alcoholic liver injury in these patients. This figure illustrates one lymphoid follicular-like infiltrate.

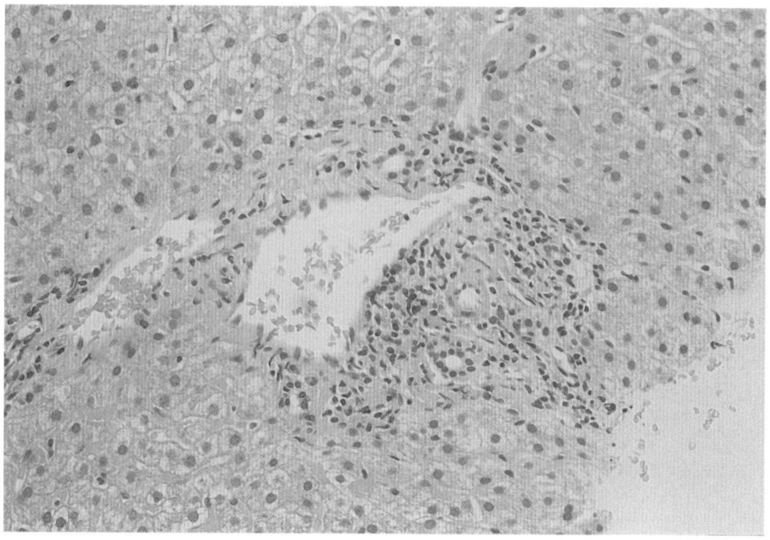

FIGURE 5-10.

This illustration depicts very mild chronic hepatitis with minimal lymphocytic inflammation confined to the portal areas.

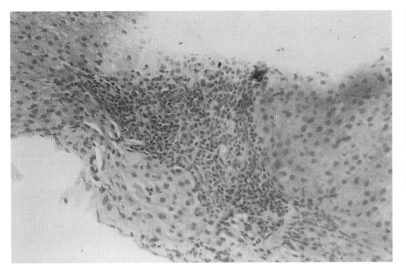

FIGURE 5-11.

This specimen reflects a more intense inflammatory response, which remains confined predominantly to the portal areas.

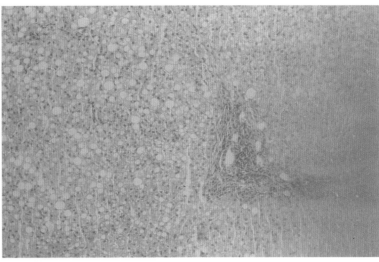

FIGURE 5-12.

A typical histologic feature of chronic hepatitis C is macrovesicular fatty infiltration, evident on this liver biopsy, which also shows mild portal inflammation.

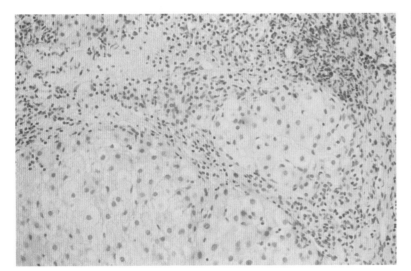

FIGURE 5-13.

The development of bridging necrosis and fibrosis, indicative of a more aggressive and advanced state of chronic hepatitis evolving towards cirrhosis, is evident in this figure.

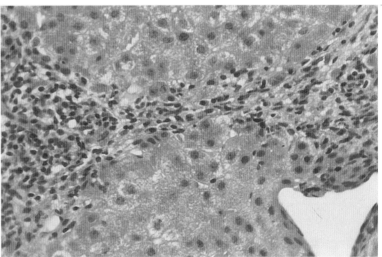

FIGURE 5-14.

This figure depicts a high-power view of bridging fibrosis.

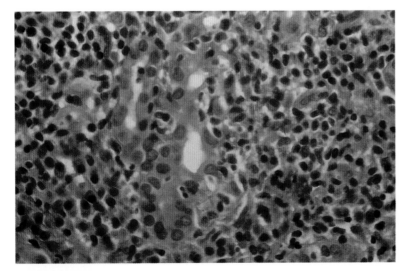

FIGURE 5-15.

Bile ductular epithelial changes are typically found in chronic hepatitis C, as seen here.

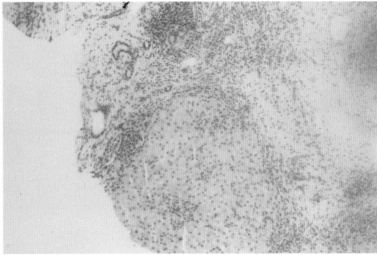

FIGURE 5-16.

This liver biopsy specimen demonstrates well-established cirrhosis secondary to hepatitis C.

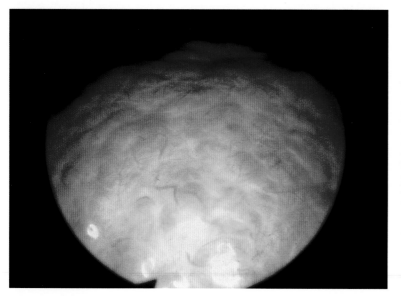

FIGURE 5-17.

Percutaneous liver biopsy with or without ultrasonic guidance is a standard diagnostic approach for establishing the presence of chronic hepatitis. Laparoscopic liver biopsy, which is used in large referral centers, has the advantage of minimizing the sample error by facilitating gross inspection of the liver and thus ensuring an adequate biopsy sample size. This figure depicts a laparoscopic view of a patient with chronic active hepatitis and early cirrhosis [25,26].

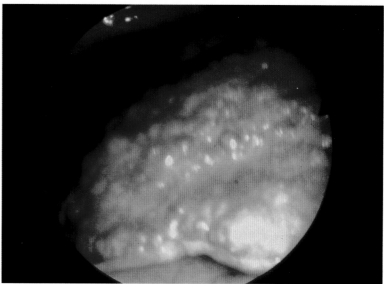

FIGURE 5-18.

The progression of chronic hepatitis C to advanced cirrhosis is associated with a significant risk for superimposed hepatocellular carcinoma. In this advanced cirrhotic patient, the numerous large nodules make it more difficult to exclude an occult carcinoma.

HEPATOCELLULAR CARCINOMA

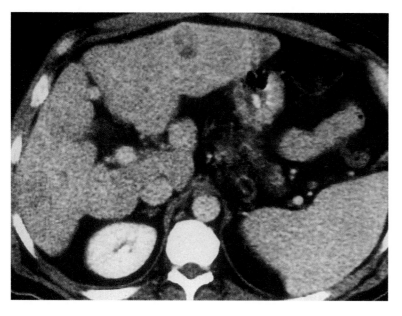

FIGURE 5-19.

Hepatocellular carcinoma. Computed tomographic scan showing a cirrhotic liver with splenomegaly. A hepatocellular carcinoma is noted in the left lobe and a second lesion is seen in the right lobe. Multicentric hepatocellular carcinoma are commonly seen in cirrhosis, secondary to hepatitis C virus.

Laparoscopy

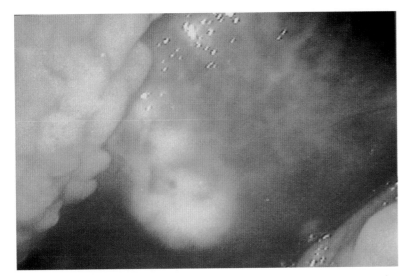

FIGURE 5-20.

Laparoscopic view of the liver revealing an hepatocellular carcinoma arising in a cirrhotic liver.

Histologic features

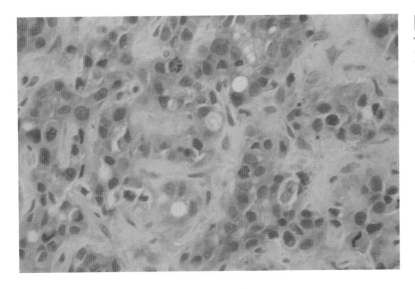

FIGURE 5-21.

The histologic documentation of a poorly differentiated hepatocellular carcinoma.

■ VASCULITIS AND CRYOGLOBULINEMIA

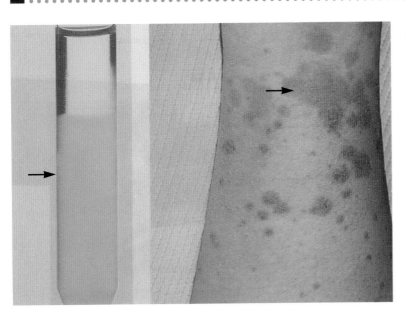

FIGURE 5-22.

Vasculitis and cryoglobulinemia related to hepatitis C virus. Mixed essential cryoglobulinemia has been associated with many chronic liver diseases. However, there appears to be an abnormally high prevalence of cryoglobulinemia in patients with hepatitis C. The figure on the **right** depicts an area of palpable purpura approximately 2 by 3 cm on the medial aspect of the lower extremity of a patient with hepatitis C (*arrow*). The photograph on the **left** shows uncentrifuged serum after 48 hours at 4°C with the *arrow* indicating cryoprecipitate [27–29].

MEMBRANOUS GLOMERULONEPHRITIS

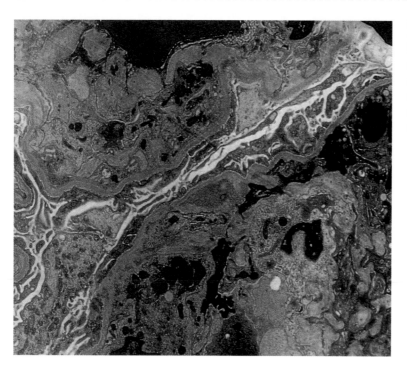

FIGURE 5-23.

Membranous glomerulonephritis is an extrahepatic manifestation associated with hepatitis C. This figure is a depiction of an electron micrograph of a nephron with swelling of the foot process, reduplication of the basement membrane, subendothelial deposits of cryoprecipitate, and infiltration of the interstitium by inflammatory cells [30].

PORPHYRIA CUTANEA TARDA

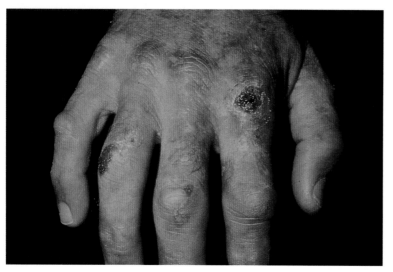

FIGURE 5-24.

Porphyria cutanea tarda. Fifty percent of cases of porphyria cutanea tarda in the United States are positive for antibodies to hepatitis C virus. Furthermore, many cases of chronic hepatitis C have histologic evidence of increased iron depositions in the liver. Preliminary studies suggest that iron overload impedes interferon therapy for chronic hepatitis [31–33].

HEPATITIS C VIRUS GENOME AND RECOMBINANT PROTEINS

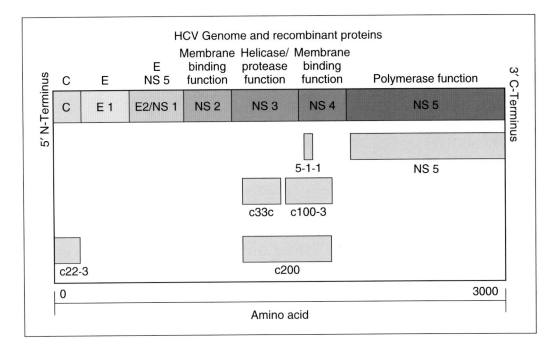

FIGURE 5-25.

Hepatitis C virus (HCV) genome and recombinant proteins. The HCV genome is approximately 3000 nucleotides in length. The HCV viral genome begins with a 5' N-terminus and contains two structural regions (core [C] and envelope [E]) and five nonstructural regions (NS 1 to 5), which extend to the 3' C-terminus. The 5' terminal region is relatively conserved and is the component used for the nested primers in polymerase chain reaction testing [34,35].

SEROLOGIC SEQUENCE

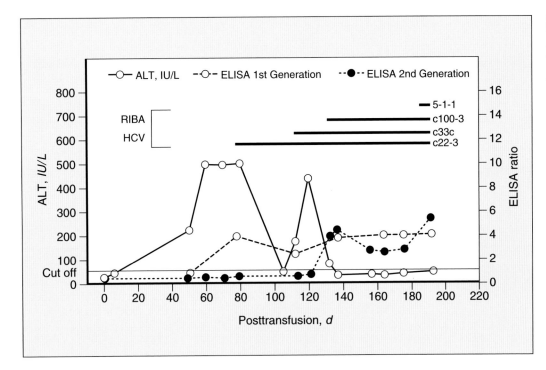

FIGURE 5-26.

Serologic sequence in recipient of hepatitis C virus (HCV)-RNA positive blood. Second generation enzyme-linked immunosorbent assay (ELISA) testing became available in 1992. This test detects the c100-3 antigen in combination with another protein from the NS 3 region, c33c (the composite antigen, c200), and the core c22-3 epitope, an HCV–nucleocapsid antigen. ELISA testing does not differentiate between acute and chronic infection nor does it indicate immunity or infectivity. The introduction of blood-donor screening of second-generation ELISA testing for HCV has resulted in the disappearance of posttransfusion HCV infection. Although second-generation ELISA testing is very sensitive, there remains a significant rate of false-positive results and therefore recombinant immunoblot assay (RIBA) testing should be considered to confirm "positivity" [36,37]. ALT—alanine aminotransferase.

RECOMBINANT IMMUNOBLOT ASSAY

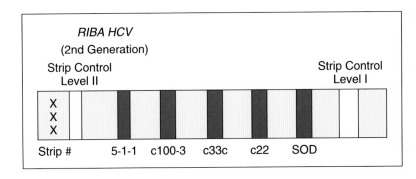

FIGURE 5-27.

Recombinant immunoblot assay (RIBA) 2.0 (Chiron Corp., Emeryville, CA). RIBA 2.0 is used as a supplemental assay for specificity for enzyme-linked immunosorbent assay–positive specimens. RIBA 2.0 testing is indicated in patients with no identifiable risk factors, in patients with normal alanine aminotransferase levels, in patients with suspected autoimmune disease, and in situations where the diagnosis is in doubt. RIBA 2.0 detects four epitopes: c100-3, 5-1-1, c33c, and c22-3. A positive result is indicated by reaction of two or more epitopes [36,38]. HCV—hepatitis C virus; SOD—human superoxide dismutase.

Frequency of immunoblot patterns in 1077 (R) sera										
Patterns	1	2	3	4	5	6	7	8	9	10
5-1-1	+	−	−	+	+	+	+	−	+	+
c100-3	+	−	+	−	+	−	+	+	+	−
c22-3	+	+	+	+	+	+	−	+	−	−
c33c	+	+	+	+	−	−	+	−	−	+
# (R)	685	195	92	75	14	7	5	2	1	1
(%)	63.6	18.1	8.5	6.9	1.3	.7	.5	.2	.1	.1

FIGURE 5-28.

Frequency of immunoblot patterns in 1077 (R) sera. The majority of recombinant immunosorbent assay–positive specimens will include reactions to c22-3 and c33c [39,40].

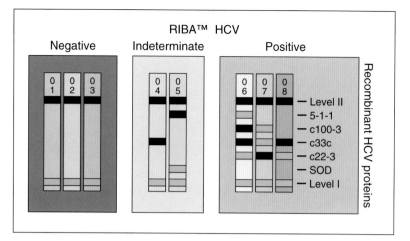

FIGURE 5-29.

Recombinant immunosorbent assay (RIBA) 2.0 (Chiron Corp., Emeryville, CA). An indeterminate result is the observation of only one positive band. Reactions to human superoxide dismutase (SOD), the substance bound to epitopes in the assay, is a false-positive one. Although most positive RIBA specimens are associated with viremia, up to 50% of RIBA–positive volunteer blood donors with normal alanine aminotransferase values will have no virus in the blood [41]. HCV—hepatitis C virus.

(R) single band	Visible band intensity, *positive (+) HCV-RNA, n /IND sera, n (%)*				
	4+	3+	2+	1+	Total
c33c	9/10 (90)	3/4 (75)	2/2 (100)	4/8 (50)	18/24 (75)
c22-3	11/16 (69)	1/4 (0)	1/5 (20)	1/8 (13)	13/33 (39)
c100-3	------	------	0/1 (0)	0/6 (0)	0/7 (0)
5-1-1	------	------	0/1 (0)	------	0/1 (0)
Total	20/26 (77)	3/8 (38)	3/9 (33)	5/22 (23)	31/65 (48)

FIGURE 5-30.

Correlation of hepatitis C virus (HCV)-RNA with single band characters in 65 indeterminate (IND) sera. Correlation of IND recombinant immunosorbent assay results with HCV-RNA activity would suggest that an IND result that involves c22-3 or c33c of 2+ or more is likely to reflect a truly positive enzyme-linked immunosorbent assay test. Conversely, a less than 2+ c100-3 band is unlikely to be associated with true positivity [39,42].

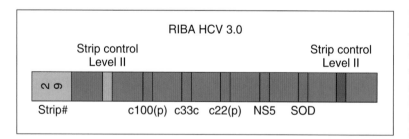

FIGURE 5-31.

Recombinant immunoblot assay (RIBA) 3.0 (Chiron Corp., Emeryville, CA). Further refinement and supplemental assay testing has led to development of a RIBA 3.0 assay with improved sensitivity and specificity. In this assay, the 5-1-1 epitope has been replaced with NS 5, and the c-100 and c-22 antigenic components are present as more sensitive peptides (p). The cost-effective superiority of RIBA 3.0 remains to be demonstrated [43–45]. HCV—hepatitis C virus.

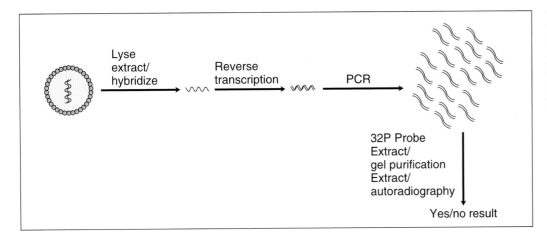

FIGURE 5-32.

Polymerase chain reaction (PCR) is an amplification technique used to detect hepatitis C virus (HCV)-RNA in both the serum and the liver. PCR is difficult to perform and contamination may occur leading to false-positive results. False-negative results may occur if there are important mismatches between the primers used in the PCR assay and the nucleotide sequences of the HCV genotype under study. This assay is tedious and difficult to perform [46,47]. (*From* Chiron Corp., Emeryville, CA; with permission.)

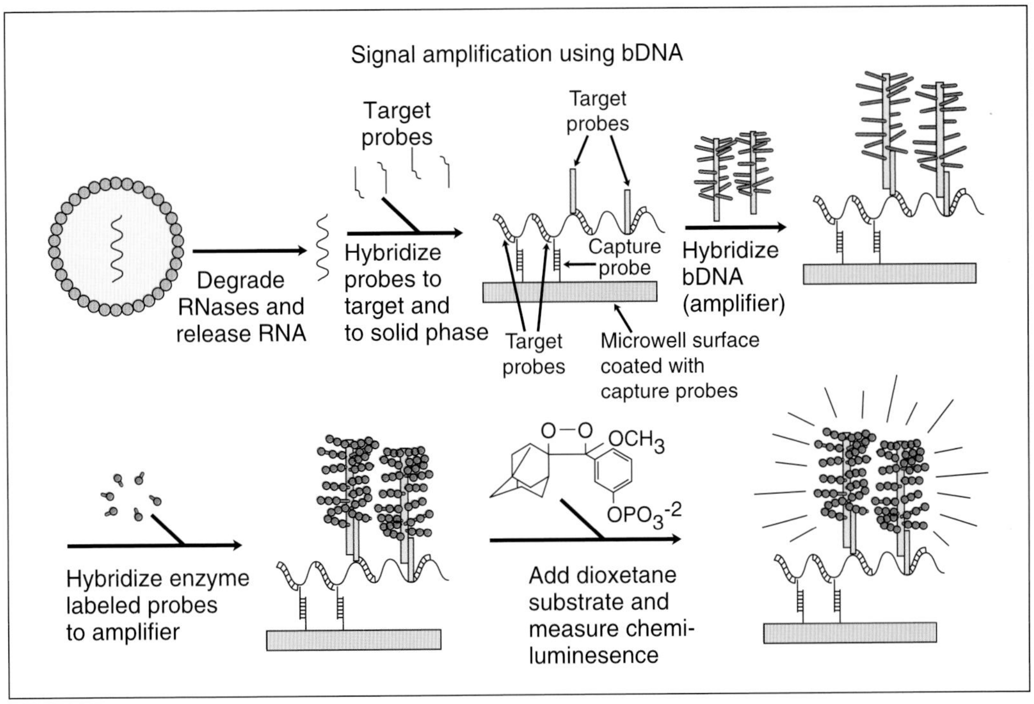

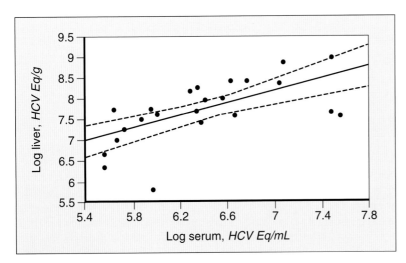

FIGURE 5-33.

Quantitative hepatitis C virus (HCV)-RNA. Quantitative HCV-RNA assays have been developed. The HCV-RNA signal amplification assay is a technique that increases detection signals of HCV-RNA, thereby permitting accurate quantitation of HCV-RNA. This test is technically easy to perform and is readily reproducible. It does, however, lack the sensitivity of polymerase chain reaction. Therefore, a negative branched DNA (bDNA) finding in the assay does not exclude lower concentrations of virus (< 3.5 × 10^5 Eq/mL) [48,49]. (*From* Chiron Corp., Emeryville, CA; with permission.)

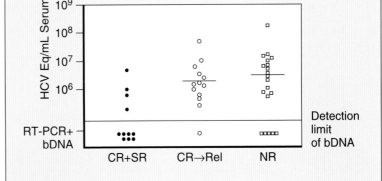

FIGURE 5-34.

Relationship of hepatitis C virus (HCV)-RNA in serum and liver tissue. HCV-RNA concentrations in the serum correlate with those in liver tissue. A negative serum HCV-RNA by polymerase chain reaction is indicative of undetectable HCV-RNA in the corresponding liver tissue in most cases [50]. (*From* Chiron Corp., Emeryville, CA; with permission.)

FIGURE 5-35.

Hepatitis C virus (HCV)-RNA level as a predictor of response to interferon. The most important predictor of response to interferon therapy in patients with chronic HCV is the serum HCV-RNA concentration. Lau *et al.* [51] have shown that patients with significantly lower levels of viremia will have a greater number of complete (CR) and sustained responses (SR) than those with high levels of viremia. bDNA—branched DNA; NR—no response; PCR—polymerase chain reaction; Rel—relapse; RT—reverse transcriptase. (*From* Lau *et al.* [51]; with permission.)

Complete and sustained response

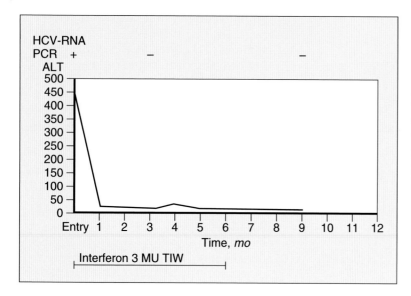

FIGURE 5-36.

Complete and sustained response. Interferon is currently the only approved therapy for chronic hepatitis C virus (HCV). Biochemical and virologic remission is achieved in 50% of patients while they are receiving interferon therapy at a dose of 3 MU three times a week (TIW) for 6 months. However, up to 80% of these patients will relapse with cessation of therapy. This figure reflects a patient with an early sustained biochemical and virologic response to interferon therapy. Prolonged remission for over 4 years only occurs in up to 15% of cases [52–55]. ALT—alanine aminotransferase; PCR—polymerase chain reaction.

Failure to respond

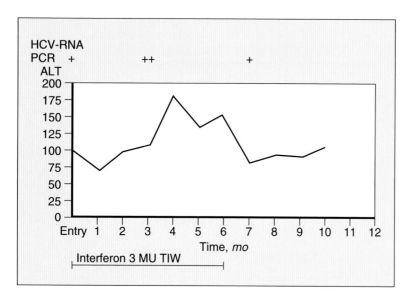

FIGURE 5-37.

Failure to respond. Failure to achieve a remission after 3 months of therapy is indicative of a need to either increase the interferon dosage or to stop therapy. Continuation of the same dose beyond 3 months is unlikely to achieve remission as demonstrated in this figure [56]. ALT—alanine aminotransferase; HCV—hepatitis C virus; PCR—polymerase chain reaction; TIW— three times a week.

Breakthrough

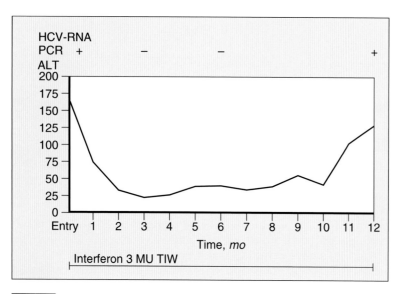

FIGURE 5-38.

Breakthrough. One explanation for the limited efficacy of interferon treatment is the changing nature of amino acid sequences within a given genotype of the virus. This phenomena is evident in a "breakthrough" during what initially appears to be successful therapy. The reappearance of viremia as interferon therapy has been associated with changes to a more resistant form of virus. In this patient, after 10 months of successful interferon therapy, in spite of continued treatment, viremia reappeared [57]. ALT—alanine aminotransferase; HCV—hepatitis C virus; PCR—polymerase chain reaction; TIW—three times a week.

Rebound

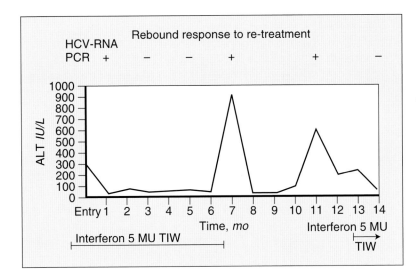

FIGURE 5-39.

Rebound. One common result of initially successful treatment is a relapse with a recurrence of viremia and alanine aminotransferase (ALT) elevation with cessation of therapy. As in this patient, the relapse is associated with higher ALT levels than baseline values. This situation is often referred to as a rebound. Fortunately, with reinstitution of interferon, a remission can once again be achieved in most cases. HCV—hepatitis C virus; PCR—polymerase chain reaction; TIW—three times a week.

Monitoring treatment

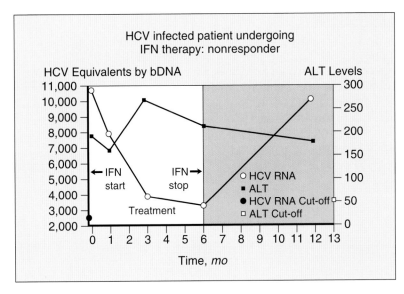

FIGURE 5-40.

Monitoring quantitative hepatitis C virus (HCV)-RNA during treatment. Monitoring therapy with quantitative HCV-RNA levels provides a more rational basis for adjustments in dose and duration of therapy. In this case, although alanine aminotransferase (ALT) levels had not decreased, indicating treatment failure, HCV-RNA levels were steadily decreasing and longer duration of therapy may have resulted in virologic and biochemical remission. bDNA—branched DNA; IFN—interferon.

Vasculitis

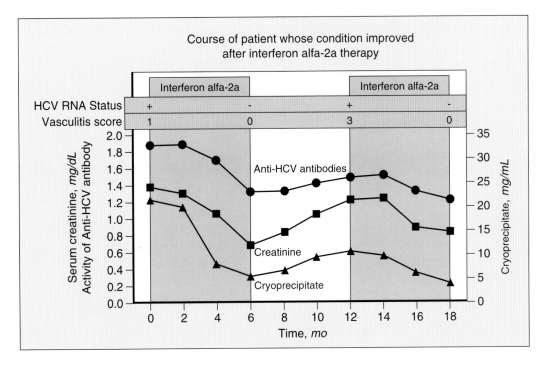

FIGURE 5-41.

Vasculitis improving with interferon therapy. Extrahepatic manifestations of hepatitis C virus (HCV) infection include cryoglobulinemia, membranous glomerulonephritis, porphyria cutanea tarda, and polyarteritis nodosa. Reduction in immune complex formation has been associated with improvement in symptoms. This patient illustrates the improvement of cryoglobulinemia with interferon therapy for HCV. The patient's vasculitis core improved as HCV-RNA levels decreased. After interferon was stopped, there was recurrence of HCV-RNA along with a worsening of the patient's vasculitis score. Anti-HCV—antibodies to HCV. (*From* Misiani *et al*. [58]; with permission.)

Side effects

TABLE 5-4. INTERFERON TREATMENT

EARLY VS LATE ADVERSE EFFECTS IN CHRONIC VIRAL HEPATITIS

EARLY (<4 WK)	LATE (>4 WK)
Fever	Malaise
Headache	Asthenia
Myalgias	Depression
Rigors	Irritability
Fatigue	Alopecia

TABLE 5-4.

Side effects of interferon. Short-term side effects of interferon are common and include fever, headache, myalgias, rigors, and fatigue. Long-term side effects, while on treatment, such as malaise, asthenia, depression, irritability, and alopecia, are less common [59].

Adverse laboratory changes

TABLE 5-5. INTERFERON ADVERSE LABORATORY EFFECTS

HEMATOLOGIC	IMMUNOLOGIC
Decreased granulocytes	Autoantibodies
Decreased platelets	Autoimmune thyroiditis
Decreased hemoglobin	Interferon antibodies

TABLE 5-5.

Adverse laboratory changes with interferon. Interferon has been associated with certain hematologic and immunologic side effects. Decreased levels of granulocytes, platelets, and hemoglobin commonly occur with interferon treatment and must be monitored. The development of autoimmune thyroiditis, autoantibodies, and interferon antibodies while on interferon therapy has been described. The majority of interferon side effects are reversible upon cessation of treatment [59].

Predictors of response

TABLE 5-6. PREDICTORS OF RESPONSE

Serum HCV-RNA levels
Genotype 1b
Hepatic iron concentration
Cirrhosis
Duration of illness
? Total dose of interferon

TABLE 5-6.

Predictors of response. Factors associated with a favorable response to interferon include the presence of a low serum hepatitis C virus (HCV)-RNA level, genotype other than 1b, normal hepatic iron concentration, the absence of cirrhosis, and a relatively short duration of chronic hepatitis. Treatment regimens with higher doses or longer durations of interferon therapy than the licensed regimen in the United States (3 MU three times a week for 6 months) have been associated with more favorable response rates [60–63].

Treatment

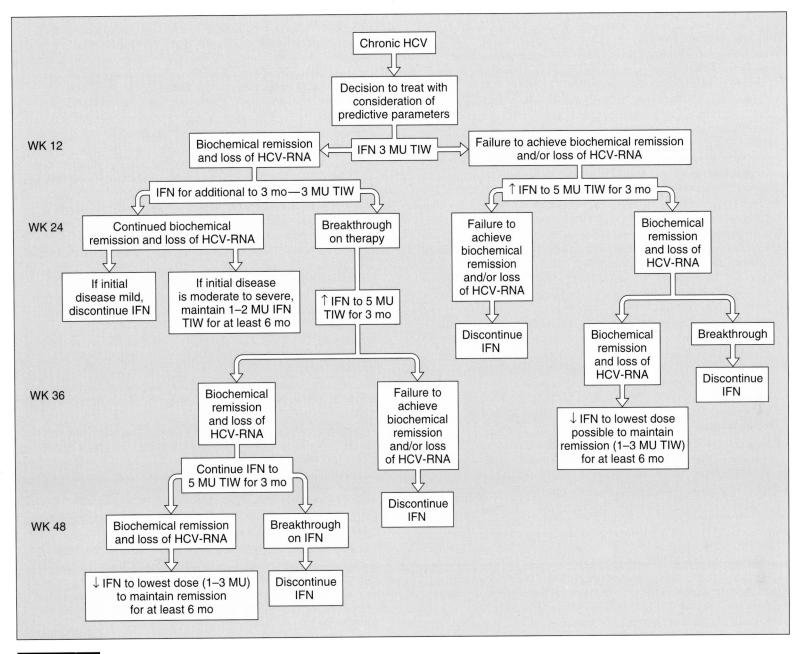

FIGURE 5-42.

A suggested algorithm for interferon (IFN) treatment of chronic hepatitis C virus (HCV) at the University of Miami. The experience with antiviral treatment for chronic HCV has been relatively limited. The ultimate goals for successful therapy are to 1) increase life expectancy, 2) improve the quality of life, 3) prevent the progression to cirrhosis and its complications, and 4) to prevent the development of hepatocellular carcinoma. Only long-term analysis will determine the success of IFN to achieve any or all of these goals. Therefore, short-term goals are to achieve biochemical, virologic, and histologic remission. Improved efficacy will depend on the development of newer antivirals as well as adjunctive agents for combination therapy with IFN. TIW—three times a week.

REFERENCES

1. *Hepatitis Surveillance Report #55*. Atlanta: Centers for Disease Control and Prevention; 1994:30–34.

2. Houghton M, Weiner AJ, Han J, *et al.*: Molecular biology of the hepatitis C viruses: Implications for diagnosis, development and control of viral disease. *Hepatology* 1991, 14:382–388.

3. Li XM, Shao LJ, de Medina M, *et al.*: Isolation and visualization of hepatitis C virion by buoyant gradient density ultra centrifugation and immunoelectron microscopy [Abstract]. *Gastroenterology* 1994, 106:A930.

4. Aach RD, Steven CE, Hollinger FB, *et al.*: Hepatitis C virus infection in post-transfusion hepatitis: An analysis of first and second generation assays. *N Engl J Med* 1991, 325:1325–1329.

5. Ohto H, Terazawa S, Sasiki N, *et al.*: Transmission of hepatitis C virus from mothers to infants. *N Engl J Med* 1994, 330:744–750.

6. Weinstock HS, Bolan G, Reingold AL, *et al.*: Hepatitis C virus infection among patients attending a clinic for sexually transmitted diseases. *JAMA* 1993, 269:392–394.

7. Alter MJ, Margolis HS, Krawezynskik K, *et al.*: The natural history of community acquired hepatitis C in the United States. *N Engl J Med* 1992, 27:1899–1905.

8. Stevens CE, Taylor PE, Pindyk J, *et al.*: Epidemiology of hepatitis C virus: A preliminary study of voluntary blood donors. *JAMA* 1990, 263:49–53.

9. Jeffers LJ, Perez GO, de Medina M, *et al.*: Hepatitis C in two urban hemodialysis units. *Kidney Int* 1990, 38:320–322.

10. Kijosawa K, Sodeyama T, Tanaka E, *et al.*: Hepatitis C in hospital employees with needle stick injuries. *Ann Intern Med* 1992, 115:367–369.

11. Mitsui T, Iwano K, Masuko K, *et al.*: Hepatitis C virus infection in medical personnel after needle stick accident. *Hepatology* 1992, 16:1109–1114.

12. Jeffers LJ, Hasan F, de Medina M, *et al.*: Prevalence of antibodies to hepatitis C virus among patients with cryptogenic chronic hepatitis and cirrhosis. *Hepatology* 1992, 15:187–190.

13. Merican I, Sherlock S, McIntyre N, *et al.*: Clinical, biochemical and histological features in 102 patients with chronic hepatitis C virus infection. *Q J Med* 1993, 86:119–125.

14. Puoti M, Zonaro A, Ravagg A, *et al.*: Hepatitis C virus RNA and antibody response in the clinical course of acute hepatitis C virus infection. *Hepatology* 1992, 16:877–881.

15. Resnick RH, Koff R: Hepatitis C related hepatocellular carcinoma. *Arch Intern Med* 1993, 17:S108–S111.

16. Kanazawa Y, Hayashi N, Mita E, *et al.*: Influence of viral quasispecies on effectiveness of interferon therapy in chronic hepatitis C patients. *Hepatology* 1994, 20:1121–1130.

17. McOmish F, Yap PL, Dow BC, *et al.*: Geographic distribution of hepatitis C virus genotypes in blood donors: An international collaborative study. *J Clin Microbiol* 1994, 32:884–892.

18. Simmonds D, Alberti A, Alter HJ, *et al.*: A proposed system for the nomenclature of hepatitis C viral genotypes. *Hepatology* 1994, 19:1321–1324.

19. Bartholomew M, Kuhns MC, Rusti V, *et al.*: Decline in HCV anti-core IgG level correlates with response to therapy [Abstract]. *Hepatology* 1994, 20:160A.

20. Tabone M, Galatola G, Secreto P, *et al.*: Serum levels of anti-hepatitis C virus IgM core antibodies may predict the response to interferon α therapy in chronic hepatitis C. *J Viral Hepatitis* 1994, 1:155–157.

21. Zaaijer HL, Mimms LT, Cuypers HTM, *et al.*: Variability of IgM response in hepatitis C virus infection. *J Med Virol* 1993, 40:184–187.

22. Alter HJ, Purcell RH, Shih JW, *et al.*: Detection of antibody to hepatitis C virus in prospectively followed transfusion recipients with acute and chronic non A, non B hepatitis. *N Engl J Med* 1989, 321:1494–1500.

23. Tremolada F, Casarin C, Tragger A, *et al.*: Antibody to hepatitis C virus in post-transfusion hepatitis. *Ann Intern Med* 1991, 114:277–281.

24. Hoofnagle J: Chronic hepatitis. In *Liver Biopsy Interpretation for the 1990's. AASLD Postgraduate Course Syllabus 1991.* Edited by Hoofnagle JH, Goodman Z. Thorofare: Slack Inc; 1991:124.

25. Phillips RS, Reddy KR, Jeffers LJ, *et al.*: Experience with diagnostic laparoscopy in a hepatology training program. *Gastrointest Endosc* 1987, 33:417–420.

26. Soloway RD, Baggenstoss AH, Schoenfield LJ, *et al.*: Observer error and sampling variability testing in evaluation of hepatitis. *Am J Dig Dis* 1971, 16:1082–1086.

27. Ferri C, Greco F, Longombardo G, *et al.*: Association between hepatitis C virus and mixed cryoglobulinemia. *Clin Exp Rheumatol* 1991, 9:621–624.

28. Lunel F, Musset L, Cacoub P, *et al.*: Cryoglobulinemia in chronic liver diseases: Role of hepatitis C virus and liver damage. *Gastroenterology* 1994, 106:1291–1300.

29. Shakil AO, DiBisceglie AM: Images in clinical medicine: vasculitis and cryoglobulinemia related to hepatitis C. *N Engl J Med* 1994, 331:1624.

30. Johnson RJ, Getch DR, Yamabe H, *et al.*: Membranous glomerulone-phritis associated with hepatitis C virus infection. *N Engl J Med* 1993, 328:465–470.

31. DeCastro M, Sanchez J, Herrera JF, *et al.*: Hepatitis C virus antibodies and liver disease in patients with porphyria cutanea tarda. *Hepatology* 1993, 17:551–557.

32. Fargion S, Piperno A, Cappellini MD, *et al.*: Hepatitis C virus and porphyria cutanea tarda: Evidence of a strong association. *Hepatology* 1992, 16:1322–1326.

33. Olynyk JK, Luxon BA, Jeffrey GP, *et al.*: Predicting phlebotomy requirements in the treatment of iron overload [Abstract]. *Hepatology* 1994, 20:A323.

34. Weiner AJ, Christopherson C, Hall JE: Sequence variation in hepatitis C viral isolates. *J Hepatol* 1991, 13:S6–S14.

35. Delisse AM, Descurieux M, Rutgers T, *et al.*: Sequence analysis of the putative structural genes of hepatitis C virus from Japanese and European origin. *J Hepatol* 1991, 13:S20–S23.

36. van der Poel CL, Cuyper HTM, Reesink HW, *et al.*: Confirmation of hepatitis C virus infection by a new four antigen recombinant immunoblot assay. *Lancet* 1991, 337:317–319.

37. van der Poel CL: Hepatitis C virus infection from blood and blood products. *FEMS Microbiol Rev* 1994, 14:241–246.

38. Prohaska W, Schroeter E, Kaars-Wiele P, *et al.*: Enzyme immuno-assays for anti-hepatitis C virus antibodies improved specificity and analytical sensitivity by combination of three different recombinant viral proteins in second generation tests. *Eur J Clin Chem Clin Biochem* 1992, 30:397–404.

39. Li XM, Reddy KR, Jeffers LJ, *et al.*: Indeterminate hepatitis [Letter]. *Lancet* 1993, 341:835.

40. Watson HG, Ludlam CA, Rebus S, *et al.*: Use of several second generation serological assays to determine the true prevalence of hepatitis C virus infection in hemophiliacs treated with non-virus inactivated factor VIII and IX concentrations. *Br J Hematol* 1992, 80:514–518.

41. Farci P, Alter HJ, Wong D, *et al.*: A long term study of hepatitis C replication in non-A, non-B hepatitis. *N Engl J Med* 1991, 325:98–104.

42. Lelie PN, Cuypers HTM, Reesink HE, *et al.*: Patterns of serological markers in transfusion transmitted hepatitis C virus infection using a second generation hepatitis C virus assay. *J Med Virol* 1992, 37:203–209.

43. Aiza I, de Medina M, Li XM, *et al.*: Evaluation of RIBA HCV 2.0 SIA indeterminate specimens by RIBA HCV 3.0 SIA and HCV-RNA by PCR [Abstract]. *Hepatology* 1994, 20:240A.

44. Chicheportiche C, Cantaloube JF, Biagini P, *et al.*: Analysis of ELISA hepatitis C virus positive blood donor population by PCR and RIBA: Comparison of second and third generation RIBA. *Acta Virol* 1993, 77:123–131.

45. Courouce AM, Le Marrec N, Girault A, *et al.*: Anti-hepatitis C virus (anti-HCV) seroconversion in patients undergoing hemodialysis: Comparison of second and third generation anti-HCV assays. *Transfusion* 1994, 34:790–795.

46. Okamoto H, Sugiyama Y, Okada S, *et al.*: Typing hepatitis C virus by PCR with type specific primer: Applications to clinical surveys and tracing infectious sources. *J Gen Virol* 1992, 73:673–679.

47. Zaaijer HL, Cuypers HTM, Reesink HW, *et al.*: Reliability of polymerase chain reaction for detection of hepatitis C virus. *Lancet* 1993, 341:722–724.

48. Davis GL, Lau JYN, Urdea MS, *et al.*: Quantitative detection of hepatitis C virus RNA with a solid phase signal amplification method: Definition of optimal conditions for specimens collection and clinical application in interferon treated patients. *Hepatology* 1994, 19:1337–1341.

49. Urdea MS: Branched DNA signal amplification. *Biotechnology* 1994, 12:926–927.

50. Jeffers LJ, Dailey PJ, Coehlo-Little E, *et al.*: Correlation of HCV-RNA quantitation in sera and liver tissue of patients with chronic hepatitis C [Abstract]. *Gastroenterology* 1993, 104:A923.

51. Lau JYN, Davis GC, Kniffen J, *et al.*: Significance of serum hepatitis C virus RNA levels in chronic hepatitis C. *Lancet* 1993, 341:1501–1504.

52. Hoofnagle JH, Mullen KD, Jones DB, *et al.*: Treatment of chronic non-A, non-B hepatitis with recombinant human α interferon: A preliminary report. *N Engl J Med* 1986, 315:1575–1578.

53. Davis GL, Balart LA, Schiff ER, *et al.*: Treatment of chronic hepatitis C with recombinant interferon alfa: A multicenter randomized controlled trial. *N Engl J Med* 1989, 321:1501–1506.

54. Lavergne J, Jeffers LJ, Reddy KR, *et al.*: Long-term follow-up of hepatitis C sustained responders to IFN-alfa 2B [Abstract]. *Hepatology* 1994, 20:169A.

55. Stoffa RJ, White H, Rice C, *et al.*: Long term followup of HCV RNA and ALT after α interferon therapy for chronic hepatitis C [Abstract]. *Hepatology* 1994, 20:169A.

56. Lindsay KL, Davis GL, Schiff ER, *et al.*: Long term response to higher doses of interferon alfa 2b treatment of patients with chronic hepatitis C [Abstract]. *Hepatology* 1993, 18:106A.

57. Finkelstein SD, Sayegh R, Uchman S, *et al.*: HCV undergoes extensive mutational change in NS5 region in association with relapse/breakthrough following α interferon therapy [Abstract]. *Hepatology* 1992, 16:132A.

58. Misiani R, Bellavita P, Fenili D, *et al.*: Interferon alfa 2a therapy in cryoglobulinemia associated with hepatitis C virus. *N Engl J Med* 1994, 330:751–756.

59. Renault PF, Hoofnagle JH: Side effects of α interferon. *Semin Liver Dis* 1989, 9:273–277.

60. Arber N, Moshkowitz M, Konikoff F, *et al.*: Iron overload in patients with chronic hepatitis C virus infection predicts a poor response to interferon therapy [Abstract]. *Gastroenterology* 1994, 106:A860.

61. Campbell C, Daley PJ, Urdea MS, *et al.*: HCV-RNA in peripheral blood mononuclear cells of chronic hepatitis C patients treated with interferon alfa 2b: Another possible indicator of response [Abstract]. *Gastroenterology* 1994, 106:A871.

62. Lam N, DeGuzman L, Pitrak D, *et al.*: Clinical and histologic predictors of response to α interferon in patients with chronic hepatitis C viral infection [Abstract]. *Gastroenterology* 1994, 106:A923.

63. Marcellin P, Castelnau C, Milotova V, *et al.*: Influence of the dose and of the duration of interferon treatment on the response to therapy according to hepatitis C virus genotype in chronic hepatitis C [Abstract]. *Hepatology* 1994, 20:A155.

Chapter 6

Drugs and the Liver

ANASTACIO HOYUMPA
STEVEN SCHENKER

Strategically located between the splanchnic and systemic circulations and equipped with a vast array of enzymes, the liver functions as a major organ of drug metabolism. Drugs presented to the liver may follow one of several possible fates. First, an inactive agent or prodrug may be biodegraded into its pharmacologically active form. Second, an already active drug may be rendered into inactive metabolites and eliminated from the body. Third, the biotransformation of a pharmalogic agent may lead to the formation of products that cause damage to the liver or other organs. Finally, drug metabolism may lead to carcinogenesis.

This chapter focuses on the effect of liver disease on the elimination of drugs and the possible mechanisms by which drugs may cause hepatocellular damage. The chapter is not meant to be an exhaustive review, rather specific drugs will be used to illustrate and stress key points. With the present tendency to use multiple drugs in the management of patients, drug-drug interactions are also discussed. In addition, because of the rising trend among patients to try alternate or nonconventional methods of treatment, hepatotoxicity associated with the use of folk medicine is discussed at some length, with emphasis on possible pathogenesis.

A better understanding of the key role of the liver in drug metabolism should lead to a more rational drug prescribing practice, especially in patients with liver disease, and a keener insight into the pathogenesis of hepatic injury may aid in devising strategies to prevent, minimize, and manage drug hepatotoxicity.

CENTRAL ROLE OF THE LIVER IN DRUG METABOLISM

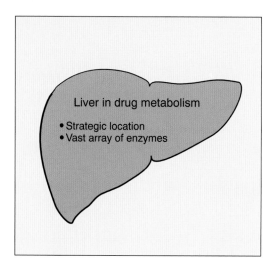

Liver in drug metabolism

- Strategic location
- Vast array of enzymes

FIGURE 6-1.

Central role of liver in drug metabolism. The liver plays a vital role in drug metabolism by virtue of its location between the splanchnic and the systemic circulations, and because it possesses a vast array of enzymes that are capable of transforming drugs into pharmacologically active compounds or of degrading them for subsequent elimination.

Entry of drugs into the hepatocyte

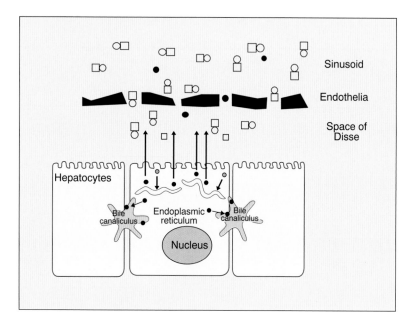

FIGURE 6-2.

Entry of drugs into the hepatocyte. Most drugs are fat soluble or lipophilic to a variable extent. Fat solubility is important because in order to reach the systemic circulation, an orally administered drug must generally diffuse across the lipid membrane of the enterocyte. A drug with little or no lipophilic property is poorly absorbed and is excreted in the stool. In contrast, a drug that is absorbed is then bound to protein, usually albumin, and distributes itself to various tissues, including fat. Unless rendered more polar or water soluble, such drugs tend to accumulate in the body over a prolonged period and may affect cellular processes. Whether given orally or parenterally, drugs eventually pass through the liver. The degree of hepatic drug extraction depends on hepatic blood flow and the activity of the drug-metabolizing enzymes. In the hepatic sinusoids the drugs (*open circles*) bound to protein (*open squares*) pass through openings (fenestrae) in the endothelium and gain access to the space of Disse, from which they enter the hepatocytes, where enzymes convert them into more polar compounds (*solid circles*). Some of these water-soluble molecules pass back to the sinusoids, whereas others enter the biliary canaliculi. (*From* Watkins [1]; with permission.)

Principal reactions in drug metabolism

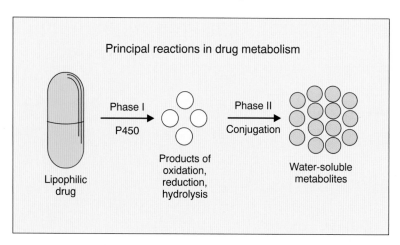

Principal reactions in drug metabolism

Lipophilic drug → Phase I P450 → Products of oxidation, reduction, hydrolysis → Phase II Conjugation → Water-soluble metabolites

FIGURE 6-3.

Principal reactions in drug metabolism. The chemical reactions involved in the biotransformation of drugs fall into two principal pathways generally referred to as phase I and phase II. Phase I reactions consist of oxidative and reductive processes that create functional chemical groups (eg, OH, COOH, NH_2, SH_2) as well as hydrolytic reactions that cleave esters and amides to uncover functional groups. In phase II, products of oxidation, reduction, and hydrolysis are coupled with endogenous substrates such as glycine, ascetic acid, and sulfuric acid. These processes that render lipophilic compounds progressively more polar may occur sequentially or concomitantly. The more polar metabolites are subsequently excreted in bile if the molecules are relatively large (> 0.4 nm) or in urine if relatively small (< 0.2 nm).

Electron flow pathway in the microsomal drug-oxidizing system

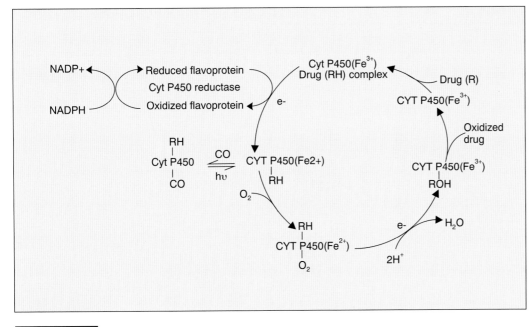

The reactions require the presence of NADPH (nicotinamide adenine dinucleotide phosphate [reduced form]) and O_2. As shown in the schematic, NADPH is oxidized by the flavoprotein NADPH–cytochrome P450 reductase to form NADP+ (nicotinamide adenine dinucleotide phosphate [oxidized form]). In the process an electron is transferred to the oxidized form of cytochrome P450 to produce a P450 drug complex. This complex undergoes a one-electron reduction. Molecular oxygen then binds to give a reduced (Fe^{2+}) cytochrome P450-dioxygen complex. Subsequently, a second electron from cytochrome P450 reductase or from NADH, through cytochrome b_5, is added to the complex. There is subsequent cleavage of the oxygen-oxygen bond along with the incorporation of an oxygen atom into a molecule of water, the transfer of the second atom to the substrate, and finally the dissociation of the oxidized product. (*From* Alvares and Pratt [2]; with permission.)

FIGURE 6-4.

Electron flow pathway in the microsomal drug-oxidizing system. Phase I reactions are catalyzed by a family of closely related hemoproteins designated as cytochromes P450.

Sequential four-electron reduction of dioxygen

$$O_2 \xrightarrow{e-} O_2^- \xrightarrow{e-} H_2O_2 \xrightarrow{e-} \cdot OH \xrightarrow{e-} H_2O$$

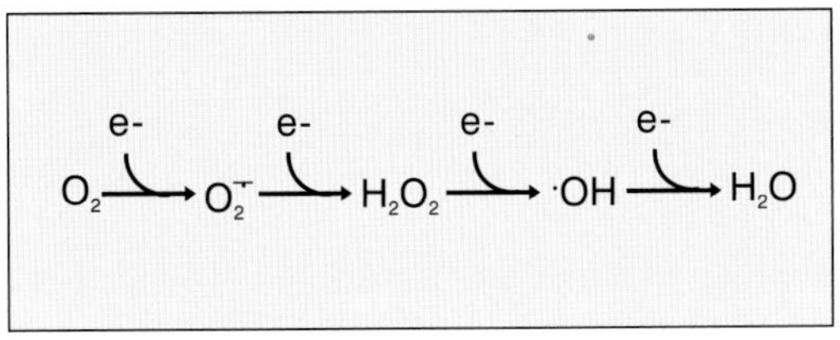

FIGURE 6-5.

Sequential four-electron reduction of dioxygen. In the process of drug metabolism, the insertion of an oxygen atom can lead to the formation of a more reactive molecule that can be toxic or carcinogenic. With the regeneration of ferric hemoprotein P450 (Fe^{3+}) RH, oxycytochrome P450 can dissociate to give superoxide, O_2^-. After superoxide has been formed, it can be reduced further to hydrogen peroxide (H_2O_2) and reactive hydroxyl radical (.OH). These three reactive oxyradicals may stimulate lipid peroxidation that can lead to the disruption of the lipid cell membrane. Therefore, these radicals are individually and collectively toxic to mammalian cells. Arrayed against these toxic oxyradicals are such protective factors as superoxide dismutase, catalase, and glutathione peroxidase. When these natural defenses are overwhelmed, toxic levels of various oxyradicals accumulate and cause tissue damage.

Catalytic specificity of P450s

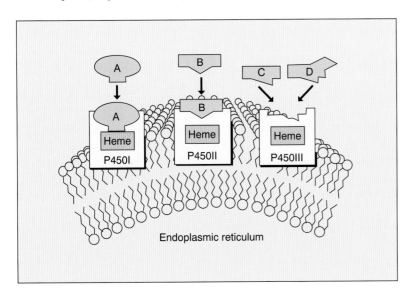

FIGURE 6-6.

Catalytic specificity of P450s. Each human P450 isoenzyme appears to be expressed by a particular gene. The *P450* genes, however, are distributed among different chromosomes. One P450 isoenzyme may be involved in the metabolism of one or more drugs and a single drug may be acted upon by multiple enzymes. Many drugs, however, are largely metabolized by a single form of P450. These findings may be explained by the observation that relative binding affinities for specific drugs vary among the different P450s. Drugs must bind to the P450 at the substrate binding site which is located close to the enzyme's heme prosthetic group. The binding affinity between certain drugs and P450 may vary so that a single P450 may be largely responsible for the metabolism of some drugs. As illustrated in the figure, drug A and drug B are metabolized individually by P450I and P450II, respectively. These drugs will not bind with the other P450s. But each P450 can metabolize more than one drug as shown by the ability of a single P450III to bind drugs C and D. (*From* Watkins [1]; with permission).

TABLE 6-1. SOME DRUGS THAT APPEAR TO BE SUBSTRATES FOR SPECIFIC CYTOCHROMES P450

IA2

Phenacetin[*]

Caffeine

Theophylline

Acetaminophen

IID[†]

Debrisoquin

Bufuralol

Dextromethorphan

Metoprolol and other β blockers

Perhexiline

Amitriptyline and other neuroleptics

Encainide

Codeine

IIC[†]

Mephenytoin

Hexobarbital

Diazepam

Tolbutamide

Sulfinpyrazole

Phenylbutazole

Sulfaphenazole

Oxyphenazole

IIEII

Acetaminophen

Ethanol

Isoniazid

IIIA

Erythromycin

Triacetyloleandomycin

Nifedipine

Cyclosporine

Steroids

Ketoconazole

Estrogens

Midazolam

Triazolam

Lidocaine

---

[*]This drug has been withdrawn from the market in the United States.

[†]Multiple subfamily members exist that may have differing catalytic properties.

TABLE 6-1.

Individual P450s and other drug substrates. (From Watkins [1]; with permission).

Formation of ether glucuronide

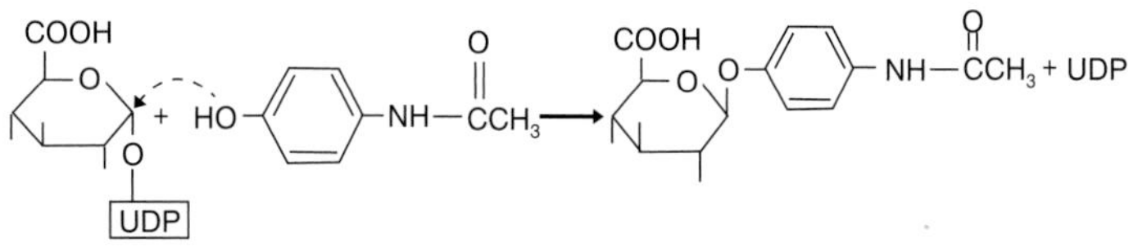

UDPGA   p-Hydroxyacetanilid   p-Hydroxyacetanilid glucuronide

FIGURE 6-7.

Formation of ether glucuronide. As previously mentioned, phase II of drug metabolism involves conjugation reactions. Shown here is one example involving the coupling of glucuronic acid with the *hydroxyl* group of a compound. The result of such conjugation is termed *ether glucuronide*. Glucuronic acid is derived from uridine diphosphate glucuronic acid (UDPGA); its synthesis is catalyzed by enzymes found in the soluble fraction of the liver, and the transfer of glucuronic acid to various acceptors is mediated by transferases that are found in the hepatic microsomes [2]. Other examples of drugs that undergo ether glucuronidation include acetaminophen, carprofen, ciramadol, dezocine, lorazepam, oxazepam, temazepam, and morphine [3].

Formation of ester glucuronide

UDPGA + Benzoic acid → Benzoyl glucuronide + UDP

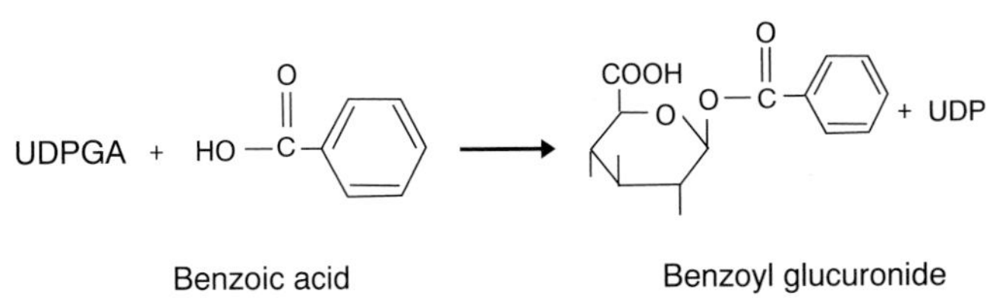

FIGURE 6-8.

Formation of ester glucuronide. This figure illustrates the conjugation of benzoic acid through the carboxylic group. This type of reaction results in the formation of ester glucuronide. A similar

reaction is involved in the metabolism of ketoprofen and zomepirac. In general, the glucuronide metabolites are polar substances and thus pharmacologically inactive. On the other hand, certain conjugates of N-hydroxyarylamines can induce the formation of tumors in the urinary bladder (*see* Fig. 6-9).

Other conjugation reactions involve endogenous amines (glycine, glutamine, ornithine), reactions with endogenous acids (acetylation, sulfation), and conjugation with glutathione. Methylation, although a relatively minor pathway, is unique, because it may lead to the generation of a compound with greater activity. One such example is the conversion of methyldopa to methylnorepinephrine.

The efficiency of drug metabolism, however, whether by the oxidative or conjugative pathway, varies from individual to individual partly because of polymorphism. UDPGA—uridine diphosphate glucuronic acid. (*From* Alvares and Pratt [2]; with permission.)

Genetic polymorphism

TABLE 6-2. GENETIC POLYMORPHISM OF CYTOCHROME P450 AND ACETYLATION

ENZYME	P450IID6	P450IIC	N-ACETYLTRANSFERASEE (NAT)
Designation	Debrisoquine/sparteine polymorphism	Mephenytoin polymorphism	Acetylation (INH) polymorphism
(Other drugs involved)	Antidepressants	Mephobarbital	Hydralazine
	Antiarrhythmics	Hexobarbital	Phenelzine
	β blockers	Omeprazole	Procainamide
	Codeine, neuroleptics		Dapsone
			Sulfamethazine
			Sulfapyride
Poor metabolism (incidence)			
Japanese	5%–10%	18%–23%	40%–70%
Chinese	0%–2%	15%–20%	10%–20%
Whites	10%–15%	2%–5%	

TABLE 6-2.

Genetic polymorphism of cytochrome P450 and acetylation [4,5]. Genetic deficiency of a drug-metabolizing enzyme leads to the division of individuals into poor or efficient metabolizers. Such a polymorphism in P450 activity was first noted with debrisoquine, an antihypertensive drug. In the white population, 5% to 10% of individuals fail to hydroxylate this drug efficiently and are at greater risk from its accumulation and its more profound hypotensive effect. The difficulty has been traced to the absence of an amino acid of P450IID protein that results in defective RNA splicing. The defect that involves not only the metabolism of debrisoquine but also of sparteine and other drugs as shown here is inherited as a recessive gene in poor metabolizers but as a homozygous or heterozygous dominant gene in efficient metabolizers. In addition to being at risk from hypotension, individuals who are debrisoquine-poor metabolizers may develop Parkinson's disease early, whereas rapid metabolizers may be more likely to develop cancer of the lung and bladder [6]. Those with two or more functional P450IID6 alleles are at

greater risk of developing primary liver cancer [7].

Other forms of polymorphism involve P450IIC (mephenytoin). Defective metabolism of mephenytoin results in increased sedation. Present as an autosomal recessive trait, this defect affects the hydroxylation of S-mephenytoin but not the methylation of R-mephenytoin.

Polymorphism also affects drug degradation by conjugation. The classic example is the difference in the acetylation of isoniazid. Isoniazid acetylation is controlled by two alleles at a single autosomal gene locus. Slow acetylating patients are homozygous for a recessive allele. Other drugs that are similarly affected are shown in this table. Peripheral neuropathy is associated with the slow acetylation of isoniazid, whereas lupus erythematosus may result from the slow acetylation of hydralazine and procainamide. Patients who are slow acetylators are also at greater risk for cancer of the urinary bladder, whereas fast acetylation may be associated with breast cancer. (*From* Meyer [4]; with permission.)

Consequences of drug biotransformation and modifying factors

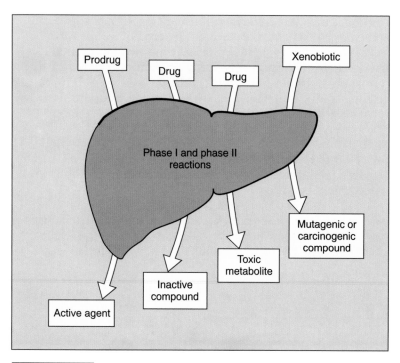

(Librium®; Hoffmann-LaRoche, Nutley, NJ) is oxidized into desmethylchlordiazepoxide, demoxepam, and oxazepam. These metabolites are themselves pharmacologically active. Oxazepam, a commercially available compound (Serax®; Wyeth-Ayerst Laboratories, Philadelphia, PA), is then conjugated with glucuronic acid to form an inactive ether glucuronide that is excreted in the urine. Like oxazepam, lorazepam (Ativan®; Wyeth-Ayerst Laboratories) does not undergo a preliminary oxidation but is directly inactivated by glucuronidation to another ether glucuronide (*see* Fig. 6-13).

3. Another important outcome of drug biotransformation is the generation of toxic metabolites as exemplified by hepatotoxicity caused by acetaminophen or isoniazid. Drug-induced liver injury is the main focus of discussion in Figures 6-21 to 6-32.

4. Oxidation of nitrosamines by cytochrome P450 plays an important role in carcinogenesis. Evidence suggests that P450IIE1, the enzyme that is involved in the metabolism of ethanol, is the most important enzyme in the activation of nitrosamines in human liver microsomes [8]. As mentioned earlier, conjugation reactions may also generate carcinogens (*see* Fig. 6-8).

Because the liver plays a vital role in drug elimination, the first two outcomes are relevant in appreciating the potential risks involved, and precautions are needed in prescribing drugs to patients with significant liver disease of various causes. If possible, an alternate and safer drug should be chosen; if the same drug is used, its dose and dosing interval should be adjusted. On the other hand, the last two outcomes are important in understanding drug-induced liver injury, as well as in providing a basis for possible carcinogenesis.

These outcomes of drug biotransformation, however, may be modified by several factors. These factors include genetic characteristics, age, gender, environmental condition, diet, and nutritional state. Another important factor is the concomitant use of another drug.

FIGURE 6-9.

Consequences of drug biotransformation. The hepatic metabolism of a pharmacologic compound may have four possible outcomes.

1. Drugs that are administered in their inactive forms are subsequently transformed into active compounds by the liver. Examples of such prodrugs include cortisone that is transformed into its active moiety cortisol, prednisone to prednisolone, and azathioprine to 6-mercaptopurine.

2. Other pharmacologic preparations, already active in their original forms, are degraded in the liver into active or inactive metabolites. For example, the benzodiazepine chlordiazepoxide

Drug-drug interactions

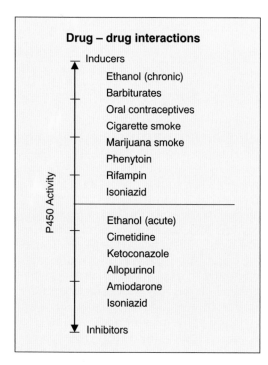

FIGURE 6-10.

Drug-drug interactions. Administration of one drug may influence the metabolism and elimination of another, depending on whether the drug-metabolizing enzyme system is induced or inhibited. This figure gives a list of certain drugs that enhance or depress the activity of P450 isozymes. Figures 6-11 and 6-12 illustrate examples of drug-drug interactions that may have clinical importance [5]. One example involves oxidation, the other conjugation.

Cyclosporine

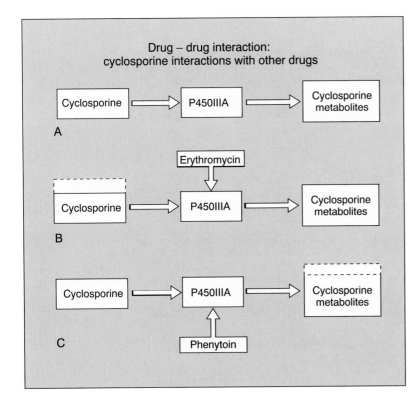

Drug – drug interaction:
cyclosporine interactions with other drugs

FIGURE 6-11.

Drug-drug interaction: inhibition of cyclosporine metabolism by erythromycin. The advent of cyclosporine, an important immunosuppressant, has revolutionized the management of rejection in organ transplantation. It has also been useful in the treatment of other conditions with altered immunity. Cyclosporine is degraded by hydroxylation and demethylation mediated by P450IIIA as shown in **panel A**. This same P450 isoenzyme also catalyzes the demethylation of erythromycin (**Panel B**). Erythromycin competes with cyclosporine for binding with P450IIIA and reduces the oxidative degradation of the latter. With erythromycin coadministration, the concentration of cyclosporine is increased (as represented by the *broken line*) leading to a greater risk of nephrotoxicity and other adverse effects. Unwanted cyclosporine interactions have also been observed with ketoconazole, oral contraceptives, androgens, and calcium channel blockers. Of the calcium channel blockers, diltiazem is a more potent inhibitor than nicardipine and verapamil; nifedipine, however, is noninhibitory. By contrast, as shown in **panel C,** coadministration of phenytoin, which induces P450IIIA, accelerates the elimination of cyclosporine, represented in the panel as the generation of a greater amount of cyclosporine metabolites. In addition to phenytoin, other drugs such as phenobarbital, rifampicin, carbamazepine, valproate, phenylbutazone, and sulfinpyrazone have the actual or potential ability to induce P450IIIA activity and thereby to decrease the overall effectiveness of cyclosporine.

Zidovudine

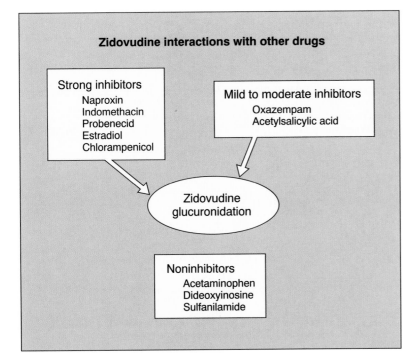

Zidovudine interactions with other drugs

FIGURE 6-12.

Interactions of zidovudine with other drugs. As with P450–mediated oxidative drug metabolism, interactions also occur among pharmacologic agents that undergo conjugative degradation. This phenomenon is exemplified by the interaction of zidovudine, a useful agent in the management of HIV infection, with other agents.

Zidovudine prevents viral replication by inhibiting HIV viral DNA–dependent polymerase (reverse transcriptase). The drug is degraded by conjugation with glucuronic acid to form an inactive ether glucuronide. The major metabolite of zidovudine, 3'azido-3' deoxy-5' O-β-D-glucupyranurosylthymidine, does not inhibit HIV replication. As indicated in this figure, several drugs that also undergo glucuronidation have been shown in vitro to inhibit the degradation of zidovudine [9]. Naproxen, indomethacin, probenecid, estradiol, and chloramphenicol are strong inhibitors, whereas oxazepam and aspirin are weaker inhibitors. Thus, the coadministration of any of these drugs has the potential of increasing zidovudine's side effects, the most frequently seen being granulocytopenia and anemia. However, the clinical significance of the in vitro interaction is still uncertain. It is also relevant to point out that dideoxyinosine, another anti-HIV agent, does not affect zidovudine's metabolism.

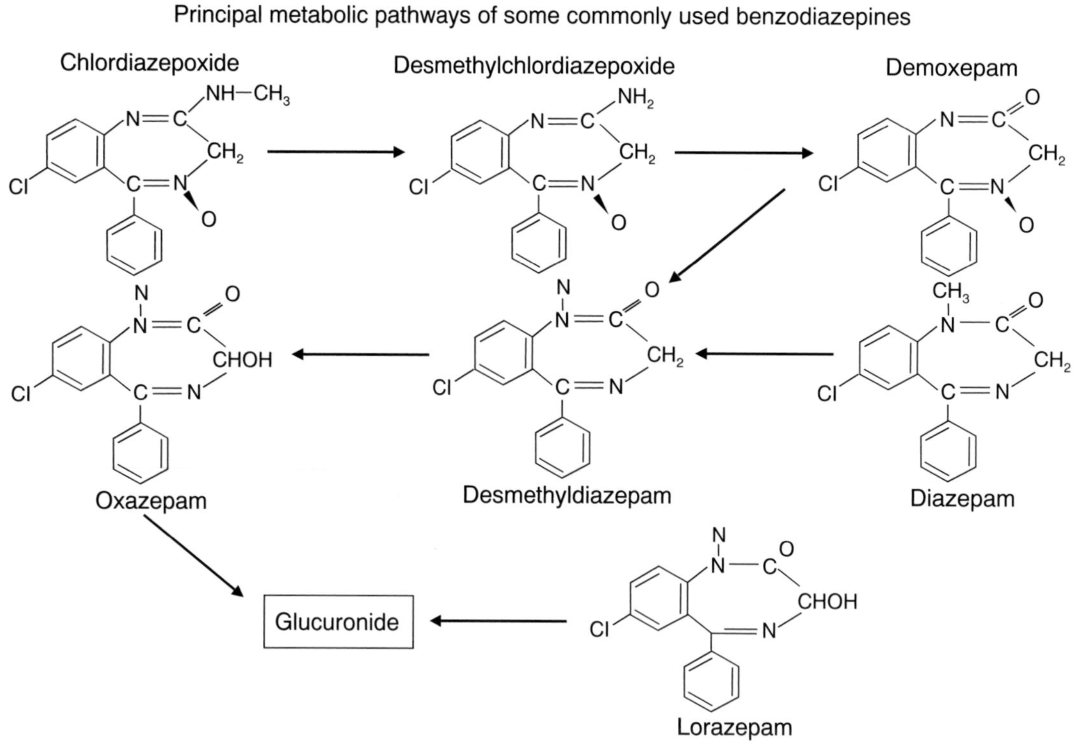

Principal metabolic pathways of some commonly used benzodiazepines

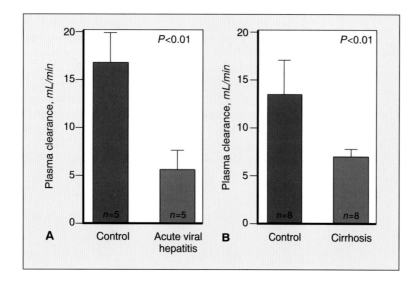

FIGURE 6-13.

Principal metabolic pathways of some commonly used benzodiazepines. Because the liver plays an essential role in the metabolism of drugs, it is not surprising that in the presence of significant liver disease, drug elimination is impaired [5]. This impairment is illustrated using some of the commonly used benzodiazapines. Often used as sedatives or tranquilizers, benzodiazepines undergo Phase I and Phase II hepatic biotransformation as shown. Chlordiazepoxide (Librium®; Hoffmann-LaRoche, Nutley, NJ) is demethylated to desmethylchlordiazepoxide, which is in turn hydroxylated to

demoxepam. Demoxepam is converted to desmethyldiazepam, which is also the principal oxidative metabolite of diazepam (Valium®; Roche Products, Manati, Puerto Rico). Desmethyl diazepam is hydroxylated to form oxazepam (Serax®; Wyeth-Ayerst Laboratories, Philadelphia, PA). These compounds are pharmacologically active. Oxazepam and lorazepam (Ativan®; Wyeth-Ayerst Laboratories) undergo conjugation with glucuronic acid to form inactive ether glucuronides that are excreted in the urine. (*From* Hoyumpa and Schenker [5]; with permission.)

FIGURE 6-14.

Effect of liver disease on the elimination of chlordiazepoxide. As shown here, the clearance of chlordiazepoxide is reduced in patients with acute viral hepatitis (**A**) and in patients with cirrhosis (**B**). In patients with liver disease, the corresponding elimination half-life of chlordiazepoxide is prolonged. Impairment of chlordiazepoxide clearance in patients with liver disease may account for the precipitation of hepatic encephalopathy when this drug is given to patients with liver disease. (*Data from* Roberts *et al.* [10]; with permission.)

Diazepam clearance

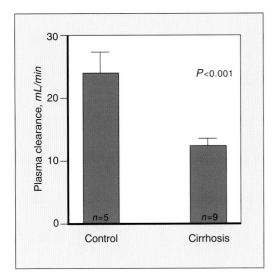

FIGURE 6-15.

Effect of cirrhosis on the plasma clearance of diazepam. As in the case of chlordiazepoxide (Librium®; Hoffmann-LaRoche, Nutley, NJ), the biotransformation of diazepam (Valium®; Hoffmann-LaRoche), another benzodiazepine that undergoes hepatic degradation by oxidation, is also impaired in patients with liver disease [11–14]. As depicted here, the plasma clearance of diazepam is greatly reduced (50%) in patients with stable alcoholic cirrhosis as compared with age-matched controls. Although not shown here, the elimination of diazepam is also impaired in patients with acute viral hepatitis. In patients with this disorder, the elimination half-life is prolonged more than twofold [9–11]. (*Data from* Klotz *et al.* [11]; with permission.)

Oxazepam metabolism

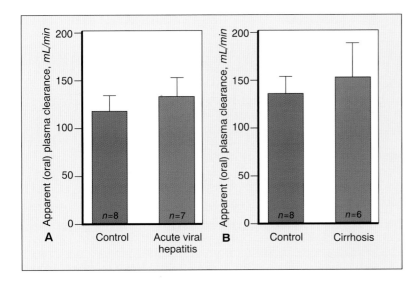

FIGURE 6-16.

Effect of liver disease on oxazepam metabolism. In contrast, the biotransformation of oxazepam (Serax®; Wyeth-Ayerst Laboratories, Philadelphia, PA) is not adversely affected in patients with liver disease [15]. As depicted here, the apparent clearance of orally administered oxazepam does not differ significantly between age-matched controls and patients with acute viral hepatitis (**A**) and between age-matched controls and patients with stable alcoholic cirrhosis (**B**). (*Data from* Shull *et al.* [15]; with permission.)

Lorazepam metabolism

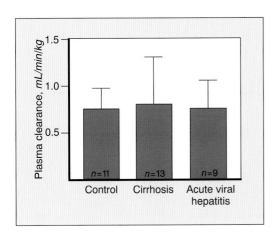

FIGURE 6-17.

Elimination of lorazepam in patients with liver disease. Lorazepam, like oxazepam, undergoes conjugation with glucuronic acid to form an ether glucuronide. As shown here in this figure, its clearance is likewise not affected in patients with compensated alcoholic cirrhosis or in patients with acute viral hepatitis [16].

These studies with benzodiazepines, as well as with other classes of drugs not illustrated here, suggest that in patients with liver disease the oxidation of drugs is generally impaired whereas glucuronidation is relatively spared [5]. This relative preservation of glucuronidation, however, may be lost when the liver disease is severe, as shown in Figure 6-18.

Drug metabolism in severe liver disease

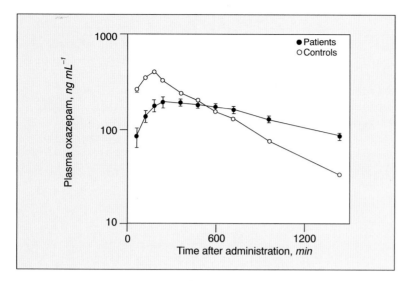

FIGURE 6-18.

Plasma concentration versus time curves of oxazepam in controls and patients with severe liver disease. Unlike the observations in Figure 6-17, elimination of oxazepam is significantly reduced in the patient whose severely decompensated alcoholic liver disease is associated with portal systemic encephalopathy. Similar impairment of glucuronidation in patients with severe alcoholic liver disease has been shown with morphine as well as with acetaminophen and zomepirac. (*From* Sonne *et al.* [17]; with permission.)

Mechanisms of impaired drug metabolism

Primary factors

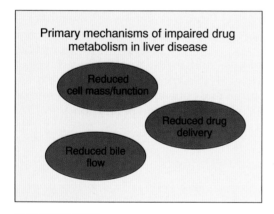

FIGURE 6-19.

Primary mechanisms of impaired drug metabolism. In patients with acute or chronic liver disease, the activities of the drug-metabolizing enzymes may be reduced in a variable and sometimes selective manner. Several factors may bring about this reduction and consequent impairment of drug

metabolism. These factors can be divided into primary and secondary. Of the primary factors, the first important consideration involves reduced parenchymal cell mass and function. The individual hepatocytes may possess a diminished complement of enzymes (sick-cell hypothesis). Alternatively, the hepatocytes, although intact, may be functionally impaired because of poor perfusion (intact hepatocyte hypothesis). Second, drug delivery to the hepatocytes may be reduced as a result of several possibilities. Blood flow to the intact hepatocytes may be decreased because of the formation of collaterals and attendant extrahepatic portacaval shunting. Apart from the obvious extrahepatic shunts, less noticeable intrahepatic shunts, which divert blood from otherwise intact hepatocytes, have also been observed. These intrahepatic shunts have been associated with reduced intrinsic drug clearance. Furthermore, in patients with chronic liver disease, reduced sinusoidal blood flow may curtail delivery of drugs to the hepatocytes (*see* Fig. 6-2).

Moreover, in cirrhosis, sinusoidal capillarization with distortion, diminution, or obliteration of the sinusoidal fenestrae may occur to further impede the diffusion of drugs from the sinusoids to the hepatocytes. Highly protein-bound drugs and those of relatively large molecules are particularly affected. Capillarization may also impair oxygen delivery, and the resulting hypoxia depresses drug metabolism. The oxidative system appears more vulnerable to hypoxia than the conjugative enzymes. The third important factor is the reduction of bile flow, either from intrahepatic inflammation or extrahepatic obstruction. This mechanism applies to those drugs that are primarily excreted in bile without undergoing biochemical changes. Examples of such drugs are nafcillin, piperacillin, mezlocillin, apalcillin, cefoperazone, ceftriaxone, and cefpiramide.

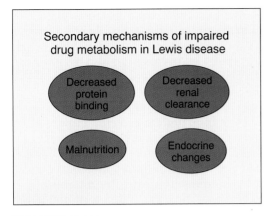

Secondary mechanisms of impaired drug metabolism in Lewis disease

- Decreased protein binding
- Decreased renal clearance
- Malnutrition
- Endocrine changes

FIGURE 6-20.

Secondary mechanisms of impaired drug reactions. Apart from primary factors, associated findings in liver disease may also affect drug metabolism secondarily. Foremost is reduced drug binding to protein due to the hypoproteinemia that is common in patients with cirrhosis. The important plasma proteins involved in drug binding are albumin, α_1-acid glycoprotein, and lipoprotein. Albumin binds acidic and neutral drugs whereas α_1-acid glycoprotein and lipoprotein bind mainly basic drugs. In cirrhosis, drug binding to plasma protein is often significantly reduced; this defect is particularly relevant to highly bound drugs (> 80%). Thus, in patients with cirrhosis, total plasma clearance of naproxen, a highly protein-bound, nonsteroidal anti-inflammatory agent, was unchanged, but the clearance of its unbound fraction was only 40% of normal.

A second factor is the presence of associated renal impairment in cirrhotic patients, in whom serum creatinine is not a reliable measurement of renal functional state. Indeed, in a prospective study, 57% of patients with cirrhosis and ascites already had renal insufficiency (creatinine clearance of 32 mL/min or less) despite normal serum creatinine levels. Moreover, sodium handling may be impaired before ascites becomes clinically apparent. In addition, subtle glomerular changes may be observed using electron microscopy and immunofluorescence microscopy in up to 95% of cirrhotic patients with no overt evidence of biochemical renal impairment. In cirrhotic patients with renal dysfunction, impaired elimination of such drugs as morphine, cimetidine, and ciramadol has been noted [3].

Inasmuch as the oxidation and conjugation of drugs are catalyzed by enzymes, which are proteins, and formation of metabolites require participation of nutrients, the patient's nutritional state is also a determinant of drug metabolism. Some nutrients involved in oxidation include such vitamins as nicotinic acid, riboflavin, and ascorbic acid, as well as minerals (iron, copper, calcium, zinc, and magnesium). For conjugation, the body provides glucuronic acid from carbohydrates, as well as glycine, cysteine, glutamine, glutathione, sulfate, and methionine from protein, and acetyl radicals from fat, carbohydrate, or protein. Malnutrition, whether caloric, protein, or a combination of both, leads to impaired drug biotransformation by either oxidation or conjugation.

Finally, endocrine changes that occur in patients with chronic liver disease may modify drug metabolism. Although direct studies are not readily available, inferences may be derived from other studies. Oral contraceptive steroids inhibit the oxidation of drugs (*eg*, chlordiazepoxide, caffeine, antipyrine, triazolam, alprazolam, prednisolone). In contrast, these oral contraceptive agents may enhance the glucuronidation of a number of drugs (*eg*, oxazepam, lorazepam, temazepam, clofibrate, morphine, acetaminophen). Because feminization occurs in male cirrhotic patients in whom the proportion of estrogen is increased relative to testosterone, biotransformation of some of these drugs may be potentially altered in a manner similar to the effects of oral contraceptive steroid administration in women.

DRUG-INDUCED LIVER INJURY

Clinicopathological types

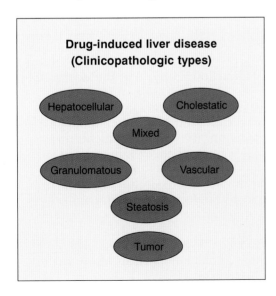

Drug-induced liver disease (Clinicopathologic types)

- Hepatocellular
- Cholestatic
- Mixed
- Granulomatous
- Vascular
- Steatosis
- Tumor

FIGURE 6-21.

One of the outcomes of drug metabolism is the induction of liver injury. This topic has been the subject of more extensive reviews [18–20]. The present discussion is more selective. The disorder can manifest in one of several ways as shown in the figure. Drug-induced liver disease may be predominantly hepatocellular in which necrosis of the hepatocytes is present. The necrosis may be diffuse, spotty, or centrilobular. Clinically, the disorder mimics viral hepatitis. Agents such as halothane, acetaminophen, α-methyldopa, and isoniazid cause hepatocellular damage and can also result in fulminant hepatic failure. On the other hand, a cholestatic disorder is produced by chlorpromazine, erythromycin, estrogen, and other C-17 alkylsteroids. The underlying mechanism is still not fully understood, but there is a general impairment of ion transport associated with changes in the hepatocyte lipid membrane and NA-K ATPase activity. Ultimately bile flow is reduced. A mixed hepatocellular and cholestatic liver disease may result from sulindac, P-amino salicylic acid, and phenytoin toxicity. The formation of granulomas has been associated with allopurinol and quinidine. Vascular abnormalities may be associated with certain drugs. Peliosis hepatitis may be produced by oral contraceptives, androgenic and anabolic steroids, tamoxifen, and danazol. Thrombosis of hepatic veins and other vessels, adenomas (which tend to bleed), and rarely, hepatocellular carcinoma may also complicate oral contraceptive use. Finally, drug-induced liver disease may be in the form of steatosis. Tetracycline and valproic acid typically produce microvesicular fat accumulation, whereas perhexiline is associated with macrovesicular phospholipidosis.

Mechanisms of drug-induced hepatocellular necrosis

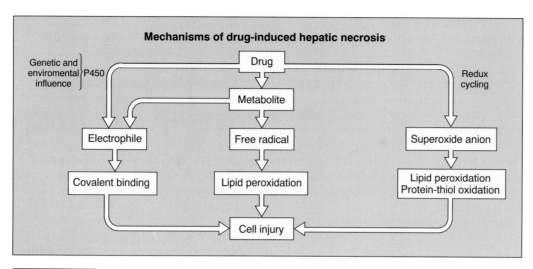

FIGURE 6-22.

Because compounds that are known to be direct toxins are not used as pharmacologic agents in clinical practice, the hepatotoxicity associated with drugs is idiosyncratic and unpredictable rather than intrinsic and predictable. Moreover, because it is idiosyncratic in nature, the drug-induced hepatotoxicity seen in clinical practice cannot be entirely eliminated based on the results of previous animal studies alone. Idiosyncratic drug toxicity may result from a metabolic derangement that leads to the production of toxic reactive metabolites. It may also result from hypersensitivity (allergy).

As shown in this figure, hepatocellular injury is usually not caused by the drug itself, but by its metabolic products [18]. The drug metabolizing enzymes (P450 system), under genetic and environmental influences, cause the generation of electrophilic substances, which seek and accept electrons from other compounds, thereby forming covalent bonds. Electrophiles may form bonds with thiol (sulfur-containing groups), as is seen in acetaminophen toxicity, or with amino groups, as evident in halothane toxicity. Covalent binding of potent alkylating, arylating, or acylating agents to hepatic molecules adversely affects normal cell function and cell necrosis ensues. This condition becomes especially true when levels of

intracellular protective substances like glutathione, which are capable of preferentially combining with toxic metabolites, are depleted. Cell necrosis can also result from the generation of free radicals (metabolites with unpaired electrons) in the course of oxidative drug metabolism. These free radicals can bind both to proteins and unsaturated fatty acids of the cell membranes, resulting in lipid peroxidation, membrane damage, and disruption of membrane and mitochondrial functions. An example of free radical–mediated injury is carbon tetrachloride hepatoxicity. Lipid peroxidation can also result from the generation of superoxide anion through redox cycling. Necrosis may be greatest in the centrilobular zone where the sinusoidal oxygen tension is lowest and where the concentration of P450 enzymes tends to be highest.

Arrayed against these mechanisms of liver injury are protective compounds. Foremost is glutathione. Some electrophiles preferentially attack the thiol of glutathione, a reaction that is catalyzed by the glutathione S-transferase. Another defense mechanism is mediated by scavengers that interfere with the free radical chain reaction of lipid peroxidation. The leading free radical scavenger against lipid peroxidation is tocopherol, but such endogenous substances as uric acid, bilirubin, ascorbic acid, and vitamin A may be important also.

Mechanisms of acetaminophen toxicity

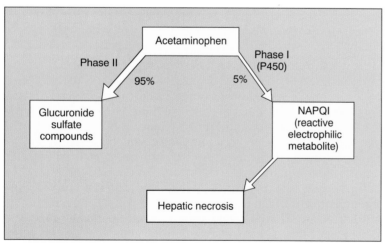

FIGURE 6-23.

Mechanisms of acetaminophen toxicity [21]. The major bulk of acetaminophen is metabolized by phase II reaction (95% or

more), mainly through glucuronidation and sulfation, whereas only 5% or less undergo oxidation that results in the formation of a reactive electrophilic metabolite, N-acetyl-P-benzoquinoneimine (NAPQI). NAPQI preferentially binds to glutathionine (GSH), and when cytosolic GSH concentration falls, NAPQI toxicity ensues. Mitochondrial function is impaired. The isoenzyme (P450IIE$_1$) that catalyzes the oxidation of acetaminophen also metabolizes ethanol, so that chronic ethanol ingestion induces this enzyme and increases the proportion of acetaminophen that undergoes oxidative degradation. Thus, in such patients the concomitant ingestion of acetaminophen, even in ordinary therapeutic doses (3 to 4 g/day), may result in serious hepatotoxicity. Depletion of GSH by starvation, alcohol ingestion, or other drugs are important contributory factors in acetaminophen toxicity. Therapy is aimed at increasing GSH synthesis by providing N-acetylcysteine.

Because isoniazid also induces P450IIE, patients taking both this antituberculosis agent and acetaminophen are also at risk for possible acetaminophen hepatotoxicity.

Isoniazid hepatitis incidence

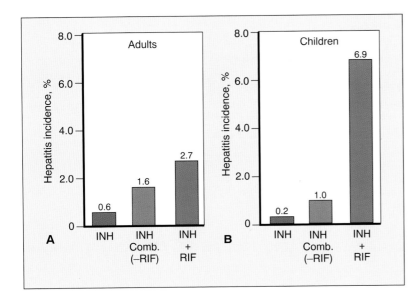

FIGURE 6-24.

Incidence of hepatitis in patients on isoniazid (INH) alone or in combination with rifampin (RIF) or other agents. Data show that the incidence of hepatitis is greater when INH is given in combination with other drugs such as para aminosalicylic acid, ethambutol, and RIF. The increase is more remarkable with the coadministration of RIF than with the other agents; particularly striking is the increase in children. However, the precise mechanism of INH toxicity is not fully elucidated. Toxicity is shown to be related to slow acetylation in some studies, but to fast acetylation in others, as discussed in Figures 6-25 to 6-28 [22]. (*Data from* Steele *et al.* [22]; with permission.)

Isoniazid metabolism

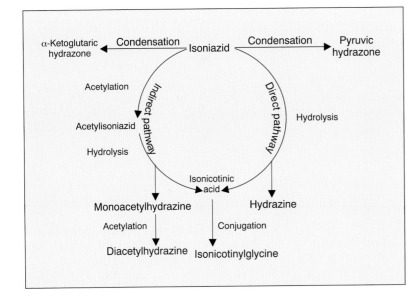

FIGURE 6-25.

Isoniazid metabolism. Isoniazid may be metabolized directly to hydrazine or indirectly to acetylisoniazid. Both pathways end with isonicotinic acid and isonicotinylglycine.

The proportion of isoniazid metabolized by the direct pathway was estimated from the ratio of total isonicotinic acid to acetylisoniazid in the urine following the administration of isoniazid or acetylisoniazid. In slow acetylators this proportion was 3% when isoniazid alone was given, but rose to 6% when rifampin was also given along with isoniazid ($P<0.001$). This finding suggested induction of isoniazid metabolism by rifampin in slow acetylators, but in rapid acetylators, this phenomenon was not observed. Furthermore, in slow acetylators, hydrazine formation through the direct pathway was increased. Thus, in some cases the greater formation of hydrazine, which has been shown to be hepatotoxic in animals, may account for the increased hepatotoxicity in slow acetylator patients treated with both isoniazid and rifampin. (*From* Sarma *et al.* [23]; with permission.)

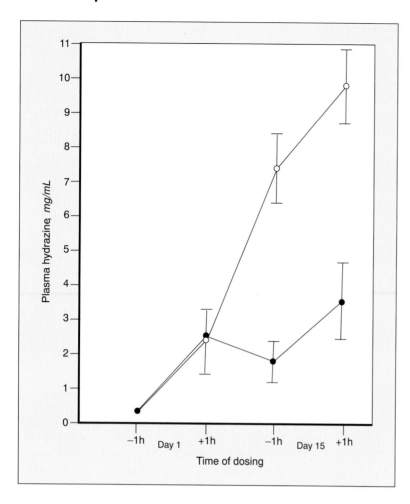

FIGURE 6-26.

Plasma hydrazine levels. This study shows that the levels of hydrazine in the plasma following the chronic administration of isoniazid are higher in slow acetylators (*open circles*) than in rapid acetylators (*closed circles*) [24]. This fact agrees with the finding presented earlier. However, a more limited study carried out in one slow acetylator and one rapid acetylator failed to confirm these observations [25]. (*From* Blair *et al.* [24]; with permission.)

Levels of acetylisoniazid and isoniazid

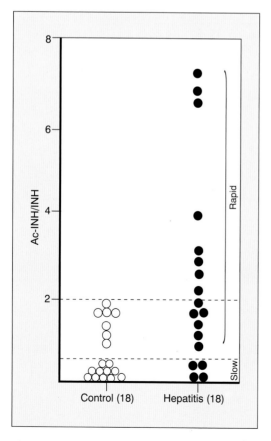

FIGURE 6-27.

Acetylisoniazid (AcINH) and isoniazid (INH) levels in a group of Japanese patients who developed no hepatitis while on antituberculosis therapy and in another group of patients who developed hepatitis while similarly treated. A high AcINH to INH ratio indicated rapid acetylation. As shown here, the rapid acetylators were at greater risk of developing hepatitis than the slow acetylators.

The observation that INH-related hepatitis is more prevalent in the fast acetylators as noted in the Japanese study is in contrast to the earlier observation of greater incidence of hepatitis in the slow acetylators in other populations. These findings suggest the presence of at least two possible mechanisms of INH hepatotoxicity, and the difference may be partly determined by genetic factors. In slow acetylators, toxicity may be related to generation of hydrazine, but in rapid acetylators, toxicity is related to the generation of acetylhydrazine as shown in Figure 6-28. (*From* Yamamoto *et al.* [26]; with permission.)

Possible mechanisms of isoniazid hepatotoxicity

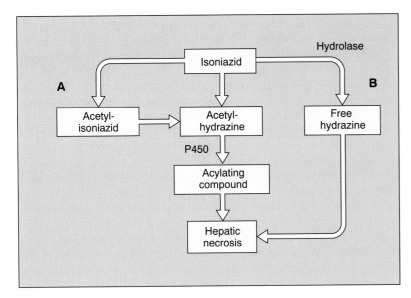

FIGURE 6-28.

Mechanisms of isoniazid hepatotoxicity. Isoniazid, as indicated previously, undergoes acetylation to acetylisoniazid with subsequent formation of acetylhydrazine by way of the indirect pathway (**A**). Action by the P450 system converts the acetylhydrazine to a potent acylating compound that is capable of producing hepatic necrosis. This situation perhaps provides a possible mechanism of hepatotoxicity in rapid acetylators. On the other hand, as indicated earlier, free hydrazine may be also directly produced from isoniazid in the presence of hydrolase (**B**). Free hydrazine is potentially hepatotoxic, as already mentioned. The studies cited previously [24] suggest that the accumulation of hydrazine may account for the toxicity noted in patients who are slow acetylators. Moreover, by inducing this pathway, the concomitant administration of rifampin increases the likelihood of isoniazid hepatotoxicity.

Cocaine-related liver injury

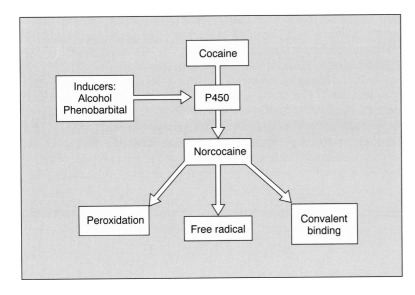

FIGURE 6-29.

Cocaine use and hepatic injury. Cocaine is another potential hepatotoxin. The hepatic lesion related to cocaine use is characterized by coagulative perivenular and midzonal necrosis with both macrovesicular and microvesicular fatty changes also being described. Hyperpyrexia and rhabdomyolysis have also been present in reported cases [27,28].

Cocaine is N-methylated to norcocaine nitroxide by P450. This reaction may be induced by chronic ethanol ingestion, as well as by phenobarbital use. Hepatic damage may be mediated through lipid peroxidation, free radical, or covalent binding. In mice the administration of cimetidine 1 hour before and 1 hour after cocaine prevented hepatotoxicity [29]. Whether a similar benefit from the use of cimetidine, a P450 inhibitor, can be obtained in clinical practice remains to be seen.

Incidentally, chronic ethanol use may enhance the toxicity, not only of acetaminophen, isoniazid, and cocaine, but also of aflotoxin, carbon tetrachloride, chloroform, vitamin A, and others [30].

Halothane hepatitis

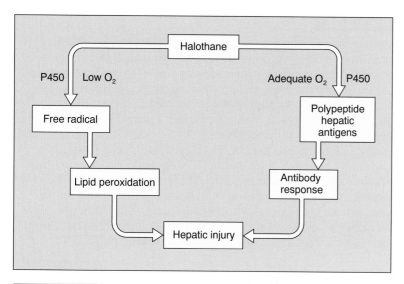

FIGURE 6-30.

Halothane hepatitis. Figures 6-21 to 6-28 stressed hepatic cell injury through the generation of electrophile or free radical and consequent covalent binding and lipid peroxidation. Another mechanism of drug hepatotoxicity involves hypersensitivity (immune or allergic) reactions. One example of drug hepatitis related to hypersensitivity is that resulting from halothane. More common in women who are middle aged and obese, halothane hepatitis is usually manifested by delayed-onset fever, rash, arthralgia, and eosinophilia. Autoantibodies are often present. The majority of patients develop this hepatitis following an earlier exposure to the anesthetic. Although the interval between exposure to the onset of jaundice is often prolonged, unlike the hepatitis caused by a direct toxin, repeated exposure within a short time is associated with greater disease severity and prompter onset of jaundice. These clinical features strongly suggest an immunologic or

hypersensitivity disorder. Although the mechanism has been subjected to close scrutiny, it is still not fully understood.

In animal studies, halothane liver injury has been reproduced in several models. These experimental models generally call for an inducing agent similar to phenobarbital, isoniazid, or other agents, given under conditions of low oxygen tension. The resulting hepatic damage is reproducible, dose-dependent, and unassociated with markers of immune disturbance. The tissue damage, as indicated in the figure, is believed to be mediated by the generation of free radical and consequent lipid peroxidation. This type of halothane hepatitis, however, does not reflect what transpires in patients as observed clinically.

On the other hand, some evidence exists, as indicated in the figure, that under normal oxygen conditions, susceptible patients develop, upon exposure to halothane, polypeptide hepatic antigens [31,32]. These antigens range in molecular weight from 54 to 100 kDa and are expressed in the livers of halothane-treated rabbits, rats, and humans but not in untreated controls. These antigens develop as a result of oxidative, cytochrome P450–mediated metabolism of halothane to CF3C0 Cl. This reactive intermediate binds covalently to the proteins, probably through the e-amino group of lysine residues to produce N_E CF_3CO-lysine side chains. The major CF_3-CO protein antigens have been purified and analyzed. Once formed, these antigens persist for many days, and this relatively long persistence may be important in enabling them to interact with the immune system of the susceptible individual and thereby initiate an immune response. Studies suggest that the P450 involved may be CYP2E1 (P450IIE$_1$). Despite the advances already achieved, important questions remain. For instance, it is not clear how the halothane-induced antigen is translocated from the endoplasmic reticulum to the hepatocyte surface membrane, how the antigen is presented to the immune system, how precisely the immune-mediated necrosis is produced, and why only a small fraction of the patients exposed to halothane manifest an immune response and develop hepatitis [31].

Drug-induced fatty liver

TABLE 6-3. AGENTS PRODUCING DRUG-INDUCED FATTY LIVER

MACROVACUOLAR

Methotrexate

Allopurinol

Halothane

Isoniazid

α-Methyldopa

MICROVESICULAR

Tetracycline

Valproic acid

Ibuprofen

Pirprofen

Amineptine

Tianeptine

Salicyclic acid

TABLE 6-3.

Although many drugs produce hepatocellular necrosis by the mechanisms discussed in Figures 6-23 to 6-29, other drugs (listed in Table 6-3) produce fatty change. The fatty change produced by these drugs can be grouped, as shown in this table, into macrovacuolar or microvesicular forms. In macrovacuolar steatosis, the hepatocyte contains a single large droplet of fat (or empty space in the hematoxylin and eosin stains) that pushes the nucleus to the side. In some instances, as in those related to ethanol ingestion, the fatty change may start as tiny droplets but eventually develop into the macrovascular form.

The apoprotein moiety of triglyceride, glycoprotein, is synthesized by the rough endoplasmic reticulum and is glycosylated there as well as in the Golgi apparatus, so that an impairment of protein synthesis, as seen with methotrexate, may also lead to steatosis. Adverse effects on the endoplasmic reticulum, Golgi apparatus, and plasma membrane by allopurinol, halothane, isoniazid, and α-methyldopa may similarly lead to macrovacuolar steatosis. In these instances, the steatosis may be associated with hepatitis or other evidence of toxic liver injury.

In microvesicular steatosis, the fat appears as tiny cytoplasmic droplets that do not displace the hepatocyte nucleus. Inhibition of the mitochondrial oxidation of fatty acids appears to be the main mechanism responsible for the steatosis of tetracycline, valproic acid, pirprofen, ibuprofen, amineptine, and tianeptine. A similar mechanism may also apply to the fatty change produced by hypoglycin, 4-pentenoic acid, and salicylic acid. The mechanism for the microvesicular steatosis of Reye's syndrome is not completely clear, but mitochondrial dysfunction and impaired β-oxidation of fatty acid have been postulated [32]. In this connection, the effect of salicylic acid on β-oxidation of fatty acids may be relevant, insasmuch as Reye's syndrome has been associated with the administration of aspirin (acetylsalicylic acid). Tetracycline microvesicular steatosis appears to result from impaired hepatic secretion of triglycerides as well as from abnormal fatty acid oxidation. In addition to causing hepatic steatosis, other drugs may also produce changes that mimic those associated with alcoholic liver disease.

TABLE 6-4. PHOSPHOLIPIDOSIS (PSEUDOALCOHOLIC LIVER DISEASE)

DRUGS

Amiodarone

Perhexilene

Hexestrol (diethylamino ethoxyhexestrol)

HISTOLOGY

Microvesicular and macrovacuolar steatosis, Mallory's bodies, necrosis, monomorphonuclear and polymorphonuclear infiltrate, fibrosis, or cirrhosis

PATHOGENESIS

Lysosomal trapping of protanated drug → formation of tight complexes with phospholipids → inhibition of phopho-lipases → accumulation of phospholipids

TABLE 6-4.

At least three drugs, all of which have antianginal or antiar-rhythmic activity, have been shown to produce hepatic lesions similar to those seen with alcoholic liver disease. For this type of lesion, the term *phospholipidosis* has been applied. These drugs are listed here along with the histologic changes that they produce and the proposed pathogenesis. The proposed mechanisms are similar for all three drugs and is illustrated in Figure 6-31 depicting perhexiline.

Metabolism of perhexiline

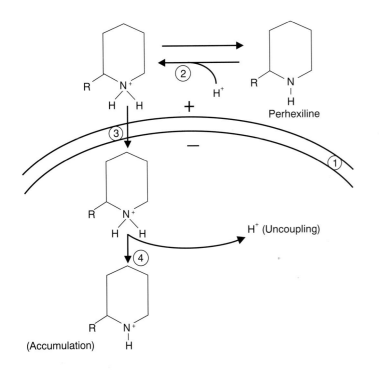

mechanism for the uptake of perhexiline by mitochondria and its effects on mitochondrial function. In the presence of respiratory substrates, transfer of electrons along complexes I, III, and IV of the respiratory chain (not shown) is associated with the release of protons from the matrix to the intermembranous space, creating a large potential difference across the inner mitochondrial membrane, with the outer side being positively charged. Uncharged perhexiline is protonated in the intermembranous space. Protonated perhexiline enters the mitochondrion along the membrane potential. This entry is facilitated by formation of an ion pair with the lipophilic anion, tetraphenylborate. Inside the mitochondria, where the pH is relatively more alkaline, protonated perhexiline dissociates into a proton, whose entry (bypassing ATP synthase) is responsible for the uncoupling effect of perhexiline, and into nonprotonated perhexiline, whose extensive accumulation (at least 20-fold) inside the mitochondrion may be responsible for inhibition of both the respiratory chain and β-oxidation.

With this sequence of events, β-oxidation is inhibited. The degree of inhibition correlates with the level of the perhexiline dose. Esterification of fatty acids to triglycerides is consequently increased, thus leading to the accumulation of tiny fat droplets in the hepatocyte cytoplasm.

Amiodarone and its principal metabolite have been shown in animal experiments to also inhibit mitochondrial β-oxidation of fatty acids. A similar mechanism for the formation of microvesicular steatosis has also been involved for hypoglycin (the toxin from unripe akee responsible for Jamaican vomiting sickness), as well as for 4-pentenoic acid and ethanol. (*From* Deschamps *et al.* [33]; with permission.)

FIGURE 6-31.

Metabolism of perhexiline. Perhexiline is metabolized in the liver mainly by hydroxylation. This process is mediated by P450IID6, the isoenzyme that is incidentally also involved in the metabolism of debrisoquine. Shown here is a proposed

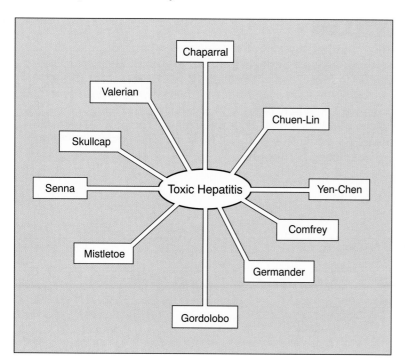

FIGURE 6-32.

Hepatotoxicity related to the use of folk medicine requires a special mention. In the 1950s, venooclusive disease was observed in patients in the West Indies who drank herbal tea [34]. A similar condition was later noted in other parts of the world, particularly in other Third World countries. The disease was later traced to the toxic effects of certain pyrrolizidine alkaloids, which are present in at least 60 different plant genera. Some of the more important of these genera include *Senecio, Crotalaria, Heliotropium,* and *Symphytum*. Another example of hepatoxicity produced by a plant is the vomiting sickness found in Jamaica, caused by the agent hypoglycin, which is present in unripe akee fruit which tends to be consumed when other food is scarce. This vomiting disorder is associated with hepatic steatosis, as already mentioned. In recent years instances of toxic hepatitis have been reported with the use of the folk remedies shown here. Details are given in Table 6-5.

TABLE 6-5. HERBAL PREPARATIONS IMPLICATED AS POSSIBLE HEPATOXINS*

COMMON NAMES	SCIENTIFIC NAMES	FOLK USES	POSSIBLE TOXIC COMPONENT	HEPATIC DISORDER
Chaparral (Creosote bush, greasewood, governadora)	Larrea tridentata Larrea divaricata	Cancer, arthritis, bruises, diarrhea, eczema, colds, bronchitis, menstrual cramps, amenorrhea, venereal disease, "blood purifier", emetic, antiseptic, diuretic	Nordihydroquaiaretic acid (DNGA) and other related compounds	Acute and subacute hepatitis
Chinese herbs Chuen-Lin (Huang-Lien, Ma Huang)	Coptis senesia Coptis japonicum	Tonic, to remove "toxic products of pregnancy" in neonates	Unknown	Unconjugated hyperbilirubinemia
Yin-Chen	Antemesia scoparia	Neonatal jaundice	Unknown	Potential kernicterus
Comfrey	Symphytum officinate	Fatigue, abdominal pain, allergy	Pyrrolizidine alkaloids	Venoocclusive disease
Germander	Teucrium chamaedrys	Weight control, bitter tonic, appetizer, choleretic, antiseptic	Furano neoclerodane deterpenoids	Reversible acute hepatitis, fatal massive hepatic necrosis
Gordolobo	Verbascum thaprus, senecio longilobus, gnaphalium macounii		Pyrrolizidine alkaloids	Potential for venoocclusive disease
Mistletoe	Viscum album, phoradendron flavescens	Infertility, asthma, epilepsy, aphrodisiac	β-Phenylethylamine, tyramine, acetylcholine, propionylcholine	Hepatitis with piecemeal necrosis and distortion of lobular architechture
Senna	Cassia angustifolia, cassia acutifolia	Laxative or cathartic	Senosides, rhein anthron	Hepatitis
Skullcap	Scuttelaria galericulata	Sedative, anticonvulsant		Hepatitis with centrilobular and bridging necrosis
Valerian (garden heliotrope)	Valerian officinalis	Sedative, hypnotic, spasmolytic, hypotensive		Hepatitis with piecemeal necrosis, chronic aggressive hepatitis with fibrosis

*Herbal teas vary widely in composition and may contain several potential toxins often containing pyrrolizidine alkaloids from Senecio, Symphytum, Crotalaria, or Heliotropum. Intrauterine damage may also result from maternal consumption of these concoctions. Babies may develop toxic liver disease from consuming herbal beverages or milk from mothers taking toxin-containing herbal drinks.

TABLE 6-5.

Herbal preparations implicated in hepatotoxicity. This table summarizes the common names, scientific names, folk uses, possible toxic components, and the hepatic disorders associated with the use of those folk remedies. Although many cases can be attributed to the toxic properties of pyrrolizidine alkaloids, some are related to other plant toxins. These preparations are ingested as infusions, other forms of liquid concoctions, tablets, or capsules. In addition, herbal preparations may be adulterated with more conventional agents, like aminopyrine, which have been banned because of toxicity, and with heavy metals like lead, arsenic, and cadmium [35].

A popular Chinese herbal preparation *Chuen-Lin* (also known as *Huang Lien* or *Ma Huang*) is frequently used as a tonic by adults and given to neonates to rid them of "various toxic products of pregnancy". It has been shown to produce indirect hyperbilirubinemia by displacing bilirubin binding from plasma protein, but the component responsible for this effect has not yet been identified. The concoction may also precipitate hemolysis in infants with a deficiency of glucose 6-phosphate dehydrogenase. In both situations, the danger of kernicterus is real [36].

Mechanisms of toxic injury

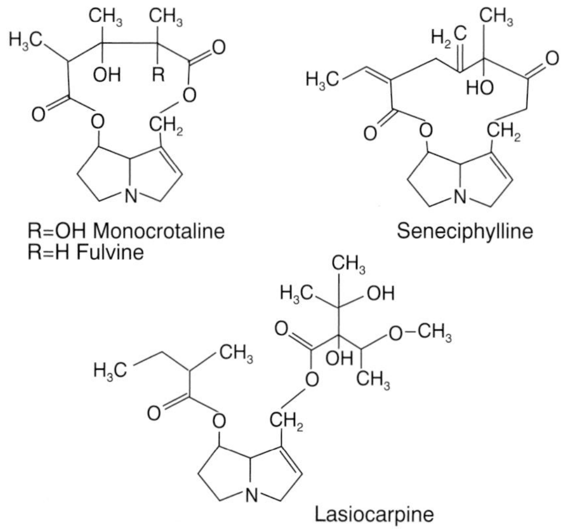

FIGURE 6-33.

Mechanisms of toxic injury. The possible mechanisms whereby these plant toxins damage tissues are not fully understood, but studies with pyrrolizidine have yielded important data. The pyrrolizidine-induced hepatic damage is dependent on the dose and can be reproduced in animals [37]. This figure shows the three typical pyrrolizidine alkaloids. Monocrotaline and fulvine represent *Crotalaria*-type alkaloids, whereas seneciphylline represents a *Senecio*-type alkaloid and lasiocarpine a *Symphytum*-type alkaloid. Pyrrolizidine alkaloids are metabolized by cytochrome P450 to two major products: the reactive and highly toxic pyrrole and the less toxic N-oxide [38]. The pyrrole may then form a conjugate with glutathione. The toxicity of pyrrolizidine is said to be a function of the $\alpha_1\beta$ unsaturation of the necic acid esters and the C1–C2 unsaturation of the necine base [38]. Susceptibility to the toxic effects of pyrrolizadine varies among different animal species. Animals that form pyrroles efficiently, such as cattle, are more likely to develop toxicity than the less efficient metabolizers, such as sheep [9]. (*From* Huxtable [39]; with permission.)

Metabolism of pyrrolizidine

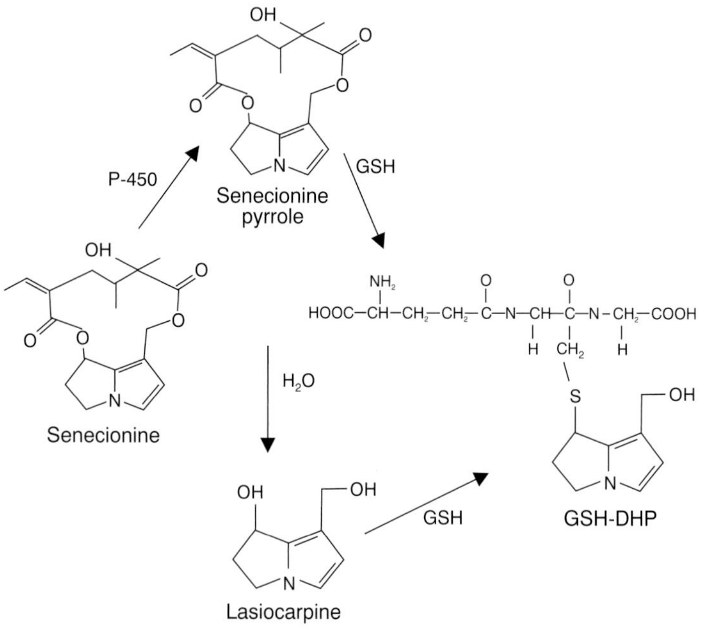

FIGURE 6-34.

Possible metabolism of the pyrrolizidine compound senecionine. This figure shows the metabolism of senecionine to a reactive metabolite, senecionine pyrrole, and the subsequent formation of a glutathione (GSH) conjugate with dehydrosenecionine or with the dehydrosenecionine hydrolysis product, DHP (6,7 dihydro-7-hydroxy-1-hydroxymethyl-5H-pyrrolizidine). GSH preferentially reacts with the strong electrophile, dehydrosenecionine, and thus plays a role in detoxification.

In rats, the oxidation of pyrrolizidine alkaloids differs between males and females. The cytochrome P450IICII, specific to male rats, is mainly involved with N-oxidation, whereas P450IIIA2 is responsible for the formation of pyrrolic metabolites [41]. (*From* Buhler *et al.* [42]; with permission.)

Hepatic metabolism and structural requirements

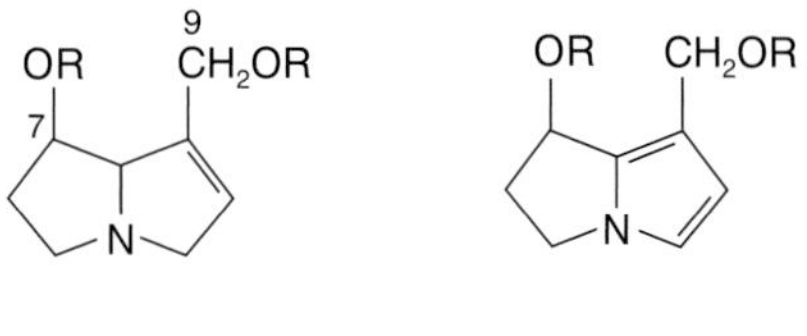

FIGURE 6-35.

Hepatic metabolism and structural requirements. This figure shows the structural requirement for hepatic metabolism, that is, the presence of 1,2-double bond or of a 2-hydroxy group. The 1,2-unsaturated pyrrolizidines are capable of hepatic oxidation to the dehydropyrrolizidines or pyrroles. The bolder bonding lines show the minimum structural unit required for toxicity.

Pyrrolizidines are toxic not only to the liver but also to the lungs and may cause pulmonary hypertension and cor pulmonale. They also possess a carcinogenic potential. Liver damage appears to be worse with the *Senecio* alkaloids, whereas lung damage is worse with the less toxic *Crotalaria* alkaloids. Hepatic or pulmonary toxicity is produced mainly by the hepatic metabolite because the lungs are incapable of metabolizing pyrrolizidines. (*From* Huxtable [39]; with permission).

Proposed mechanism of hepatic and pulmonary toxicity of pyrroles

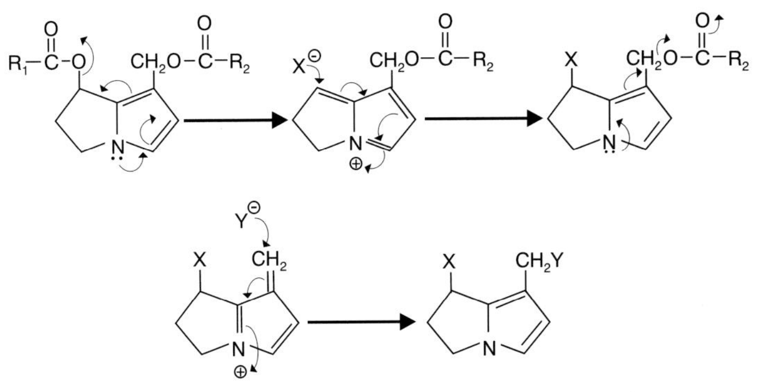

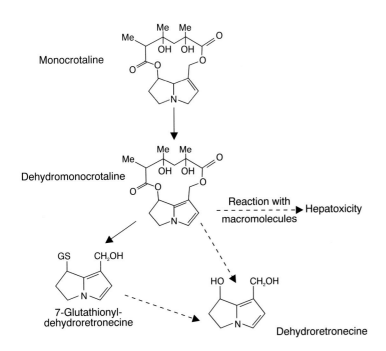

FIGURE 6-36.

Proposed mechanism of hepatic and pulmonary toxicity of pyrroles. Certain pyrroles are bidentate alkylating agents because of their ability to form stabilized carbonium ions at positions 7 and 9. Formed by an S_N1 process, these ions react with nucleophiles, such as sulhydryl groups on cell macromolecules or low molecular weight molecules such as glutathione to form two covalent bonds as shown. (*From* Huxtable [39]; with permission.)

Monocrotaline metabolism and possible hepatotoxicity

FIGURE 6-37.

A proposed scheme for monocrotaline metabolism and possible hepatotoxicity. The pneumotoxic alkaloid, monocrotaline, is oxidized by a P450–mixed function oxidase system in the liver to the pyrrole, dehydromonocrotaline. Dehydromonocrotaline either reacts with macromolecular constituents of the cell, thus producing hepatotoxicity, or undergoes hydrolysis to the relatively inocuous secondary pyrrole, dehydroretronecine. A third pathway, conjugation with glutathione to produce glutathionyldehydroretronecine, may be responsible for the pneumotoxicity. The differing pneumotoxicity of the various pyrrolizidines may be a function of the proportion of the primary pyrrole diverted into the conjugation pathway. (*From* Huxtable *et al.* [43]; with permission.)

Possible mechanism of germander hepatotoxicity

FIGURE 6-38.

Possible mechanism for the hepatotoxicity of germander. Germander (*see* Fig. 6-32) has been used as a bitter tonic, appetizer, choleretic, and for weight control. The pathogenesis of the hepatic injury produced by germander has been studied in mice using lyophilisate of germander tea, furano neoclerodane diterpenoids. These compounds may be activated particularly by cytochrome P450IIIA into reactive metabolites, probably epoxides. The metabolites are in turn inactivated by glutathione conjugate formation (and probably by epoxide hydrolase as well) or they may react with hepatic proteins resulting in toxic hepatitis. (*From* Loeper *et al.* [44]; with permission.)

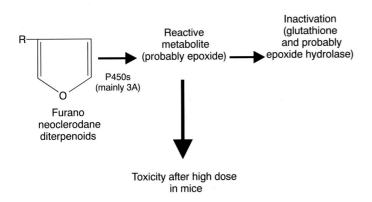

REFERENCES AND RECOMMENDED READING

1. Watkins PB: Role of cytochrome P450 in drug metabolism and hepatotoxicity. *Semin Liver Dis* 1990, 10:235–250.

2. Alvares A, Pratt WB: Pathways of drug metabolism. In *Principles of Drug Action. The Basis of Pharmacology.* Edited by Pratt WB, Taylor P. New York: Churchill-Livingstone; 1990:365–422.

3. Hoyumpa A, Schenker S: Is glucuronidation truly preserved in patients with liver disease? *Hepatology* 1991, 13:786–795.

4. Meyer UA: Drug metabolism in health and disease. In *Extrahepatic Manifestations in Liver Diseases.* Edited by Schmid R, Bianchi L, Gerok W, Maier KP. Dordrecht/Boston/London: Kluwer Academic Publishers; 1993:286–295.

5. Hoyumpa A, Schenker S: Influence of liver disease in the disposition and elimination of drugs. In *Diseases of the Liver.* Edited by Schiff L, Schiff E. Philadelphia: J. B. Lippincott; 1993:784–824.

6. Caporaso N, Landi MT, Vineis P: Relevance of metabolic polymorphisms to human carcinogenesis: Evaluation of epidemiologic evidence. *Pharmacogenetics* 1991, 1:4–9.

7. Agundez JAG, Ledesma MC, Benitez J, et al.: CYP2D6 genes and risk of liver cancer. *Lancet* 1995, 345:830–831.

8. Yamazaki H, Inui Y, Yun CH, et al.: Cytochrome P450 2E1 and 2A6 enzymes as major catalysts for metabolic activation of N-nitrosodialkylamines and tobacco-related nitrosamines in human liver microsomes. *Carcinogenesis* 1992, 13:1789–1794.

9. Sim SM, Back DJ, Breckenridge AM: The effect of various drugs on the glucuronidation of zidovudine (azidothymidine, AZT) by human liver microsomes. *Br J Clin Pharmacol* 1991, 32:17–21.

10. Roberts R, Wilkinson GR, Branch RA, et al.: Effect of age and parenchymal liver disease on the disposition and elimination of chlordiazepoxide. *Gastroenterology* 1978, 75:479–485.

11. Klotz U, Avant GR, Hoyumpa A, et al.: The effects of age and liver disease on the disposition and elimination of diazepam in adult man. *J Clin Invest* 1975:347–359.

12. Greenblatt DJ, Allen MD, Harmatz JS, et al.: Diazepam disposition determinants. *Clin Pharmacol Ther* 1980, 27:301–312.

13. Andreasen PB, Hendel J, Greisen G, et al.: Pharmacokinetics of diazepam in disordered liver function. *Eur J Clin Pharmacol* 1976, 10:115–120.

14. Branch RA, Morgan MH, James J, et al.: Intravenous administration of diazepam in patients with chronic liver disease. *Gut* 1976, 17:975–983.

15. Shull HS, Wilkinson GR, Johnson R, et al.: Normal disposition of oxazypam in acute viral hepatitis and cirrhosis. *Ann Intern Med* 1976, 84:420–425.

16. Kraus JW, Desmond PV, Marshall JP, et al.: Effects of age and liver disease on disposition of lorazepam. *Clin Pharmacol Ther* 1978, 24:411–419.

17. Sonne J, Andreason PB, Loft S, et al.: Glucuronidation of oxazepam is not spared in patients with hepatic encephalopathy. *Hepatology* 1990, 11:951–956.

18. Kaplowitz N: Drug metabolism and hepatotoxicity. In *Liver and Biliary Diseases.* Edited by Kaplowitz N. Baltimore: Williams & Wilkins; 1992:82–97.

19. Desmet VJ: Drug-induced liver disease: Pathogenetic mechanisms and histopathological lesions. *Medical Intelligence* 1994, 2:36–47.

20. Lee: Review article: Drug-induced hepatotoxicity. *Alim Pharmacol Ther* 1993, 7:477–483.

21. Nelson SD: Molecular mechanisms of the hepatoxicity caused by acetaminophen. *Semin Liver Disease* 1990, 10:267–278.

22. Steele MA, Burk RI, Des Prez RM: Toxic hepatitis with isoniazid and rifampin. *Chest* 1991, 99:465–471.

23. Sarma GR, Immanuel C, Kailsam S, et al.: Rifampin-induced release of hydralazine from isoniazid. *Am Rev Resp Dis* 1986, 133:1072–1075.

24. Blair IA, Tinoco RM, Brodie MJ, et al.: Plasma hydrazine concentrations in man after isoniazid and hydrazine administration. *Hum Toxicol* 1985, 4:195–202.

25. Jenner PJ, Ellard GA: Isoniazid-related hepatotoxicity: A study of the effects of rifampin administration of the metabolism of acetylisoniazid in man. *Tuberculosis* 1989, 70:93–101.

26. Yamamoto T, Suou T, Hirayama C: Elevated serum aminotransferase induced by isoniazid in relation to isoniazid autylator phenotype. *Hepatology* 1986, 6:295–298.

27. Kanel GC, Cassidy W, Shuster L, et al.: Cocaine-induced liver injury: comparison of morphological features in man and in experimental models. *Hepatology* 1990, 11:646–651.

28. Wanless IR, Dore S, Gopinath N, et al.: Histopathology of cocaine hepatoxicity. *Gastroenterology* 1990, 98:497–501.

29. Peterson FJ, Knodell RG, Lindemann NJ, et al.: Prevention of acetaminophen and cocaine hepatoxicity in mice by cimetidine treatment. *Gastroenterology* 1983, 85:122–129.

30. Bay MK, Schenker S: Interactions between alcohol and other hepatotoxins. In *Alcoholic Liver Disease. Pathology and Pathogenesis.* Edited by Hall P, Arnold E. London, Boston, Melbourne, Auckland; 1995:260–278.

31. Kenna JG, VanFelt FN: The metabolism and toxicity of inhaled anaesthetic agents. *Anaesthetic Pharmacol Rev* 1994, 2:29–42.

32. Elliot RH, Strunin L: Hepatotoxicity of volatile anaesthetics. *Brit J Anaesthesia* 1993, 70:339–348.

33. Deschamps D, DeBeco V, Fisch C, et al.: Inhibition by perhexiline of oxidative phosphorylation and the beta-oxidation of fatty acids: possible role in pseudoalcoholic liver lesions. *Hepatology* 1994, 19:948–961.

34. Stuart KL, Bras G: Veno-occlusive disease of the liver. *Quart J Med* 1957, 26:291–315.

35. Chan TY: The prevalence, use and harmful potential in some Chinese herbal medicines in babies and children. *Vet Hum Toxicol* 1994, 36:238–240.

36. Yeung CY, Lee FT, Wong HN: Effect of a popular Chinese herb on neonatal bilirubin protein binding. *Biol Neonate* 1990, 58:98–103.

37. Yeong ML, Wakefield ST, Ford HC: Hepatocyte membrane injury and bleb formation followed by low comfy toxicity in rats. *Int J Exp Path* 1993, 74:211–217.

38. Kim H-Y, Stermitz FR, Molyneaux RJ, et al.: Structural influences on pyrrolizadine alkaloid-induced cytopathology. *Toxicol and Appl Pharmacol* 1993, 122:61–69.

39. Huxtable RJ: Activation and pulmonary toxicity of pyrrolizidine alkaloids. *Pharmacol Ther* 1990, 47:371–389.

40. Cheeke PR: A review of the functional and evolutionary roles of the liver in the detoxification of poisonous plants, with special reference to pyrrolizidine alkaloids. *Vet Hum Toxicol* 1994:240–247.

41. Williams DE, Reed R, Kedzierski B, et al.: The role of flavin-containing monooxygenase in the N-oxidation of the pyrrolizidine alkaloid senecionine. *Drug Metab Disp* 1989, 17:380–386.

42. Buhler DR, Miranda CL, Kedzierski B, et al.: Mechanisms for pyrrolizidine alkaloid activation and detoxification. In *Biol Reactive Intermediates IV.* Edited by Witmer CM, et al.. New York: Plenum Press; 1990:597–603.

43. Huxtable RJ, Bowers R, Mattocks AR, et al.: Sulfur conjugates as putative pneumotoxic metabolites of the pyrrolizidine alkaloid, monocrotaline. In *Biological Reactive Intermediates IV.* Edited by Witmer CM, et al.. New York: Plenum Press; 1990:605–612.

44. Loeper J, Descatoire V, Letteron P, et al.: Hepatotoxicity of Germander in mice. *Gastroenterology* 1994, 106:464–472.

Chapter

7

Acute Liver Failure

WILLIAM M. LEE

When liver failure occurs in a previously healthy individual, its onset is often so rapid that it takes even experienced physicians by surprise. The terms *hyperacute* or *fulminant* hepatic necrosis are used to emphasize the rapidity and severity of the condition. The onset of acute liver failure is heralded by an altered mental state, agitation and confusion proceeding to coma, and evidence of a coagulopathy [1–3]. Acute liver failure patients may be subdivided into groups according to rapidity of onset— either from the presentation of first symptoms or from the onset of jaundice—because prognosis, in part, appears to depend on how rapidly the condition evolves. Paradoxically, patients with a slower evolution carry a poorer prognosis. The primary causes of acute liver failure are viral infections of the liver and drug reactions, although there is a large miscellaneous group of rare causes that lead to extensive loss of hepatocyte mass and functional capacity. These etiologies include Wilson's disease, ischemic liver injury secondary to congestive heart failure or drugs, venoocclusive disease following conditioning for bone marrow transplantation, and fatty liver of pregnancy [4–9]. The viruses implicated vary in prevalence in different parts of the world, and the use of certain agents, such as acetaminophen, is more common in the United Kingdom and the United States than in Africa or Asia.

Unique clinical features of acute liver failure that occur in more than 50% of patients include altered mental status and the evolution of cerebral edema [10–12]. Although a prominent feature of acute liver failure, cerebral edema is virtually never seen in cirrhotic patients. However, hypotension and peripheral vasodilation similar to that in cirrhosis is observed. The loss of intravascular fluid volume into the interstitial tissues results in renal failure and lactic acidosis if volume status is not carefully maintained. Bleeding from the gastrointestinal tract, increased susceptibility to a variety of nosocomial infections, adult respiratory distress syndrome, and occasionally cardiac arrhythmias are observed, testifying to the widespread organ involvement engendered by the loss of hepatocyte function [13].

A liver biopsy in these very ill patients is seldom possible because of coagulopathy. When tissue is available, the typical findings are massive necrosis of hepatocytes with varying degrees of inflammation. Replacement of cells by tumor deposits is occasionally seen, and microvesicular fatty infiltration of hepatocyte without loss of membrane integrity is characteristic of the acute fatty liver syndrome observed in late pregnancy in association with eclampsia.

Initial diagnostic efforts are directed at confirming the presence of coagulation changes, elevated ammonia levels, and a central nervous system–mediated respiratory alkalosis. Equally important is the determination of the etiology, because prognosis and possible use of antidotes hinge on this finding. Historic evidence for specific ingestion of acetaminophen in excess, either as an intentional suicidal overdose or in more modest doses concurrent with excessive alcohol abuse, should be of paramount concern because N-acetylcysteine administered by nasogastric tube may prove to be lifesaving [14–17]. Similarly, mushroom poisoning must be specifically indicated historically so that the proper antidotes are obtained [18]. Most cases that appear to be viral in origin (ie, no ingestion history) are usually diagnosed as hepatitis B, or occasionally hepatitis D in a hepatitis B–positive individual, or possibly a virus as yet unidentified, sometimes referred to as *hepatitis F*. Hepatitis A, C, and E are less frequently implicated, except that hepatitis E, a disease common in underdeveloped countries, seems to have a predilection to severity in pregnant women [19].

The hallmark of treatment consists of good intensive care and support because no specific therapy has yet been discovered to provide the required rapid hepatic regeneration. Attention to careful fluid management, surveillance for infection, and prompt resuscitation for evidence of gastrointestinal bleeding are important. Platelets and plasma may be required but are usually only administered with evidence of hemorrhage. Increases in intracranial pressure may lead to brain-stem herniation and death. Specific therapy with intravenous mannitol may be used to abort signs of increased intracranial pressure such as decerebrate posturing, pupillary dilatation, and respiratory pattern changes [20]. Gastrointestinal bleeding can be prevented by prophylactic use of histamine$_2$-receptor blockers such as cimetidine [21].

The use of transplantation over the past 10 years has produced remarkable patient rescues, with a 1-year survival figure of greater than 70% [22,23]. However, difficulties in timing of transplantation and in predicting prognosis, as well as the lack of readily available donor organs, has limited use of this technique. Future options will include liver-support devices employing animal organs or liver cells in culture cartridges as well as temporary auxiliary transplants and partial organs derived from relatives [24–26]. The crisis that evolves rapidly in acute liver failure can quickly dissipate once the failing liver begins to recover its own intrinsic function, but the overall survival rates (fewer than 20% of patients) testify to the gravity of this relatively rare condition.

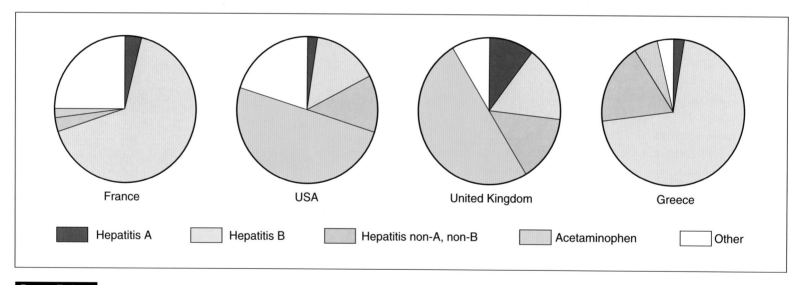

France   USA   United Kingdom   Greece

■ Hepatitis A   ▢ Hepatitis B   ▨ Hepatitis non-A, non-B   ▨ Acetaminophen   ▢ Other

FIGURE 7-1.

Estimated prevalence of the most common causes of acute liver failure worldwide. Great variation is observed between the United Kingdom (high prevalence of acetaminophen toxicity) and Greece (predominantly hepatitis B). Overall, viral hepatitis is the most common cause of acute liver failure outside the United Kingdom. Nevertheless, an increasing number of cases of acetaminophen toxicity is occurring in the United States. Although generally less severe, these cases may account for more than 50% of patient hospital admissions for acute liver failure in certain urban areas [3]. No extensive epidemiologic data concerning this condition are available.

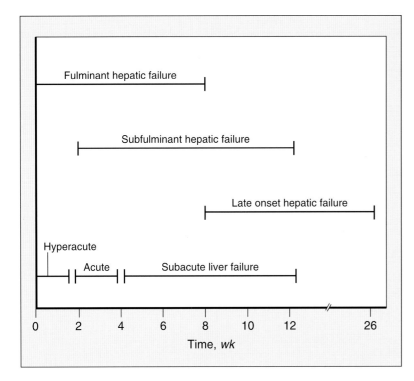

FIGURE 7-2.

Terms used to define acute liver failure. These terms are determined by the length of time from onset of illness to development of encephalopathy. Not all observers agree on even these definitions; some groups follow time of onset of jaundice rather than illness and others use diminution of factor V levels below 50% to define the onset of liver failure. A very short hyperacute evolution from illness to encephalopathy appears to carry a better prognosis than more slowly evolving cases. Patients with the longest duration of illness prior to the onset of encephalopathy usually have the poorest prognosis. These patients tend to have less cerebral edema, more ascites and renal failure, and less likelihood of full recovery.

ETIOLOGY

TABLE 7-1. PRINCIPAL CAUSES OF ACUTE LIVER FAILURE

VIRAL HEPATITIS
A, B, D, E, F, herpes simplex virus

DRUG-RELATED LIVER INJURY
Acetaminophen, idiosyncratic drug reactions

TOXINS
CCl_4, *Amanita phalloides*, phosphorus

VASCULAR
Ischemic, venoocclusive, heat stroke, malignant infiltration

MISCELLANEOUS
Wilson's disease, acute fatty liver of pregnancy

TABLE 7-1.

Etiology of acute liver failure is important because it determines prognosis (*see* Fig. 7-11 and Table 7-8). In many instances, radically differing initial management is required for each. Disease-specific treatments include antidotes to acetaminophen and mushroom poisoning that must be given immediately upon patient admission to the hospital. Identification of severe heart failure as the cause of acute liver failure will lead to proper resuscitation and correction of any fluid balance disturbance. Likewise, recognition of acute fatty liver of pregnancy will lead to consideration of delivery of the mother as the logical treatment for this condition. Patients with fulminant Wilson's disease carry such a bad prognosis that urgent consideration for transplantation must be immediately undertaken after diagnosis is made.

TABLE 7-2. PRESENTATIONS OF ACUTE LIVER FAILURE ASSOCIATED WITH HEPATITIS B

	HBsAg	Anti-HBc IgM	Anti-delta	HBeAg
Acute viral hepatitis B	+	+	−	+/−
Acute viral hepatitis B (early clearance)	−	+	−	−
Acute delta hepatitis (chronic hepatitis B carrier)	+	−	+	+/−
Hepatitis B mutant	+	+/−	−	−
Hepatitis B and C (Anti-HCV positive)	+	−	−	+/−

TABLE 7-2.

Several different forms of hepatitis B virus infection lead to liver failure. Each differs in serologic pattern from other presentations in the table. The most common forms in most areas of the world are the first three. Hepatitis B surface antigen (HBsAg) may be negative in certain patients with early clearance. This situation is presumed to result from the active immune response observed and is often a good prognostic sign. Such patients can only be diagnosed by obtaining immunoglobulin M (IgM) antibodies to hepatitis B core antigen (Anti-HBc) which will be positive in the absence of other markers. If liver transplantation is required for these early clearance patients, their prognosis is good because infection of the new liver graft rarely occurs. Many intravenous drug users are found to have combined hepatitis B and D or hepatitis B and C infections. The combination of these infections carries a higher morbidity than either alone, although hepatitis C rarely causes true acute liver failure. The combination of acute hepatitis B with acute hepatitis D infection is also uncommon; clearance of hepatitis B infection aborts any continued delta infection, and each virus appears to inhibit replication of the other to some extent, thus facilitating clearance of both. Anti-delta—antibodies to delta; Anti-HCV—antibodies to hepatitis C virus; HBeAg—hepatitis B e antigen.

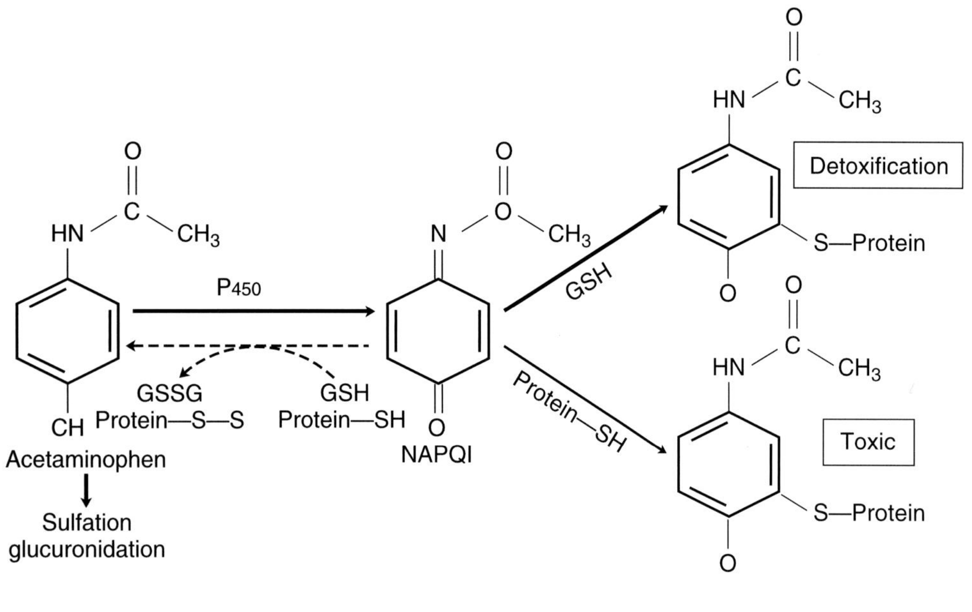

FIGURE 7-3.

Acetaminophen metabolic pathway. The main metabolic pathways for xenobiotic metabolism by the liver are divided into phase I (employing cytochrome P450), phase II (sulfation and glucuronidation), and the glutathione-S-transferase system. Acetaminophen is a prime example of a well-understood metabolic pathway and employs all three mechanisms. Acetaminophen in therapeutic doses undergoes sulfation and glucuronidation (phase II reactions) but is metabolized by cytochrome P450 2E1 (phase I reaction) to N-acetyl-p-benzoquinoeimine (NAPQI) if the capacity of the phase II reactions is exceeded or if the cytochrome is induced. Glutathione-S-transferase is capable of detoxifying NAPQI to mercapturic acid if glutathione is available. N-acetylcysteine is an excellent source of glutathione substrate. Acetaminophen serves as an excellent example of a direct toxin, one in which toxicity occurs in all individuals, is dose related, and wherein all animal models demonstrate the same or similar reactions. In alcoholic patients or individuals who are malnourished, glutathione depletion accentuates the liver injury. In addition, P450 2E1 is induced by alcohol and some other drugs, whereas cimetidine inhibits acetaminophen metabolism through P450 2E1. GSH—reduced glutathione; GSSG—oxidized glutathione. (*Adapted from* Kaplowitz [27]; with permission.)

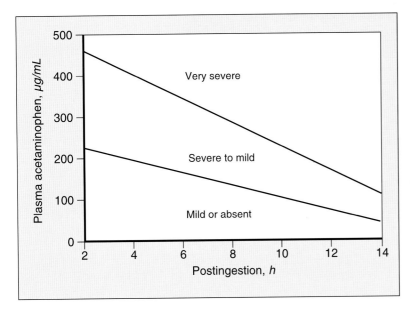

FIGURE 7-4.

Acetaminophen toxicity nomogram. This nomogram aids in determining the likelihood of serious acetaminophen hepatotoxicity using plasma levels and the estimated time of the ingestion-to-sampling interval. Levels falling in the lower zone indicate that the liver damage should be mild and those falling in the upper zone indicate that the damage will be severe. Use of N-acetylcysteine (NAC) as an antidote is indicated in either case, because it is quite safe and acetaminophen toxicity is sometimes unpredictable, particularly when the interval from ingestion to clinical presentation is long or unknown. NAC may still have some value 48 hours or more following ingestion. (*Adapted from* Zimmerman [28]; with permission.)

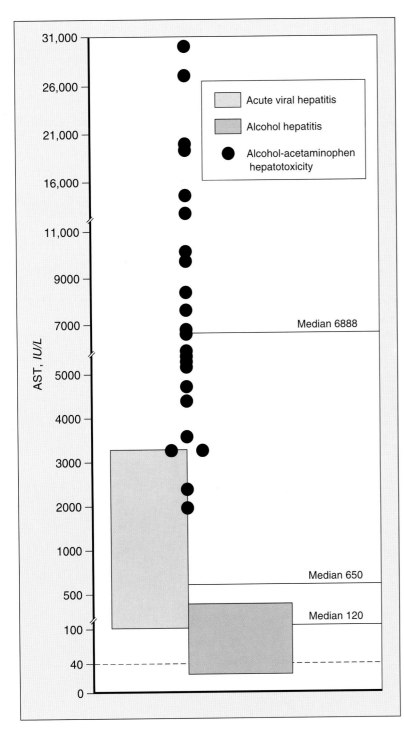

FIGURE 7-5.

Values for peak aspartate aminotransferase (AST) in patients with combined alcohol-acetaminophen toxicity. Strikingly elevated values are found in the alcohol-acetaminophen syndrome, in distinction to those seen in viral hepatitis (median 650) or alcoholic hepatitis (median 120). AST values above 4000 IU/L are seen almost exclusively in this condition and only rarely in viral hepatitis or ischemic hepatic injury (following cardiac arrest or congestive heart failure). Similar values may be observed in suicidal acetaminophen ingestions. (*Adapted from* Seeff *et al.* [17]; with permission.)

TABLE 7-3. DRUGS IMPLICATED IN IDIOSYNCRATIC LIVER INJURY LEADING TO ACUTE LIVER FAILURE

INFREQUENT BUT NOT RARE	RARE	COMBINATION AGENTS WITH ENHANCED TOXICITY
Isoniazid	Carbamazepine	Alcohol-acetaminophen
Valproate	Ofloxacin	Trimethoprim-sulfamethoxazole
Halothane	Ketoconazole	Rifampicin-isoniazid
Phenytoin	Lisinopril	Amoxicillin-clavulanic acid
Sulfonamides	Nicotinic acid	
Propylthiouracil	Labetalol	
Amiodarone	Etoposide (VP-16)	
Disulfiram	Imipramine	
Dapsone	α-Interferon	
	Flutamide	

TABLE 7-3.

Virtually every drug has been implicated at one time or another as the cause of acute liver injury, but there are also many drugs that have never been associated and still others in which the occasional occurrence of significant liver damage is well known. Frequency of such reactions may vary from one in 100 patients with isoniazid to one in 10,000 patients with halothane and rarer with many other compounds. Implicating a drug requires that the physician make a careful listing of the drugs being taken by the patient, the time period involved, and the quantity ingested. Most examples of hepatotoxicity occur within the first 4 to 8 weeks of beginning use. Combination agents often have enhanced toxicity in comparison to that experienced with either agent alone.

PHYSICAL AND LABORATORY FEATURES

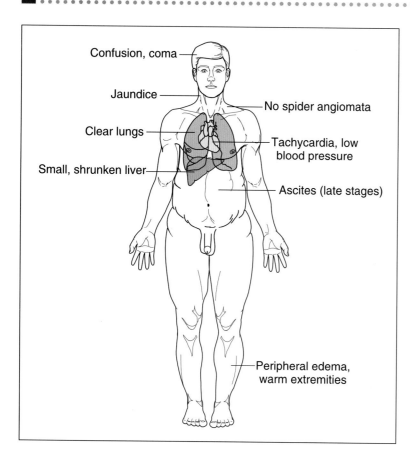

Confusion, coma

Jaundice

Clear lungs

Small, shrunken liver

No spider angiomata

Tachycardia, low blood pressure

Ascites (late stages)

Peripheral edema, warm extremities

FIGURE 7-6.

Basic physical findings in acute liver failure. Typical features observed in the patient with acute liver failure include confusion, agitation, or even hallucination. Mental status often deteriorates to coma soon after presentation, making history-taking impossible. Most patients will be icteric, although some barely so, and spider angiomata as seen in cirrhotic patients should be absent. Tachycardia, tachypnea, and relative hypotension are common. Asterixis, so commonly observed in chronic hepatic encephalopathy, is rarely seen. *Fetor hepaticus*, a sweet odor caused by mercaptans excreted in the breath, is often observed. Percussion over the rib cage to detect hepatic dullness reveals that the liver span is considerably decreased, and there may be no dullness appreciated, as evidence of the loss of hepatic mass. At autopsy, the normal liver mass of approximately 1600 g may be reduced to as little as 600 g. Edema is not observed initially but may develop in the hospital. Although the extremities are often cold, after resuscitation "warm shock" is the rule.

TABLE 7-4. NORMAL TESTS AND RESULTS ORDERED FOR PATIENTS WITH ACUTE LIVER FAILURE

COMPLETE BLOOD COUNT

Leukocyte count	Normal unless elevated because of infection
Hemoglobin/hematocrit	Normal unless gastrointestinal bleeding
Platelet count	Low in nearly 80%; frequently less than 100,000/mm^3

SERUM CHEMISTRIES

Sodium	Normal or low because of excess water intake
Potassium	Usually low because of renal loss of K$^+$
Chloride	Normal
Carbon dioxide	Low because of central hyperventilation
Blood urea nitrogen	Low
Glucose*	May be dangerously low, causing mental changes
Aspartate aminotransferase	Typically > 1000, may be > 10,000 IU/L
Alanine transaminase	Typically > 1000, may be > 10,000 IU/L
Albumin	Low because of poor synthetic function
Total protein	Low because of poor synthetic function; high globulins suggest chronicity
Ca^{++}	Low because of low albumin
PO$_4^-$	Often very low requiring replacement
Bilirubin	Typically high; less so in some hyperacute cases; very high in Wilson's disease because of hemolysis or in longstanding disease or renal failure
Alkaline phosphatase	Normal to slightly increased

COAGULATION STUDIES

Prothrombin time*	Typically at least 4 s prolonged
Partial thromboplastin time	Typically prolonged

ARTERIAL BLOOD GASSES

pH*	Often 7.5 or greater; acidosis a very bad sign
pCO$_2$ (partial pressure of carbon dioxide in the artery)	Low because of hyperventilation
pO$_2$ (partial pressure of oxygen in the artery)	Normal; low also a bad prognostic sign

VIRAL SEROLOGIES

Hepatitis A IgM	Positive only in acute hepatitis A cases
HBsAg	Positive in many different settings (see Table 7-3)
Hepatitis C antibody	Positive test may be seen; rarely causes acute liver failure
Hepatitis D antibody	Order in patients positive for HBsAg

TOXICOLOGY SCREENING TESTS

Acetaminophen*	Negative; when positive, quantitation useful
Ethanol	Negative; when positive, suspect other agents
Drug screen	Cocaine may cause acute liver failure; positive drug screen also indicates virus exposure (intravenous drug use confirmed)

OTHER ETIOLOGIC TESTS

Ceruloplasmin*	Should be strikingly low in Wilson's disease; otherwise low normal or normal

TABLE 7-4.

Normal tests and results ordered for patients with acute liver failure. Usually, these tests are requested by the clinician upon patient's admission to the hospital. Those marked with an *asterisk* are considered to be of utmost diagnostic importance. Initial emergency room tests should include measurement of prothrombin time, glucose, arterial blood gases, complete blood count, a toxicology screen, and a liver profile. Glucose should be given after blood is drawn in the patient with altered mental status until a clear etiology and blood glucose level are determined. HBsAg—hepatitis B surface antigen; IgM—immunoglobulin M.

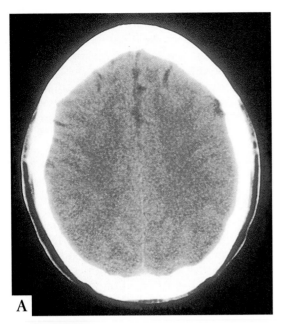

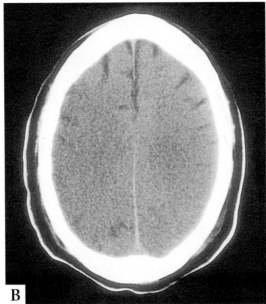

B, A similar section showing obliteration of gray and white matter demarcation caused by increased cerebral water. Obliteration of brain sulci is also seen but is a less consistent finding. Evidence of edema using CT is a late and inconstant finding in cerebral edema patients and thus is not a reliable guide to therapy. The presence of edema has two possible adverse effects. First, it decreases cerebral blood flow and may result in brain anoxia. The cerebral perfusion pressure (systemic blood pressure minus intracerebral pressure) should be maintained above 40 mm Hg to preserve adequate brain oxygenation. Second, herniation of the brain stem through the *falx cerebri* caused by cerebral edema is uniformly fatal. Erratic changes in blood pressure, temperature, or breathing pattern imply impending herniation.

FIGURE 7-7.

Cerebral edema on computerized tomographic (CT) scanning in a patient with acute liver failure. **A**, CT of a normal brain showing clear demarcation between gray and white matter.

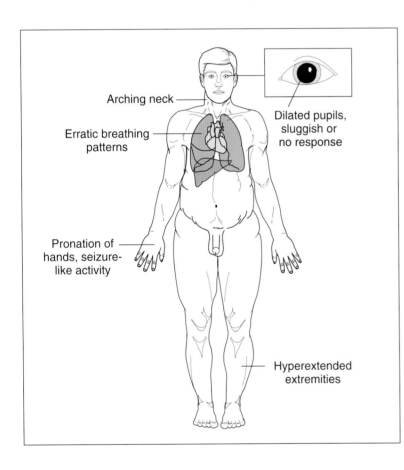

Arching neck

Dilated pupils, sluggish or no response

Erratic breathing patterns

Pronation of hands, seizure-like activity

Hyperextended extremities

FIGURE 7-8.

Physical findings in patients with advanced hepatic encephalopathy and cerebral edema. Typically, patients will experience a brief period of agitation before the development of coma. Hepatic coma is usually graded as I through IV—grade I is signified by altered personality and subtle changes in cognition; grade II typically demonstrates confusion, slurred speech, and possibly asterixis, but the patient remains able to follow commands; grade III is characterized by deepening coma responsive to strong stimuli with some purposeful movements; grade IV patients are totally unresponsive. Hyperventilation is universal in all stages of hepatic coma. In grade IV coma, decerebrate posturing, changes in breathing patterns, seizures, and pupillary abnormalities all occur in the presence of cerebral edema. These signs, alone or in association with systemic hypertension, warrant immediate intervention with mannitol and pursuit of transplantation, if available. Corticosteroids, hyperventilation, and use of phenobarbital, although recommended for head trauma patients to decrease cerebral edema, are of little benefit in acute liver failure. Diuretics have been used in addition to mannitol but are of uncertain value.

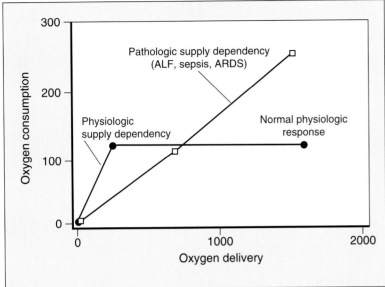

FIGURE 7-9.

Oxygen delivery curve. Patients with acute liver failure (ALF) develop a pathologic oxygen supply–dependency curve and extract oxygen over a wider range of delivery than normal. Hypoxia occurs in peripheral tissues frequently leading to lactic acidosis. Changes in peripheral oxygenation are poorly understood but appear to be the result of vasodilatation, low perfusion pressure caused by low systemic arterial pressure, platelet plugging of capillaries, and interstitial edema, all of which result in shunting of blood and subsequently, tissue hypoxia. The same abnormalities in oxygen delivery can be observed in adult respiratory distress syndrome (ARDS) and in sepsis. To optimize fluid intake in these patients, it is important to perform pulmonary artery pressure monitoring. Use of α-adrenergic agents is discouraged because it may worsen peripheral oxygen delivery. (*Adapted from* MacNaughton and Evans [29]; with permission.)

TABLE 7-5. RENAL PARAMETERS IN ACUTE LIVER FAILURE

CARDIAC CHANGES
Hypotension
High cardiac output
Low systemic vascular resistance
Tachycardia
Possible lactic acidosis

SERUM FACTORS ELEVATED
Renin
Aldosterone
Tumor necrosis factor$_\alpha$
Prostaglandins

URINE FINDINGS
Low urine volume
Low urinary sodium
Increased potassium
Increased urinary urobilinogen

Presence of high urinary volume suggests tubular necrosis

TABLE 7-5.

Massive changes in hemodynamics occur in acute liver failure and the exact mechanisms underlying these are unknown (*see* Fig. 7-9). In many respects, these patients resemble those with hepatorenal syndrome caused by advanced cirrhosis. Fluid deficits occur initially because of altered mental status leading to decreased per os intake, transudation of fluid into the extravascular space, and possibly gastrointestinal bleeding; most patients require extensive fluid resuscitation on hospital admission. Low systemic vascular resistance exacerbates this problem, and it is usually necessary to place a pulmonary artery catheter to properly assess fluid needs. Fluid replacement should emphasize colloid rather than crystalloid, although intravenous glucose may also be required for maintenance of satisfactory blood glucose levels. Diuretics should only be considered if intravascular volume has been fully restored and pulmonary or cerebral edema is a consideration. Direct renal toxicity is sometimes observed in acetaminophen overdose and will manifest as oliguria. Few patients die as a result of renal failure alone, but it often contributes to mortality (*see* Fig. 7-10).

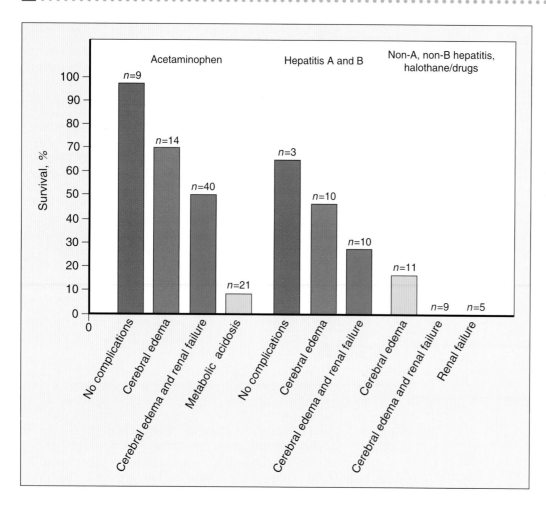

FIGURE 7-10.

Survival rates in acute liver failure correlate with the etiology and the number of complications present. Marked differences in survival are observed according to the underlying etiology determined on patient hospital admission. The level of coma is also a determinant of survival. Renal failure and metabolic acidosis, however, appear to be particularly ominous complications in all categories. (*Adapted from* O'Grady *et al.* [30]; with permission.)

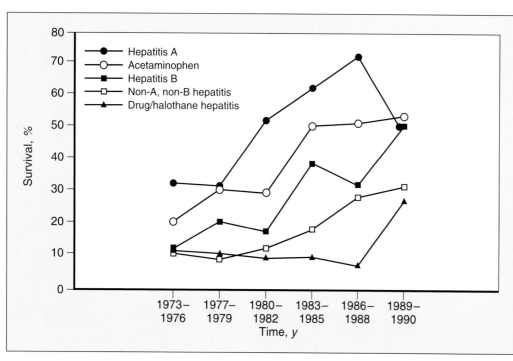

FIGURE 7-11.

Improvements in survival over 17 years, separated according to etiology. This graph depicts the survival rates of more than 750 patients admitted in grade III or IV coma to King's College Hospital in London over 17 years. Certain diagnoses are associated with good survival (hepatitis A, acetaminophen), whereas those patients with no discernible etiology or with idiosyncratic drug reaction fare particularly badly. Improvement in patient survival occurred in virtually every group—probably the result of improvement in the intensive care management of these critically ill patients. Because these results reflect the experience of a group dedicated to the care of acute liver failure, similar results may be difficult to obtain in the average community hospital. (*From* Hughes *et al.* [31]; with permission.)

TREATMENT

TABLE 7-6. INEFFECTIVE TREATMENTS FOR ACUTE LIVER FAILURE

Corticosteroid therapy	Spouse cross-perfusions	Dialysis and activated charcoal
Exchange transfusions	Heparin infusions	Insulin or glucagon infusions
Pig cross-perfusions	Hemodialysis and hemoperfusions	Prostaglandin infusions
Total body washout with saline (cardiopulmonary bypass)	Charcoal hemoperfusion	

TABLE 7-6.

In most instances, heroic measures have been used with little success. In each, initial reports of successful patient recovery gave encouragement for further use, although later controlled trials failed to show any efficacy. Professor Jean-Pierre Benhamou stated in 1972 that "...authors tend to publish isolated cases with a favorable outcome attributed to a given therapy, but not to publish cases in which therapy has failed. In fact it might be argued that the best future one can wish for a sufferer from SAHF [acute liver failure] is to undergo a new treatment and have his case published—'be published or perish!'"[3]. This advice is still good today and should provide a word of caution to those physicians who wish to promote new forms of treatment.

TABLE 7-7. NEW THERAPIES IN VARIOUS STAGES OF TESTING

ORTHOTOPIC TRANSPLANTATION
May be very effective; problems are related to logistics and timing

AUXILIARY HETEROTOPIC TRANSPLANTATION
Used as a temporary bridge while the native liver recovers

HEPATOCYTE TRANSPLANTATION
Still in experimental stage in animals; cells may be infused into the peritoneum or splenic pulp and take up some liver function until they are rejected by the host

EXTRACORPOREAL LIVER ASSIST DEVICES
A variety of columns or cartridges employing living hepatocytes from other species or tissue culture lines hold promise for providing temporary liver support without committing the patient to life-long immunosuppression

HEPATOCYTE GROWTH FACTORS
A number of growth factors have been identified that might aid hepatic regeneration; preliminary studies do not show significant efficacy

TABLE 7-7.

A variety of new therapies have been introduced and are in various stages of testing. Orthotopic liver transplantation is now considered the accepted treatment for acute liver failure. However, only approximately 10% of all patients receive transplantations as a result of logistic problems, including late arrival in hospital because of failure to recognize the severity of the problem, difficulty in transporting the patient to a transplantation center, and failure to obtain an organ donor within a suitable time. Furthermore, transplantation is costly and carries with it the problems of life-long immunosuppression for a condition that may well be self-limited. Patients who recover from acute liver failure usually do so completely. Therefore, other less drastic modes are more preferable if safe and effective. For example, auxiliary heterotopic transplantations, which provide the placement of a graft elsewhere in the abdomen without removal of the native liver, may serve as a temporary bridge, thus allowing liver support for 4 to 6 months as the native liver recovers (see Fig. 7-12). In the absence of successful immunosuppression, the transplanted organ will eventually be rejected. Partial organ transplants, in which a left or right lobe is replaced in the orthotopic position, may also enable liver function to occur for several months until the patient's own liver returns to normal function. This form of transplant, similar to auxiliary heterotopic grafts, would not require life-long immunosuppression. Extracorporeal liver-assist devices, consisting of columns or cartridges employing living hepatocytes from other species or tissue culture lines, hold promise for providing temporary liver support as well. Initially seen as a bridge to transplantation, these machines may allow time for hepatic regeneration and thus obviate the need for transplantation.

By contrast, hepatocyte transplantation is still in the early experimental stages in animals. With this form of treatment, liver cells are infused into the peritoneum or splenic pulp and can be shown to take up some liver functions until they are rejected by the host. Similarly, several hepatocyte growth factors have been identified that may aid in hepatic regeneration; however, preliminary studies do not show significant efficacy. Because growth factor levels tend to be elevated in acute liver failure, the likelihood of real benefit is small.

TABLE 7-8. PROGNOSTIC CRITERIA FOR NONSURVIVAL AND CONSIDERATION OF LIVER TRANSPLANTATION (LIKELIHOOD OF SURVIVAL CONSIDERED TO BE <20%) AT KING'S COLLEGE HOSPITAL IN LONDON

ACETAMINOPHEN	PATIENTS WITHOUT ACETAMINOPHEN SYNDROME
pH < 7.3 (irrespective of grade of encephalopathy)	Prothrombin time > 100 s (irrespective of grade encephalopathy)
Prothrombin time > 100 s and serum creatinine > 300 µmol/L (> 3.4 mg/dL) in patients with grade III or IV encephalopathy	Any three of the following variables (irrespective of grade of encephalopathy) Age < 10 y or > 40 y Etiology hepatitis non-A, non-B, halothane hepatitis, idiosyncratic drug reactions Duration of jaundice before onset of encephalopathy > 7 d Prothrombin time 50 s Serum bilirubin > 300 µmol/L (17 mg/dL)

TABLE 7-8.

These criteria are the most widely used for the establishment of prognosis in acute liver failure and the need for transplantation. The discriminant function shown here was derived from the results achieved between 1973 and 1985 in 588 patients with grade III or IV coma evaluated at King's College Hospital in London.

Prognosis is clearly different between patients with acetaminophen overdose and those with other etiologies. Note that age, etiology, and duration of disease are all important prognostic factors in this condition. (*From* O'Grady *et al.* [32]; with permission.)

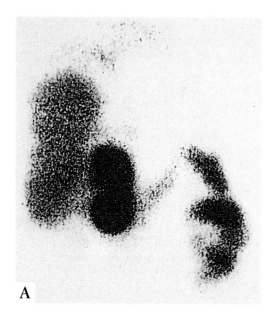
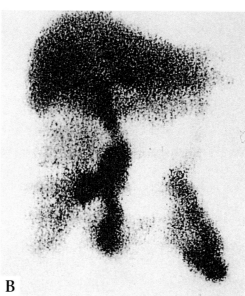

A   B

FIGURE 7-12.

Auxiliary heterotopic liver transplant. Diisopropyliminodiacetic acid (DISIDA) scintigraphy performed 1 and 6 months after auxiliary partial liver transplantation. At 1 month (**A**), uptake is achieved by the graft, whereas at 6 months (**B**), the regenerated host liver takes up the DISIDA and the auxiliary graft appears to have atrophied and virtually disappeared. This form of treatment employs a simpler operative procedure and the chance for full recovery of the native liver so that immunosuppression is not required in the long term. (*From* Metselaar *et al.* [33]; with permission.)

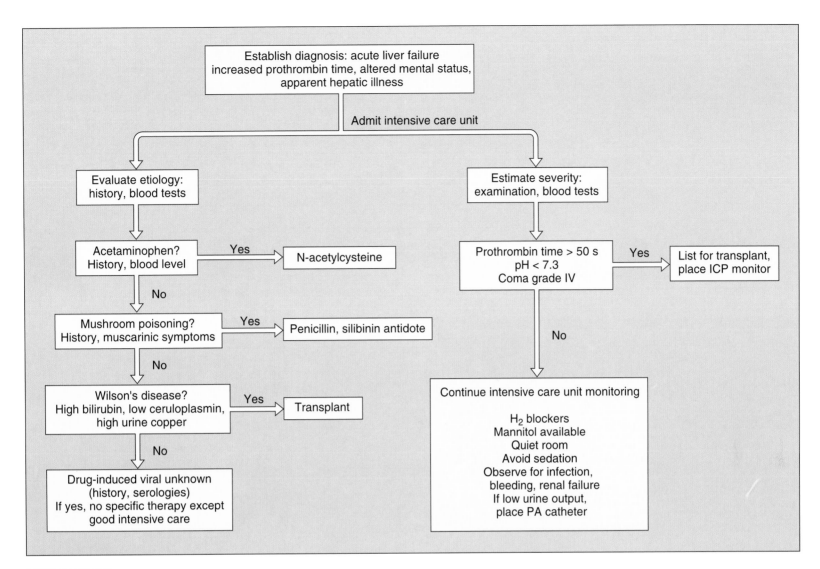

FIGURE 7-13.

Algorithm for triage, diagnosis, and treatment of the patient with acute liver failure. It is first necessary to perform the three E's—*establish* the diagnosis, *evaluate* the etiology, and *estimate* the severity of the illness. ICP—intracranial pressure; PA—pulmonary artery.

PATHOLOGIC FINDINGS

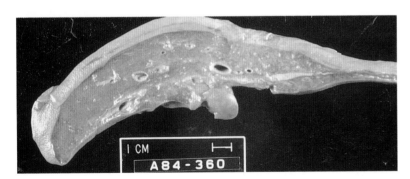

FIGURE 7-14.

Massive liver necrosis secondary to halothane anesthesia. This 55-year-old woman died 35 days after halothane anesthesia for a cholecystectomy. Twenty years prior, she had undergone a hysterectomy with halothane. The patient became ill 2 weeks after her surgery and became comatose 2 weeks later, never regaining consciousness. The liver was small and shrunken, with a wrinkled capsule, and weighed only 680 g (normal liver weight 1400–1600 g). This finding was formerly referred to as *acute yellow atrophy*.

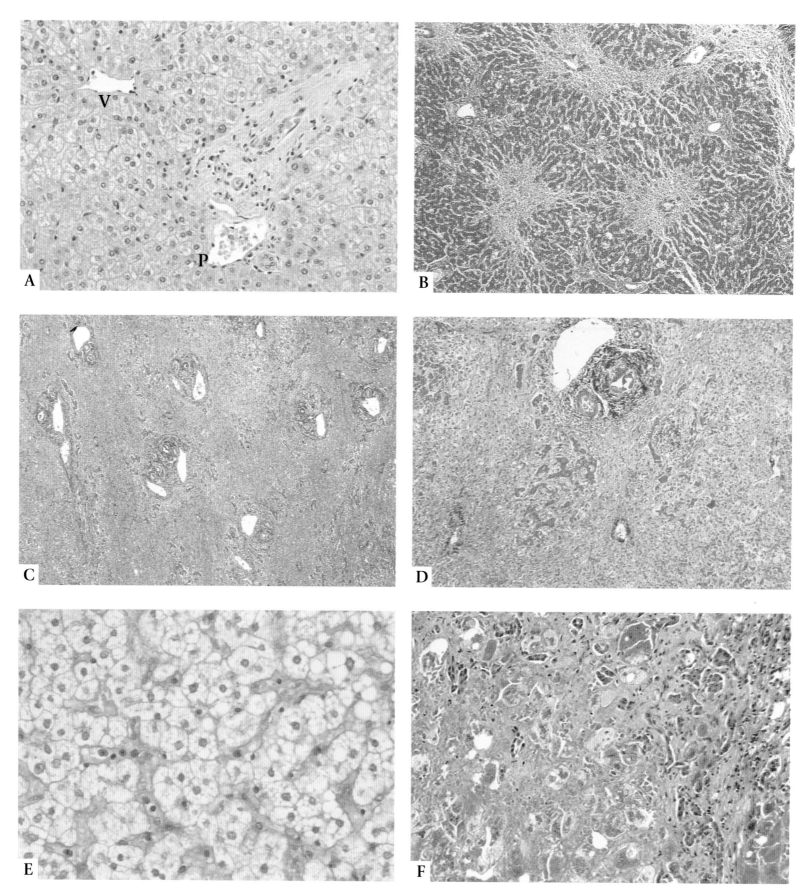

FIGURE 7-15.

Histologic findings in a selection of patients with acute liver failure. **A**, Normal liver for comparison. In this photomicrograph of a normal hepatic lobule, a portal tract (*P*) and hepatic venule (*V*) are highlighted. The liver cells appear uniform and cuboid in single-cell plates lining the sinusoids. Very few inflammatory cells are present and no signs of hepatocyte regeneration exist (hematoxylin and eosin, ×145). **B**, Autopsy specimen from a young girl who died of cerebral edema 7 days after an apparent acetaminophen ingestion. Moderately severe centrilobular necrosis is present but viable hepatocytes are seen in the periportal regions (hematoxylin and eosin, ×145). **C** and **D**, Massive hepatic necrosis caused by halothane. The patient (whose liver is shown in Fig. 7-14) died 35 days after a cholecystectomy during which she had

(Continued on next page)

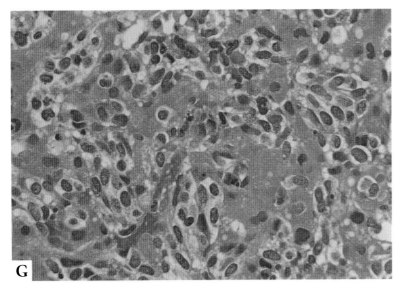

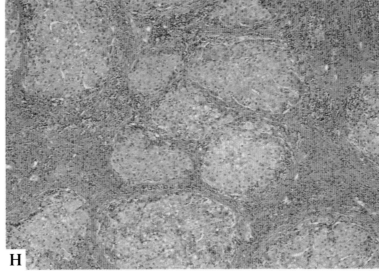

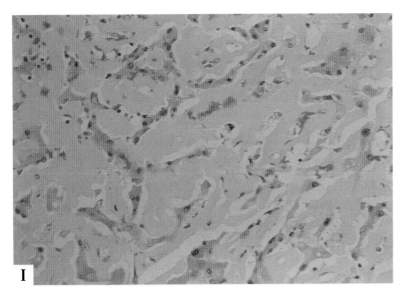

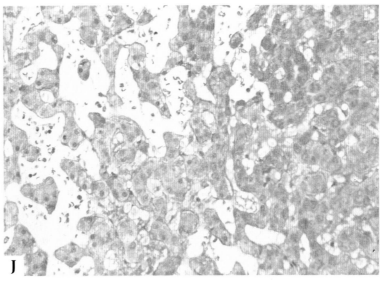

FIGURE 7-15. (CONTINUED)

received halothane anesthesia, probably representing her second exposure to the drug. Virtually the entire hepatic lobule appears necrotic with fibrinoid cellular debris interspersed between portal tracts that appear to be in close proximity because of massive collapse of the intervening hepatocytes (Masson's trichome, C, ×145, D, ×185). **E**, Reye's syndrome. This infant was admitted with liver failure shortly after developing an upper respiratory infection that was treated with aspirin. Massive infiltration of hepatocytes with microvesicular fat is seen as pale areas within cells. There is little inflammation or evidence of necrosis. The finding of microvesicular fat is characteristic of Reye's syndrome as well as of fatty liver of pregnancy and exposure to certain nucleoside analogues (fialuridine, didanosine, and possibly zidovudine) (hematoxylin and eosin, ×185). **F**, Wilson's disease. This autopsy photomicrograph is of a 16-year-old girl with a 2-week illness characterized by fatigue, confusion, and deep jaundice. Bilirubin level on admission to the hospital was 38 mg/dL, and she died on the 5th hospital day. Widespread hepatocyte necrosis and bile staining are present. There is evidence of some increased fibrosis and early cirrhosis in other sections. As in the halothane case, few remaining viable hepatocytes are seen (hematoxylin and eosin, ×185). **G**, Metastatic melanoma. This 58-year-old man presented with altered mental status, hepatomegaly, and jaundice 6 months after enucleation of

his right eye for melanoma. The sinusoids are packed with malignant cells that appear to contain pigment (melanin). Ischemic necrosis of hepatocytes is presumed to result from sinusoidal obstruction. Liver biopsy is indicated in fulminant hepatic failure if the liver is massively enlarged, thus suggesting an infiltrative process. Transplantation would be inappropriate here and biopsy would therefore clarify the diagnosis (hematoxylin and eosin, ×145). **H**, Advanced tuberculosis. This 63-year-old man presented with a febrile illness of 2 weeks' duration, accompanied by jaundice and obtundation. At autopsy, massive replacement of the liver by granulomas containing tubercle bacilli was present. The patient had no other associated illnesses (hematoxylin and eosin, ×145). **I**, Amyloidosis. Massive infiltration of the hepatic sinusoids with amyloid appears to displace hepatocytes and cause atrophy of cells (hematoxylin and eosin, ×185). **J**, Ischemic myocardiopathy causing ischemic necrosis of hepatocytes. This 54-year-old overweight man complained of fatigue and somnolence but was not found to be short of breath or in heart failure. Prothrombin time was 16 seconds, alanine transaminase was 1830 IU/L, serum ammonia was 135 mg/dL (normal < 30), and the ejection fraction was determined to be 16%. The centrilobular region shows dilated sinusoids and considerable necrosis of hepatocytes. His symptoms resolved with a cardiotonic regimen.

REFERENCES AND RECOMMENDED READING

1. Trey C, Davidson CS: The management of fulminant hepatic failure. In *Progress in Liver Diseases*. Edited by Popper H, Schaffner F. New York: Grune and Stratton; 1970:282.

2. Schalm SW, de Knegt RJ: Acute liver failure: Definitions and pathological variants. In *Acute Liver Failure: Improved Understanding and Better Therapy*. Edited by Williams R, Hughes RD. London: Miter Press; 1991:11–13.

3. Lee WM: Medical progress: Acute liver failure. *N Engl J Med* 1993, 329:1862–1874.

4. McCullough AJ, Fleming R, Thistle JL, *et al.*: Diagnosis of Wilson's disease presenting as fulminant hepatic failure. *Gastroenterology* 1983, 84:161–167.

5. Hoffman BJ, Pate MB, Marsh WH, Lee WM: Cardiomyopathy unrecognized as a cause of hepatic failure. *J Clin Gastroenterol* 1990, 12:306–309.

6. Silva MO, Roth D, Reddy KR, *et al.*: Hepatic dysfunction accompanying acute cocaine intoxication. *J Hepatol* 1991, 12:312–315.

7. Hodis HN: Acute hepatic failure associated with the use of low-dose sustained-release niacin. *JAMA* 1990, 264:181.

8. McDonald GB, Hinds MS, Fisher LD, *et al.*: Veno-occlusive disease of the liver and multi-organ failure after bone marrow transplantation: A cohort study of 355 patients. *Ann Intern Med* 1993, 118:255–267.

9. Rolfes DB, Ishak KG: Acute fatty liver of pregnancy: A clinicopathological study of 35 cases. *Hepatology* 1985, 5:1149–1158.

10. Ware AJ, D'Agostino AN, Combes B: Cerebral edema: A major complication of massive hepatic necrosis. *Gastroenterology* 1971, 61:877–884.

11. Williams R, Gimson AES: Intensive liver care and management of acute hepatic failure. *Dig Dis Sci* 1991, 36:820–826.

12. Anonymous: The brain in fulminant hepatic failure. *Lancet* 1991, 338:156–157.

13. Rolando N, Harvey F, Brahm J, *et al.*: Prospective study of bacterial infection in acute liver failure: An analysis of fifty patients. *Hepatology* 1990, 11:49–53.

14. Smilkstein MJ, Knapp GL, Kulig KW, Rumack BH: Efficacy of oral N-acetyl-cysteine in the treatment of acetaminophen overdose. *N Engl J Med* 1988, 319:1557–1562.

15. Harrison PM, Keays R, Bray GP, *et al.*:Improved outcome of paracetamol-induced fulminant hepatic failure by late administration of acetylcysteine. *Lancet* 1990, 335:1572–1573.

16. Licht H, Seeff LB, Zimmerman HJ: Apparent potentiation of acetaminophen hepatotoxicity by alcohol. *Ann Intern Med* 1980, 92:511–515.

17. Seeff LB, Cuccerina BA, Zimmerman HJ, *et al.*: Acetaminophen toxicity in alcoholics. *Ann Intern Med* 1986, 104:399–404.

18. Klein AS, Hart J, Brems JJ, *et al.*: *Amanita* poisoning: Treatment and the role of liver transplantation. *Am J Med* 1989, 86:187–193.

19. Fagan EA, Williams R: Fulminant viral hepatitis. *Br Med Bull* 1990, 45:462–480.

20. Canalese J, Gimson AES, Davis M, *et al.*: Controlled trial of dexamethasone and mannitol for the cerebral oedema of fulminant hepatic failure. *Gut* 1982, 23:625–629.

21. Macdougall B, Williams R: H$_2$ receptor antagonists in the prevention of acute upper gastro-intestinal hemorrhage in fulminant hepatic failure. *Gastroenterology* 1978, 74:464–465.

22. Bismuth H, Didier S, Gugenheim J, *et al.*: Emergency transplantation for fulminant hepatitis. *Ann Intern Med* 1987, 107:337–341.

23. Campbell DA, Ham JM, McCurry KR, *et al.*: Liver transplant for fulminant hepatitis. *Am Surg* 1991, 57:546–549.

24. Sussman NL, Chong MG, Koussayer T, *et al.*: Reversal of fulminant hepatic failure using an extracorporeal liver assist device. *Hepatology* 1992, 16:60–65.

25. Demetriou AA, Rozga J, Mosconi AD: Liver cell transplantation. In *Acute Liver Failure: Improved Understanding and Better Therapy*. Edited by Williams R, Hughes RD. London: Miter Press, 1991:66–69.

26. Metselaar HJ, Hesselink EJ, de Rave S, *et al.*: Recovery of failing liver after auxiliary heterotopic liver transplantation. *Lancet* 1990, 335:1156–1157.

27. Kaplowitz N: Drug metabolism and hepatotoxicity. In *Liver and Biliary Diseases*. Edited by Kaplowitz N. Baltimore: Williams & Wilkins; 1991:82–97.

28. Zimmerman HJ: The adverse effects of drugs on the liver. In *Hepatotoxicity*. New York: Appleton Century Crofts; 1978:289.

29. MacNaughton PD, Evans TW: Management of adult respiratory distress syndrome. *Lancet* 1992, 339:469–471.

30. O'Grady JG, Gimson AES, O'Brien CJ, *et al.*: Controlled trials of charcoal hemoperfusion and prognostic factors in fulminant hepatic failure. *Gastroenterology* 1988, 94:1186–1192.

31. Hughes RD, Wendon J, Gimson AES: Acute liver failure. *Gut* 1991, S86–S89.

32. O'Grady JG, Alexander GJM, Hayllar KM, Williams R: Early indicators of prognosis in fulminant hepatic failure. *Gastroenterology* 1989, 97:439–445.

33. Metselaar HJ, Hesselink EJ, de Rave S, *et al.*: Recovery of failing liver after auxiliary heterotopic liver transplantation. *Lancet* 1990, 335:1156–1157.

Chapter 8

Hemochromatosis and Wilson's Disease

BRUCE R. BACON

There are many similarities and some differences between the major disorders of iron overload (*ie*, hereditary hemochromatosis) and copper overload (*ie*, Wilson's disease). The liver plays an integral role in the whole body metabolism of both metals and is the principal organ affected when an excess of either metal is stored. Both hereditary hemochromatosis and Wilson's disease are inherited disorders and if diagnosed early, are fully treatable with prevention of long-term sequelae. Hereditary hemochromatosis is found in approximately one in 250 to 300 individuals, whereas Wilson's disease affects approximately one in 30,000 individuals. Both iron and copper overload affect organs other than the liver, but the distribution of the two metals differs with iron toxicity occurring primarily in the pancreas, heart, joints, and endocrine organs, whereas copper toxicity occurs in erythrocytes, kidneys, and the brain. The liver is the principal organ affected with overload by both metals; however, the mechanism by which the liver becomes overloaded differs. In hereditary hemochromatosis, the liver is the passive recipient of excess amounts of absorbed iron. In Wilson's disease, the genetic defect lies in a failure of biliary excretion of copper resulting in excess hepatic deposition. Although hepatic overload of both metals causes cirrhosis, there are many different hepatic responses to copper excess ranging from steatosis to chronic hepatitis to fulminant failure; with iron excess, the predominant pathology is portal fibrosis and cirrhosis. Patients with untreated hereditary hemochromatosis frequently develop hepatocellular cancer, but this development is a distinctly unusual finding in patients with Wilson's disease. This chapter highlights the major clinical, biochemical, histologic, and therapeutic aspects of hereditary hemochromatosis and Wilson's disease.

HEREDITARY HEMOCHROMATOSIS

History

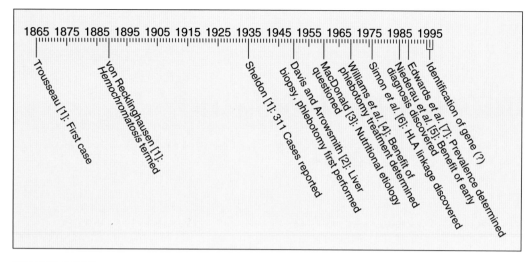

FIGURE 8-1.

History of hemochromatosis. Trousseau was the first to describe a case of hemochromatosis in the French pathology literature in 1865 [1]. In 1889, von Recklinghausen in the German literature, coined the term *hemochromatosis*, thinking that it was a blood disorder that caused pigmentation [1]. However, it was not until 1935 that Sir Wilfred Sheldon, a British gerontologist, published a monograph describing all 311 cases of the disease that were reported in the world's literature to that point, including several from his own records [1]. He concluded that hemochromatosis was an inborn error of iron metabolism and that all of the pathologic manifestations were caused by increased iron deposition.

Davis and Arrowsmith [2] performed the first liver biopsy on a patient with hemochromatosis and then treated the individual with aggressive phlebotomy. In the 1960s, a controversy developed when MacDonald [3] questioned the inherited nature of the disease, thinking instead that it was related to nutritional changes often associated with alcoholism. The benefits of phlebotomy were first shown by Williams and coworkers [4] in 1969 and were later confirmed by Niederau and coworkers [5] in 1985. The benefits of early diagnosis were also demonstrated in 1985 [5]. Simon and coworkers [6] demonstrated that the gene for hemochromatosis was linked to the HLA region on chromosome 6 in 1976. In a classic study screening 11,065 blood donors, Edwards and coworkers [7] demonstrated the high prevalence of the disease (one in 220), and it is anticipated that, over the next several years, the specific location of the gene will be identified and it will be cloned. Hopefully, this identification will lead to a genetic test rather than the phenotypic markers.

Classification

TABLE 8-1. CLASSIFICATION OF IRON OVERLOAD

Hereditary hemochromatosis

Secondary iron overload

   Anemia caused by ineffective erythropoiesis

   Liver disease

   Increased oral intake of iron

   Congenital atransferrinemia

Parenteral iron overload

Neonatal iron overload

African iron overload

TABLE 8-1.

Classification of iron overload syndromes. *Hereditary hemochromatosis* is the term used to describe individuals who have inherited two abnormal alleles for the hemochromatosis gene [1]. Individuals who absorb excess amounts of iron, as a result of some underlying cause other than the inherited defect, have secondary iron overload. There are many causes for secondary iron overload. Parenteral iron overload is always iatrogenic and comes from the administration of either iron-dextran injections or multiple transfusions of erythrocytes. Neonatal iron overload is a rare syndrome in which modest iron deposition in the neonatal liver results in a fatal outcome without transplant [8]. Finally, African iron overload is now thought to be a non-HLA–linked inherited form of iron loading that has been identified in sub-Saharan Africans [9,10]. It is exacerbated by the ingestion of beverages with a high iron content.

TABLE 8-2. PATHOGENETIC MECHANISMS

Genetic factors
  HLA associations A3 (B7,B14)
  Gene location, chromosome 6; frequency 5%
  Autosomal recessive
Pathophysiology
  Inappropriate gastrointestinal iron absorption
  2–4 mg/d; 1000 mg/y
  Clinical evidence of toxicity at >20 g total body iron stores

TABLE 8-2.

Pathogenetic mechanisms. The genetic factors in hereditary hemochromatosis indicate that it is an autosomal recessive disorder with the gene located on the short arm of chromosome 6. The gene frequency is 5% with the prevalence of homozygosity being approximately one in 250 with a heterozygote frequency of approximately one in 10 individuals. The disease is seen predominantly in white patients of Northern European descent. The inherited disorder results in an inappropriate gastrointestinal absorption of iron, and instead of the usual 1 to 2 mg/d, patients with hemochromatosis absorb 2 to 4 mg/d.

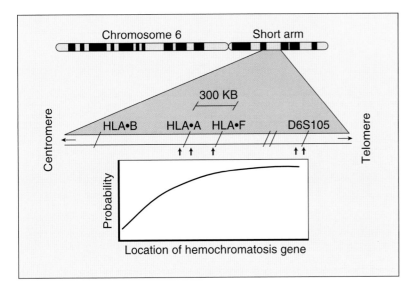

FIGURE 8-2.

The genetics of hereditary hemochromatosis. This schematic depicts chromosome 6. The small vertical *arrows* represent the areas within the chromosome where various laboratories are searching for the hemochromatosis gene. Current thought is that the most likely location for the hemochromatosis gene is near the D6S105 region.

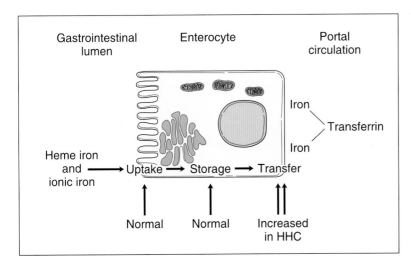

FIGURE 8-3.

Iron absorption in hereditary hemochromatosis (HHC). Iron absorption across the gastrointestinal mucosa is divided into phases called *uptake, storage,* and *transfer.* Iron absorption occurs predominantly in the duodenum and proximal jejunum. Both ionic and heme iron are found in the gastrointestinal lumen and uptake occurs across the mucosal surface of the enterocyte. Intracellular iron is found either in an intracellular transit pool of iron or in a storage compartment, both of which are poorly defined in the enterocyte. Transfer of iron from the serosal surface to the portal circulation (where it is picked up by apotransferrin) occurs by an unknown mechanism. In HHC, there is an increase in the transfer phase, suggesting that there may be an abnormal transport protein on the serosal surface of the enterocyte.

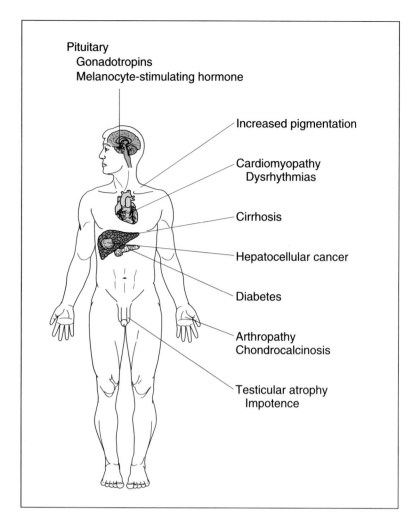

Pituitary
Gonadotropins
Melanocyte-stimulating hormone

Increased pigmentation

Cardiomyopathy
Dysrhythmias

Cirrhosis

Hepatocellular cancer

Diabetes

Arthropathy
Chondrocalcinosis

Testicular atrophy
Impotence

FIGURE 8-4.

Clinical manifestations of hereditary hemochromatosis. The clinical manifestations of hereditary hemochromatosis are protean. The most common abnormalities are found in the liver, and the development of hepatocellular carcinoma is 200 times more common in patients with untreated hemochromatosis than in the general population. In the 1990s, it is distinctly unusual to identify someone with the original triad of pigmentation, cirrhosis, and diabetes. With the advent of screening iron studies on routine chemistry panels, hemochromatosis is now often identified in asymptomatic individuals.

Clinical findings

TABLE 8-3. TYPICAL SYMPTOMS IN PATIENTS WITH HEREDITARY HEMOCHROMATOSIS

SYMPTOMS	OCCURRENCE, %
Weakness, lethargy, fatigue	40–85
Apathy, lack of interest	40–85
Abdominal pain	30–60
Weight loss	30–60
Arthralgias	40–60
Loss of libido, impotence	30–60
Amenorrhea	20–60
Congestive heart failure symptoms	0–40

TABLE 8-3.

Typical symptoms in patients with hereditary hemochromatosis. Despite the fact that many patients are now diagnosed before they develop symptoms, it is important to recognize the common characteristics that are exhibited in patients who are symptomatic, as listed in this table [11,12].

TABLE 8-4. COMMON PHYSICAL FINDINGS IN HEREDITARY HEMOCHROMATOSIS

FINDINGS	OCCURRENCE, %
Hepatomegaly	60–85
Cirrhosis	50–95
Skin pigmentation	40–80
Arthritis (second and third metacarpophalangeal joints)	40–60
Clinical diabetes	10–60
Splenomegaly	10–40
Loss of body hair	10–30
Testicular atrophy	10–30
Dilated cardiomyopathy	0–30

TABLE 8-4.

Common physical findings in hereditary hemochromatosis. As more patients are identified before developing symptoms, they may not have physical findings or they may be limited to the development of hepatomegaly. It is unusual to see someone with end-stage manifestations of liver or heart disease in the 1990s.

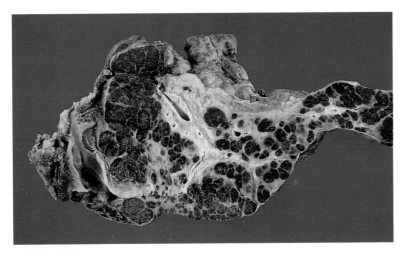

FIGURE 8-5.

Gross specimen of cirrhosis of the liver. The most serious manifestation of hereditary hemochromatosis is the development of cirrhosis of the liver. This figure is an example of a cirrhotic liver taken at the time of transplantation.

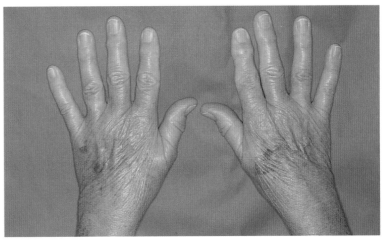

FIGURE 8-6.

The hands of a 63-year-old woman with newly diagnosed hereditary hemochromatosis. The manifestations to be noted here are increased pigmentation and the typical arthropathy with joint swelling at the second and third metacarpophalangeal joints.

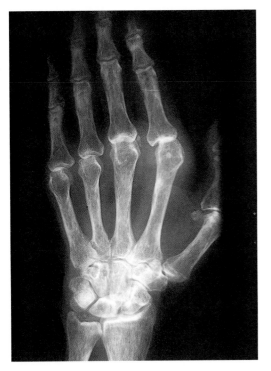

FIGURE 8-7.

Radiograph of a hand showing typical arthritis of hereditary hemochromatosis. Joint space narrowing and sclerotic changes can be seen in the second and third metacarpophalangeal joints.

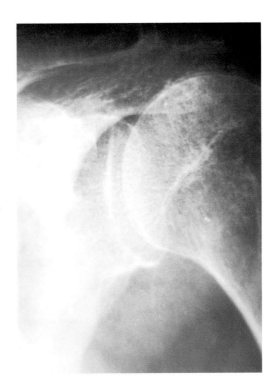

FIGURE 8-8.

Shoulder radiograph. The other arthritic changes seen in hereditary hemochromatosis are the development of chondrocalcinosis or pseudogout. This condition is depicted in this radiograph from a patient with hemochromatosis.

Diagnosis

TABLE 8-5. REPRESENTATIVE IRON MEASUREMENTS

	NORMAL	HEREDITARY HEMOCHROMATOSIS
Serum iron, μg/dL	50–150	180–300
Transferrin, mg/dL	250–370	200–300
Transferrin saturation, %	20–50	80–100
Serum ferritin, ng/mL		
Men	20–300	500–6000
Women	15–250	500–6000

TABLE 8-5.

Once the clinician's suspicion is aroused by symptoms and physical findings discussed previously, iron studies should be obtained to determine if any phenotypic expression of the disease exists. Increased transferrin saturation is the most specific abnormality, and a combination of increased transferrin saturation and increased ferritin is both highly specific and highly sensitive. The serum iron concentration is subject to a diurnal variation and is also increased following meals; therefore, iron studies are best obtained in the morning when patients are fasting. All patients with either an elevated transferrin saturation or an elevated ferritin should be further evaluated for hemochromatosis [7].

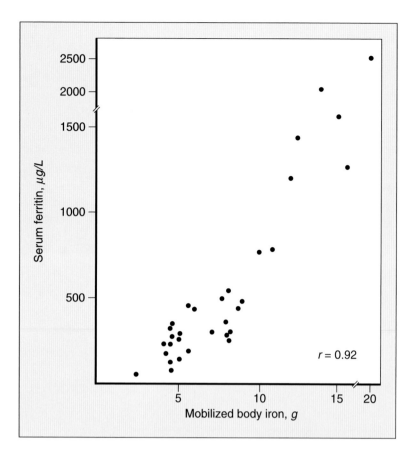

FIGURE 8-9.

Serum ferritin versus mobilized body iron stores. In patients with uncomplicated hemochromatosis, the serum ferritin level directly relates to the total body iron burden. This concept is illustrated here where ferritin measurements were taken and plotted against total body iron burden, determined retrospectively by quantitative phlebotomy. In patients with necroinflammatory liver disease (*eg,* viral hepatitis, alcoholic liver disease, and nonalcoholic steatohepatitis), the serum ferritin level can be elevated as a result of release of tissue ferritin into the circulation. In this setting, serum ferritin levels are not representative of total body iron stores. (*From* Bassett *et al.* [13]; with permission.)

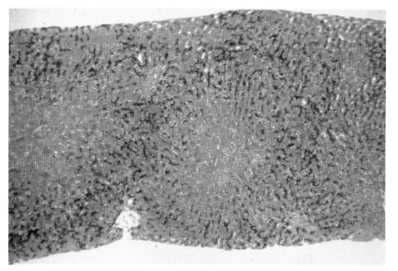

FIGURE 8-10.

A liver biopsy specimen shown at low power. The liver biopsy procedure is essential to establish the diagnosis of hemochromatosis. Histochemical staining with Perls' Prussian blue reagent stains storage iron blue against the counterstain which is red. Shown here is a liver biopsy specimen from a 34-year-old man with newly diagnosed hereditary hemochromatosis. At low power, the iron deposition is seen predominantly in a periportal distribution.

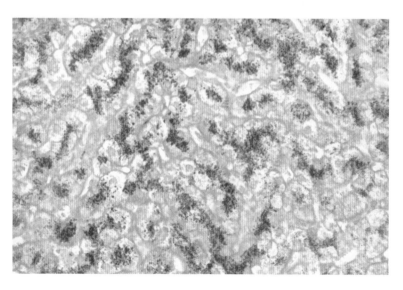

FIGURE 8-11.

A liver biopsy specimen shown at high power. At higher power, it is apparent that all iron deposition is in hepatocytes with little or none in reticuloendothelial cells (Kupffer cells). The hepatic iron concentration from this biopsy was 17,350 µ/g dry weight.

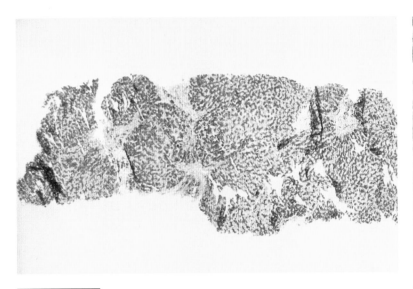

FIGURE 8-12.

A liver biopsy specimen at low power. This figure demonstrates a Perls' Prussian blue stain of a liver biopsy specimen taken from a 60-year-old man with hereditary hemochromatosis. The hepatic iron concentration is 41,040 µ/g dry weight.

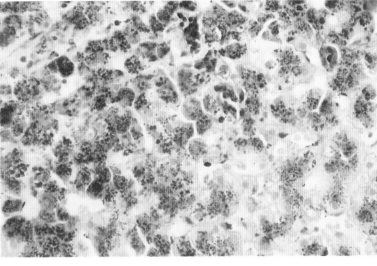

FIGURE 8-13.

A liver biopsy specimen at high power. At higher power, this figure shows that at higher iron concentration (same specimen as in Fig. 8-12) most of the iron deposition is still in hepatocytes.

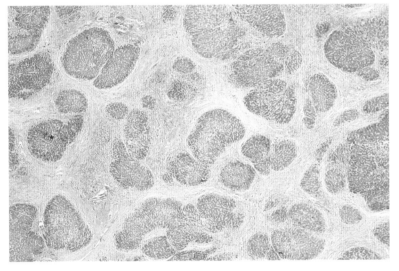

FIGURE 8-14.

A liver biopsy specimen of cirrhosis. When untreated, hemochromatosis can progress to the development of micronodular cirrhosis. This Masson trichrome stain at low power demonstrates broad fibrous bands in this explant liver from a patient who had successful liver transplantation.

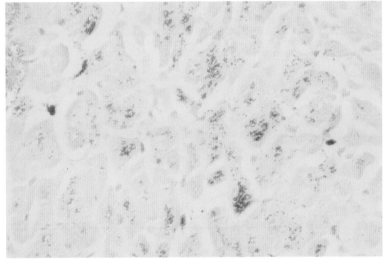

FIGURE 8-15.

A heart with Perls' stain. Iron deposition in the heart shown in a patient who was not known to have hemochromatosis before death. Iron deposition was found in subendocardial myocytes.

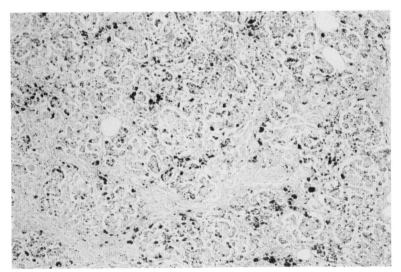

FIGURE 8-16.

A pancreas with Perls' stain. In the same patient whose heart is shown in Figure 8-15, the pancreas was also heavily iron loaded as demonstrated on this Perls' stain of a section from the pancreas. Iron deposition is predominantly found in acinar cells.

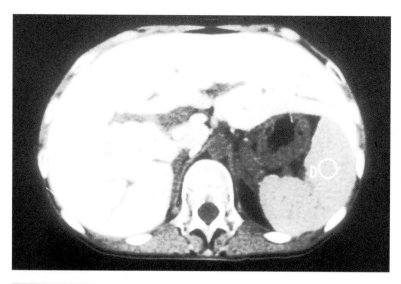

FIGURE 8-17.

Computed tomographic scan. A noninvasive means for detecting hepatic iron deposition has been sought for many years. Hepatic density measured on computed tomographic scanning can be helpful in heavily iron-loaded individuals, where the image of the iron-loaded liver has the same (or greater) density of bone, as shown here. Unfortunately, the reliability of this method is poor, especially in mild-to-moderate iron overload.

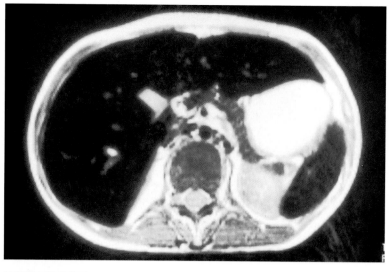

FIGURE 8-18.

Magnetic resonance imaging scan. Magnetic resonance imaging can be used to identify a markedly iron-loaded liver in patients with hemochromatosis. Again, magnetic resonance imaging is only useful in heavily loaded patients and does not replace performance of percutaneous liver biopsy for histochemical staining and biochemical determination of hepatic iron concentration.

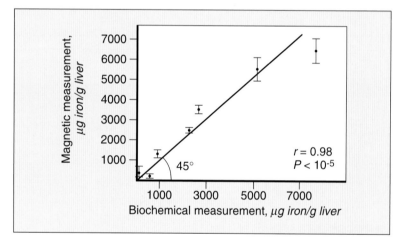

FIGURE 8-19.

Magnetic susceptibility in hemochromatosis. In research laboratories in Cleveland and Germany [14], magnetic susceptibility testing has been demonstrated to show excellent correlation with biochemical iron determination from biopsy samples. This technique uses a superconducting quantum interference device and is used as a research tool. (*From* Brittenham *et al.* [14]; with permission.)

Differential diagnosis

TABLE 8-6. DEVELOPMENT OF HEPATIC IRON INDEX

Distinguish patients with hereditary hemochromatosis from patients with alcoholic liver disease and secondary iron overload

Distinguish homozygotes from heterozygotes

Progressive increase in iron in homozygotes with age

TABLE 8-6.

Development of hepatic iron index. When biochemical iron determinations are performed on liver tissue obtained during liver biopsy, elevated levels can be found in young and old homozygotes, in some heterozygotes, and in patients who have alcoholic liver disease with mild secondary iron overload. In the latter two situations, iron concentration does not progressively increase with age as it does in patients with homozygous hereditary hemochromatosis. The hepatic iron index was developed in 1986 [15], based on the principle that hepatic iron concentration progressively increased in homozygotes with increasing age. It has been used to distinguish patients with hereditary hemochromatosis from patients with alcoholic liver disease and secondary iron overload, and it has been used to distinguish homozygotes from heterozygotes.

TABLE 8-7. EQUATIONS FOR CALCULATION OF HEPATIC IRON INDEX

μg iron/g dry liver / 56 = μmol iron/g dry liver

Hepatic iron index = μmol iron/g dry liver / age, y

TABLE 8-7.

Calculation of hepatic iron index. Hepatic iron concentration results are reported as μg of iron/g of dry liver. To calculate the hepatic iron index, it is necessary to take the value of the hepatic iron concentration and divide by the molecular weight of iron (which is 56) to yield the μmol of iron/g of dry liver. The hepatic iron index is then this number divided by the patient's age in years.

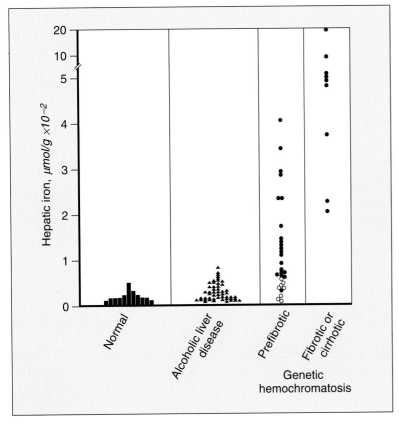

FIGURE 8-20.

Hepatic iron concentration. This figure compares the hepatic iron concentrations for four groups of patients: normal controls, patients with alcoholic liver disease, patients with prefibrotic hemochromatosis, and patients with fibrosis and cirrhosis caused by hemochromatosis. In the third panel, *open circles* represent heterozygotes, and *closed circles* represent homozygotes. There is overlap between some heterozygotes, some homozygotes, and patients with alcoholic liver disease. (*From* Bassett *et al.* [15]; with permission.)

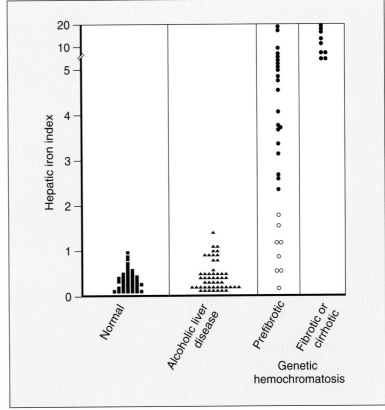

FIGURE 8-21.

Hepatic iron index. The hepatic iron index has been calculated by dividing the hepatic iron concentration (shown in Figure 8-20) by the patient's age in years. All patients with homozygous hereditary hemochromatosis, whether prefibrotic or not, have an hepatic iron index greater than 2, and all normal individuals, patients with alcoholic liver disease, and heterozygotes have an hepatic iron index less than 2. (*From* Bassett *et al.* [15]; with permission.)

TABLE 8-8. HEPATIC IRON INDEX IN HEMOCHROMATOSIS

TABLE 8-8.

Study	Normal	Alcoholic liver disease	Heterozygotes	Homozygotes
Bassett *et al.* [15]	< 1.0	< 1.4	< 1.8	> 2.0
Summers *et al.* [16]	—	—	< 1.5	> 1.9
Olynyk *et al.* [17]	< 1.1	< 1.6	—	> 2.1
Bonkovsky *et al.* [19]	< 0.7	< 1.1	< 1.8	> 2.0
Sallie *et al.* [18]	—	< 1.6	—	> 2.0
Deugnier *et al.* [20]	—	—	< 1.5	> 1.9

There have now been at least six studies evaluating the hepatic iron index in patients with hemochromatosis. In patients with alcoholic liver disease and in heterozygotes, the hepatic iron index was always less than 1.8. In contrast, in homozygotes, the hepatic iron index was always greater than 1.9. Four of these six studies were from Australia [15–18], one was from the United States [19], and one was a combined French and Australian study [20]. In my personal experience, approximately 10% of patients with hereditary hemochromatosis (identified by shared HLA haplotype with a proband) can have an hepatic iron index less than 1.9.

TABLE 8-9. TREATMENT OF HEREDITARY HEMOCHROMATOSIS

1-U Phlebotomy = 250 mg iron

Weekly phlebotomy until hematocrit ↓

Ferritin < 50 ng/mL; transferrin saturation < 50%

TABLE 8-9.

After the diagnosis of hereditary hemochromatosis has been fully established by liver biopsy with determination of hepatic iron concentration and calculation of hepatic iron index, therapy should be initiated. Treatment is with weekly or biweekly phlebotomy of 1 unit of whole blood (500 mL). Regular, aggressive phlebotomy should be continued until the hematocrit drops below 35%. Periodic measurement of ferritin and transferrin saturation is useful to predict the return to normal iron stores. Each unit of blood contains approximately 250 mg of iron; thus, after a phlebotomy program is completed, a retrospective determination of the total body iron burden can be made. Maintenance phlebotomy requirements should be individualized, but usually consist of a 1-U phlebotomy every 2 to 4 months.

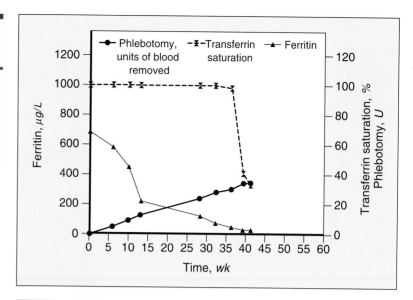

FIGURE 8-22.

Iron studies with phlebotomy therapy. Typically, with cumulative phlebotomies, the ferritin level decreases gradually, but the transferrin saturation does not drop until patients become either normal or almost iron deficient.

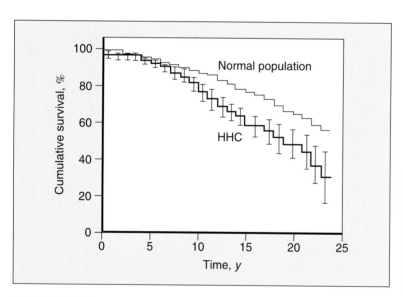

FIGURE 8-23.

Hereditary hemochromatosis (HHC) survival rates. In a large German study, Niederau and coworkers [5] showed that the cumulative survival rate for patients with HHC was less than that of an age- and gender-matched German population. (*From* Niederau *et al.* [5]; with permission.)

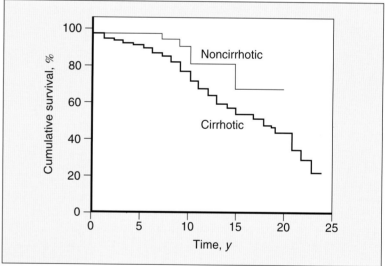

FIGURE 8-24.

Hereditary hemochromatosis: survival with cirrhosis. When Niederau and coworkers [5] looked at the presence or absence of cirrhosis as related to cumulative survival rates, it was determined that decreased survival was related to cirrhosis. (*From* Niederau *et al.* [5]; with permission.)

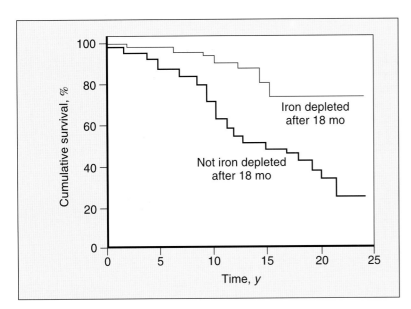

FIGURE 8-25.

Survival in hereditary hemochromatosis versus iron removal. When the total amount of excess iron could be removed within 18 months (indicating less severe iron overload), the survival was equivalent to the control population. However, when the iron burden was such that the excess iron could not be removed within 18 months of phlebotomy therapy, survival was decreased. These heavily iron-loaded patients also presented with cirrhosis and diabetes. (*From* Niederau *et al.* [5]; with permission.)

Family screening

TABLE 8-10. SCREENING REGIMEN FOR PRECLINICAL DISEASE (HEREDITARY HEMOCHROMATOSIS)

Serum iron, transferrin saturation, and serum ferritin should be tested in all first-degree relatives of proband

If any one is abnormal, a liver biopsy should be performed for stainable and biochemical iron

If two HLA haplotypes are shared with proband, then screening should be performed yearly

TABLE 8-10.

After therapy is initiated for the proband, it should be remembered that hemochromatosis is an inherited disease and screening should be performed on all first-degree relatives. Screening studies should include measuring serum iron, transferrin saturation, and ferritin levels. If any of these are abnormal, a liver biopsy should be performed for histochemical staining and biochemical iron determination. HLA studies are only useful to evaluate siblings of an affected proband or when performing pedigree analysis. HLA studies should not be used in individual patients.

WILSON'S DISEASE

History

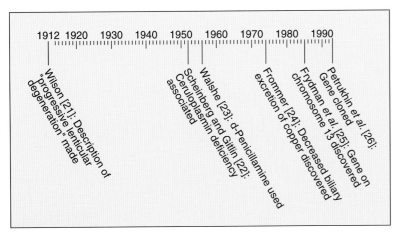

FIGURE 8-26.

History of Wilson's disease. The first description of Wilson's disease was published in 1912 as a case of "progressive lenticular

degeneration" by the British neurologist, Kinnear Wilson [21]. Occasional descriptions of the disease appeared over the years, but it was not until 1952 that Scheinberg and Gitlin [22] demonstrated a deficiency in ceruloplasmin in patients with Wilson's disease. Shortly after, in 1956, Walshe [23] demonstrated the beneficial effects of the copper chelating drug, d-penicillamine. In 1974, Frommer [24] provided evidence of decreased biliary excretion of copper, and in 1985, Frydman and coworkers [25], using linkage studies, demonstrated that the gene was on chromosome 13. Finally, Petrukhin and coworkers [26] cloned the gene and went on to demonstrate that the gene encodes a membrane spanning protein that contains copper-binding regions and P-type ATPase motifs with similarity to other heavy metal transport proteins. It is suggested that the transport protein inhibits the entry of copper into biliary excretory pathways either by reducing copper flux across lysosomal membranes or by acting directly at the bile canaliculus. Eventually, it is expected that this knowledge will lead to a genetic test for Wilson's disease.

Pathophysiology

TABLE 8-11.

TABLE 8-11. WILSON'S DISEASE PATHOPHYSIOLOGY

Chromosome 13

Copper transport protein

Decreased hepatic excretion of copper into bile

Pathophysiology of Wilson's disease. The gene has been specifically localized to chromosome 13 and has been found to code for a copper transport protein with homology to the abnormal gene responsible for Menke's disease. The abnormal gene results in decreased hepatic excretion of copper into bile either because of a defect at the lysosomal membrane or because of a defect in transporting copper across the cell membrane into bile.

Clinical features

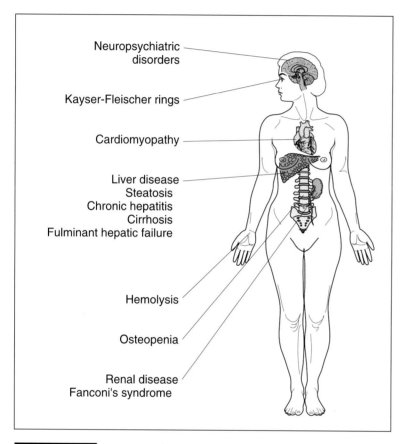

Neuropsychiatric disorders

Kayser-Fleischer rings

Cardiomyopathy

Liver disease
Steatosis
Chronic hepatitis
Cirrhosis
Fulminant hepatic failure

Hemolysis

Osteopenia

Renal disease
Fanconi's syndrome

FIGURE 8-27.

Clinical manifestations of Wilson's disease. There are numerous clinical manifestations of Wilson's disease including the presence of Kayser-Fleischer rings. Many psychiatric symptoms and disorders are typical of Wilson's disease. Rarely, cardiomyopathy ensues. All patients with Wilson's disease have hepatic involvement that can range from fairly mild steatosis to the insidious development of cirrhosis or the often fatal fulminant hepatic failure. The renal disease that occurs in Wilson's disease is comparable with that seen in Fanconi's syndrome. Hemolysis is caused by copper toxicity; many patients have significant osteopenia [21,27,28].

FIGURE 8-28.

Kayser-Fleischer rings. This young man has classical Kayser-Fleischer rings, identified as the golden-brown pigment deposits in Descemet's membrane in the periphery of the iris. These rings can be seen with the naked eye, but occasionally, a slit-lamp examination is necessary to identify them. Another unusual ophthalmologic manifestation of Wilson's disease is sunflower cataracts.

TABLE 8-12. NEUROLOGIC PRESENTATION OF WILSON'S DISEASE

Personality disturbances
Tremor
Dystonia
Choreic movements
Hypokinesis, drooling

TABLE 8-12.

There are several characteristic neurologic findings in Wilson's disease, which are only manifested after someone has presented with cirrhosis, and so the presence of these neurologic abnormalities with liver disease should prompt the physician to consider a diagnosis of Wilson's disease. Subtle personality changes are often difficult to identify in adolescents and young adults. Tremor, dystonic, and choreic movements are more profound manifestations and should lead to a quick evaluation.

TABLE 8-13. HEPATIC PRESENTATION OF WILSON'S DISEASE

Steatosis
Chronic hepatitis
Cirrhosis
Fulminant hepatic failure

TABLE 8-13.

Most patients with symptomatic Wilson's disease present with cirrhosis that has developed insidiously. All young individuals who present with abnormal liver enzymes and either have chronic hepatitis or hepatic steatosis should have a serum ceruloplasmin level measured to screen for Wilson's disease. Rarely, patients present with fulminant hepatic failure; this presentation is uniformly fatal without transplantation.

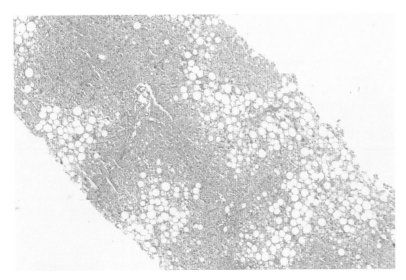

FIGURE 8-29.

Hepatic steatosis. This liver biopsy specimen shows macro- and microvesicular steatosis that can be seen in Wilson's disease. These are early manifestations and patients are more likely to present with cirrhosis.

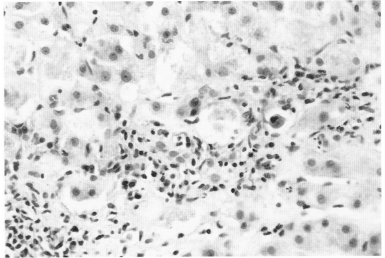

FIGURE 8-30.

This figure shows chronic active hepatitis with piecemeal necrosis and parenchymal inflammation. Some studies have suggested that as many as 25% of young individuals with nonviral chronic hepatitis have Wilson's disease.

TABLE 8-14. INDICATIONS FOR TESTING IN DIAGNOSIS OF WILSON'S DISEASE

Liver disease in children and young adults

Neurologic disease in adolescents and young adults

Hemolysis with liver disease

Presence of Fanconi's syndrome

Presence of hypouricemia

Kayser-Fleischer rings discovered

Siblings of affected patient

TABLE 8-14.

Because Wilson's disease is relatively rare (1 in 30,000 individuals), a high index of suspicion is necessary to make the diagnosis. Therefore, diagnosis should be considered in all children, adolescents, and young adults who have either liver disease or neurologic disease. In patients with liver disease complicated by hemolysis or Fanconi's syndrome, Wilson's disease should also be considered. Finally, hypouricemia can be a tip-off to Wilson's disease. All siblings of affected patients should be tested [21,27,28].

TABLE 8-15. DIAGNOSIS OF WILSON'S DISEASE

Serum ceruloplasmin

Urinary copper

Hepatic copper

Hepatic histology

Glucosuria, hemolysis

TABLE 8-15.

Diagnosis of Wilson's disease. Once clinical suspicion is raised, a serum ceruloplasmin level should be obtained. It must be remembered that approximately 15% of patients with Wilson's disease have ceruloplasmin levels within the lower limit of normal. Twenty-four–hour urine collections for copper should be examined next, and if urinary copper levels are elevated, a liver biopsy should be performed for routine histology, histochemical stains for copper, and hepatic copper determination.

TABLE 8-16. CHARACTERISTIC LABORATORY FEATURES OF WILSON'S DISEASE

	NORMAL	WILSON'S DISEASE
Serum copper, $\mu g/dL$	80–140	< 80
Urine copper, $\mu g/24\,h$	< 40	> 100
Serum ceruloplasmin, mg/dL	20–40	< 20
Hepatic copper concentration, $\mu g/g$ dry weight	15–50	250–3000

TABLE 8-16.

Characteristic laboratory features of Wilson's disease. Serum copper levels are typically depressed, but this feature is not a highly sensitive and specific laboratory finding. Twenty-four–hour urine copper excretion is the best confirmatory test, along with hepatic copper concentration as determined by liver biopsy. Serum ceruloplasmin levels are depressed in the majority of patients with Wilson's disease but can be depressed in severe malabsorption and malnutrition.

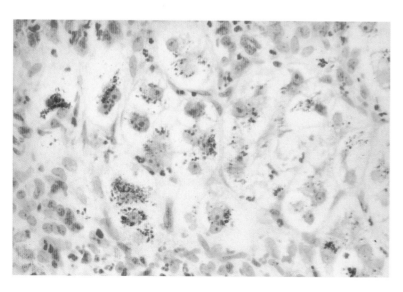

FIGURE 8-31.

A rhodanine stain of a liver biopsy for diagnosis of Wilson's disease. There are several histochemical stains for copper that can be used to help identify Wilson's disease. This figure is an example of a test that stains the copper-associated protein a golden-brown color against the blue counterstain.

TABLE 8-17. HEPATIC COPPER LEVELS IN WILSON'S DISEASE AND OTHER CHOLESTATIC LIVER DISEASES

DISEASE	MEAN HEPATIC COPPER CONCENTRATION, µg/g DRY WEIGHT
Wilson's disease	730
Primary biliary cirrhosis	410
Primary sclerosing cholangitis	245
Extrahepatic biliary obstruction	130
Indian childhood cirrhosis	1830
Alcoholic and cryptogenic cirrhosis	40
Normals	30

TABLE 8-17.

Hepatic copper concentration can be increased in other cholestatic liver diseases. The highest levels are seen in Indian childhood cirrhosis, but increased levels can be found in primary sclerosing cholangitis and primary biliary cirrhosis. The clinical settings and other supporting biochemical, clinical, and histologic features allow for easy distinction from Wilson's disease. (*From* Vierling [29]; with permission.)

Treatment

TABLE 8-18. TREATMENT OF WILSON'S DISEASE

d-Penicillamine

Trientine

Zinc supplementation

Ammonium tetrathiomolybdate

Family screening

TABLE 8-18.

Treatment for Wilson's disease usually consists of d-penicillamine [26]. If patients are intolerant to d-penicillamine or develop side effects, then treatment with trientine, another copper-chelating agent, can be given [30]. Some authors advocate the use of zinc supplementation, which interferes with copper absorption in the gastrointestinal tract and induces metallothionein to increase binding of copper to detoxify the copper [31]. Ammonium tetrathiomolybdate is an experimental agent that is being tested for treatment of Wilson's disease. As with hemochromatosis, it must be remembered that Wilson's disease is an inherited disorder; thus, family screening is exceptionally important. All first-degree relatives should be screened with serum ceruloplasmin levels, clinical history, and physical examination.

■ REFERENCES AND RECOMMENDED READING

1. Bacon BR, Tavill AS: Hemochromatosis and the iron overload syndromes. In *Hepatology. A Textbook of Liver Disease*, edn 3. Edited by Zakim D, Boyer TD. Philadelphia: WB Saunders; in press.

2. Davis WD, Arrowsmith WR: The effect of repeated bleeding in hemochromatosis. *J Lab Clin Med* 1950, 36:814–815.

3. MacDonald RA: Hemochromatosis and Hemosiderosis. Springfield: Charles C. Thomas; 1964.

4. Williams R, Smith PM, Spicer EJF, *et al.*: Venesection therapy in idiopathic haemochromatosis. *Q J Med* 1969, 38:1–16.

5. Niederau C, Fischer R, Sonnenberg A, *et al.*: Survival and causes if death in cirrhotic and noncirrhotic patients with primary hemochromatosis. *N Engl J Med* 1985, 313:1256–1262.

6. Simon M, Bourel M, Fauchet R, *et al.*: Association of HLA A3 and HLA B14 antigens with idiopathic hemochromatosis. *Gut* 1976, 17:332–334.

7. Edwards CQ, Griffen LM, Goldgar D, *et al.*: Prevalence of hemochromatosis among 11,065 presumably healthy blood donors. *N Engl J Med* 1988, 318:1355–1362.

8. Knisely AS: Neonatal hemochromatosis. *Adv Pediatrics* 1992, 39:383–403.

9. Gordeuk V, Mukiibi J, Hasstedt SJ, *et al.*: Iron overload in Africa: Interaction between a gene and dietary iron content. *N Engl J Med* 1992, 326:95–100.

10. Bacon BR: Causes of iron overload. *N Engl J Med* 1992, 326:126–127.

11. Nichols GN, Bacon BR: Hereditary hemochromatosis: Pathogenesis and clinical features of a common disease. *Am J Gastroenterol* 1989, 84:851–862.

12. Edwards CQ, Cartwright GE, Skolnick MH, *et al.*: Homozygosity for hemochromatosis: Clinical manifestations. *Ann Intern Med* 1980, 93:511–525.

13. Bassett ML, Halliday JW, Ferris RA, *et al.*: Diagnosis of hemochromatosis in young subjects: Predictive accuracy if biochemical screening tests. *Gastroenterology* 1984, 87:628–633.

14. Brittenham GM, Farrell DE, Harris JW, *et al.*: Magnetic-susceptibility measurement of human iron stores. *N Engl J Med* 1982, 307:1671–1675.

15. Bassett ML, Halliday JW, Powell LW: Value of hepatic iron measurements in early hemochromatosis and determination of the critical iron level associated with fibrosis. *Hepatology* 1986, 6:24–29.

16. Summers KM, Halliday JW, Powell LW: Identification of homozygous hemochromatosis subjects by measurement of hepatic iron index. *Hepatology* 1990, 12:20–25.

17. Olynyk J, Hall P, Sallie R, *et al.*: Computerized measurement of iron in liver biopsies: A comparison with biochemical iron measurement. *Hepatology* 1990, 12:26–30.

18. Sallie RW, Reed WD, Shilkin KB: Confirmation of the efficacy of hepatic tissue iron index in differentiating genetic haemochromatosis from alcoholic liver disease complicated by alcoholic haemosiderosis. *Gut* 1991, 32:207–210.

19. Bonkovsky HL, Slaker DP, Bills EB, *et al.*: Usefulness and limitations of laboratory and hepatic imaging studies in iron storage disease. *Gastroenterology* 1990, 99:1079–1091.

20. Deugnier YM, Turlin B, Powell LW, *et al.*: Differentiation between heterozygotes and homozygotes in genetic hemochromatosis by means of a histological hepatic iron index: A study of 192 cases. *Hepatology* 1993, 17:30–34.

21. Scheinberg IH, Sternlieb I: Wilson's disease. In *Major Problems in Internal Medicine Series*. Edited by Smith LH. Philadelphia: WB Saunders; 1984.

22. Scheinberg IH, Gitlin D: Deficiency of ceruloplasmin in patients with hepatolenticular degeneration (Wilson's disease). *Science* 1952, 116:484–485.

23. Walshe JM: Penicillamine, a new oral therapy for Wilson's disease. *Am J Med* 1956, 21:487–495.

24. Frommer DJ: Defective biliary excretion of copper in Wilson's disease. *Gut* 1974, 15:125–129.

25. Frydman M, Bonne-Tammir B, Farrer LA, *et al.*: Assignment of the gene for Wilson's disease to chromosome 13: Linkage to the esterase D locus. *Proc Natl Acad Sci U S A* 1985, 82:1819–1821.

26. Petrukhin K, Fischer SG, Pirastu M, *et al.*: Mapping, cloning and genetic characterization of the region containing the Wilson disease gene. *Nature Genet* 1993, 5:338–343.

27. Sternlieb I: Perspectives on Wilson's disease. *Hepatology* 1990, 12:1234–1239.

28. Stremmel W, Meyerow KW, Niederau C, *et al.*: Wilson's disease: Clinical presentation, treatment, and survival. *Ann Intern Med* 1991, 115:720–726.

29. Vierling J: Copper metabolism and primary biliary cirrhosis. *Sem Liver Dis* 1981, 1:293–308.

30. Scheinberg IH, Jaffe ME, Sternlieb I: The use of trientine in preventing the effects of interrupting penicillamine therapy in Wilson's disease. *N Engl J Med* 1987, 317:209–213.

31. Hill GM, Brewer GJ, Prasad AS, *et al.*: Treatment of Wilson's disease with zinc. I. Oral zinc therapy regimens. *Hepatology* 1987, 7:522–528.

Chapter 9

Alcohol-induced Liver Disease

CHARLES S. LIEBER

Originally, it was believed that liver disease in the alcoholic patient resulted exclusively from malnutrition. Subsequently, as reviewed elsewhere [1], the hepatotoxicity of ethanol has been established by the demonstration that, in the absence of dietary deficiencies, and even in the presence of protein-, vitamin-, and mineral-enriched diets, ethanol produces fatty liver with striking ultrastructural lesions in both rats and human volunteers, and fibrosis with cirrhosis in nonhuman primates. The fact remains, however, that alcohol is rich in energy (7.1 kcal/g) and that a large intake of alcohol can have profound effects on nutritional status, in part as a consequence of alcoholic hepatotoxicity. The demonstration that alcohol exerts some intrinsic hepatotoxicity led to a broadly based search for the mechanism involved. One of the most fruitful leads was the realization that many of the metabolic and toxic effects of alcohol are, in fact, linked to its metabolism.

SPECTRUM OF ALCOHOLIC LIVER INJURY: TRANSITION OF FATTY LIVER TO ALCOHOLIC HEPATITIS AND CIRRHOSIS

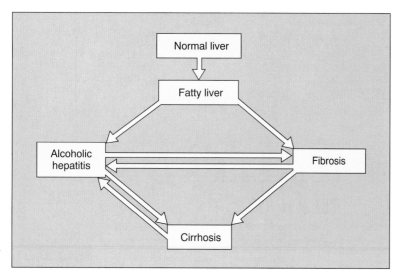

FIGURE 9-1.

As reviewed elsewhere [1], fatty liver invariably develops after heavy alcohol intake; it can progress to alcoholic hepatitis and cirrhosis. In some patients, alcoholic hepatitis is a necessary step in the development of alcohol-induced cirrhosis. However, in some other patients alcohol may stimulate the production of fibrosis and cirrhosis without requiring alcoholic hepatitis as an intermediate lesion. Furthermore, in the alcohol-fed baboon model, fibrosis and cirrhosis also developed in the absence of alcoholic hepatitis [2]. Only a minority of heavy drinkers develop cirrhosis and, experimentally, only one third of baboons fed a high dose of alcohol developed lesions more severe than those of fatty liver. The reason for this individual susceptibility to the development of these more severe complications is not known. Hereditary predisposition may play a role. For the transition of the more benign to the more severe stages of the disease, autoimmune mechanisms have been postulated and cytotoxicity of lymphocytes documented. At present, the mechanism of the transition between fatty liver and alcoholic

hepatitis and cirrhosis and the reasons for the difference in individual susceptibility are not settled. It is unclear how alcoholic hepatitis eventually develops into cirrhosis. In addition to fibrogenesis as a response to necrosis and inflammation, it is conceivable that alcohol affects collagen metabolism directly either through increased production or decreased disposition or both, and acetaldhyde has been shown to stimulate collagen production in cultured lipocytes (Ito cells) and myofibroblasts and fibroblasts. At the earliest stages, in the so-called simple or uncomplicated fatty liver, collagen is detectable by chemical means only. When collagen deposition is sufficient to become visible by light microscopy, usually it appears first around the central (also called terminal) hepatic venules, resulting in so-called "pericentral" or "perivenular" fibrosis or sclerosis which extends into the lobule (perisinusoidal and pericellular fibrosis). In cases of alcoholic hepatitis, an increased number of mesenchymal cells and polymorphonuclear leukocytes are present (*see* Fig. 9-54), but even in the absence of alcoholic hepatitis, and prior to any fibrosis, there can be an increased number of mesenchymal cells. Sequential biopsies revealed that, already at the early fatty liver stage, an increased number of myofibroblasts appear in the perivenular areas, and cells transitional between lipocytes and fibroblasts in the perisinusoidal space of Disse. This is eventually accompanied by deposition of abundant collagen bundles, first in the perivenular areas, leading to perivenular, perisinusoidal, and pericellular fibrosis and ultimately to septal fibrosis and cirrhosis. The progression of alcohol-induced injury is not orderly. Alcoholic hepatitis is often found superimposed on already established cirrhosis and the clinical manifestations result both from acute alcoholic hepatitis and from problems arising as complications of cirrhosis. Alcoholic hepatitis is considered at least partially reversible. Alcohol steatosis is considered largely reversible. Even at the stage of alcoholic hepatitis when there is early fibrosis, the possibility exists that some (if not most) of the injury may be reversible. Many patients have coexistence of fatty liver, alcoholic hepatitis, and cirrhosis.

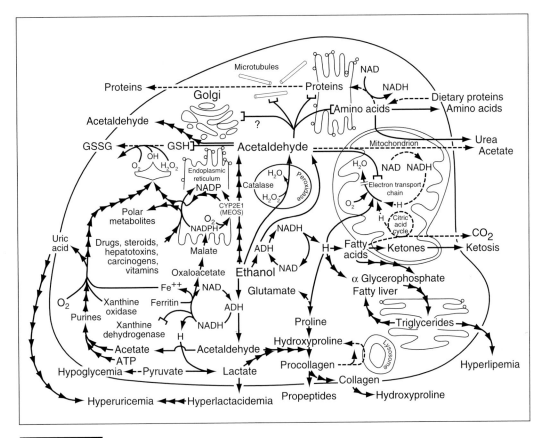

FIGURE 9-2.

Oxidation of ethanol in the hepatocyte. The hepatocyte contains three main pathways for ethanol metabolism, each located in a different subcellular compartment: 1) the alcohol dehydrogenase (ADH) pathway of the cytosol or the soluble fraction of the cell; 2) the microsomal ethanol-oxidizing system (MEOS) located in the endoplasmic reticulum; and 3) the catalase located in the peroxisomes. Each of these pathways produces specific metabolic and toxic disturbances.

Many disturbances in intermediary metabolism and toxic effects can be linked to the ADH–mediated generation of reduced nicotinamide-adenine dinucleotide (NADH) as well as acetaldehyde. ADH also occurs in extrahepatic tissues and the contribution of gastric ADH to the first-pass metabolism of ethanol and alcohol-drug interactions has been recently recognized (*see* Figs. 9-12 and 9-13). Of special significance is the fact that it is now generally accepted that acetaldehyde is also produced by an accessory pathway, the MEOS, containing P450 2E1 (CYP2E1) which, in addition, generates oxygen radicals and activates many xenobiotics to toxic metabolites, thereby explaining a corresponding increased vulnerability of heavy drinkers (*see* Table 9-2). Catalase may become significantly involved when there is ample H_2O_2, which occurs only in exceptional circumstances with an unusual supply of substrate generating the H_2O_2. The influences of hepatitis C, cytokines, gender, genetics, and age are also now emerging. Furthermore, alcohol alters the degradation of key nutrients, thereby promoting deficiencies as well as toxic interactions, such as those with vitamin A and β-carotene (*see* Figs. 9-24 to 9-33). Conversely, nutritional deficits may affect the toxicity of ethanol and acetaldehyde, as illustrated by the depletion in glutathione (GSH) (*see* Fig. 9-38). Other "supernutrients" include polyunsaturated lecithin, shown to correct the alcohol-induced hepatic phosphatidylcholine depletion and to prevent alcoholic cirrhosis in nonhuman primates (*see* Fig 9-44). Thus, a better understanding of the pathology induced by ethanol is now generating improved prospects for therapy (*see* Table 9-3). The *broken lines* indicate pathways that are depressed by ethanol, whereas *repeated arrows* reflect stimulation or activation. The *lines ending in brackets* denote interference or binding [3]. ATP—adenosine triphosphatase; GSSG–oxidized glutathione; NAD—nicotinamide-adenine dinucleotide; NADP—NAD phosphate.

MALNUTRITION VERSUS HEPATOTOXICITY OF ETHANOL

TABLE 9-1. CALORIC VALUE OF ETHANOL

ETHANOL	CALORIES
1 g	7.1
1 oz (86 proof)	71
1 "drink"	100–150
1 pt (86 proof)	1141
1 L wine (12%)	673

TABLE 9-1.

Caloric value of ethanol and alcoholic beverages. Unlike other drugs, ethanol has a large energy content: gram for gram, it provides more calories than either carbohydrates or fat. However, alcoholic beverages are devoid of substantial amounts of minerals, vitamins, proteins, and other nutrients and therefore displace other nutrients in the diet and act as "empty calories," thereby causing primary malnutrition (*see* Fig 9-3).

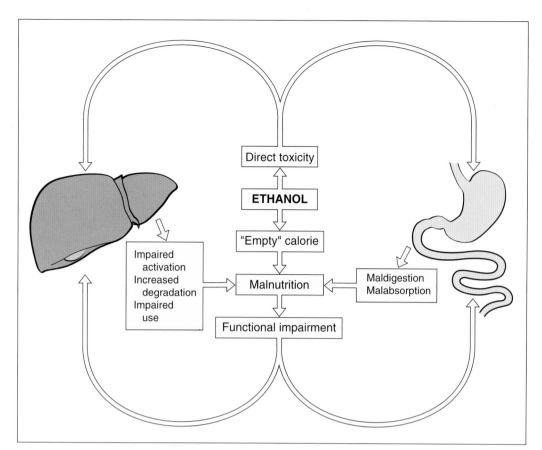

FIGURE 9-3.

This figure illustrates the role of primary malnutrition (dietary deficiencies) and that of secondary malnutrition, resulting from the interaction of direct toxicity of ethanol on the liver and gut with associated maldigestion and malabsorption, as well as impaired hepatic activation or increased degradation of nutrients [3].

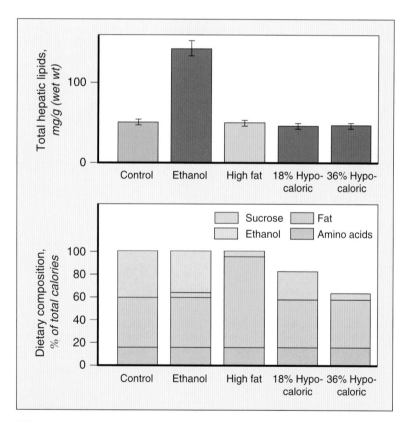

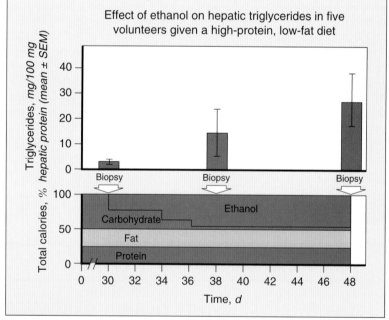

FIGURE 9-5.

Effect on ethanol on hepatic triglycerides in five volunteers given a high-protein, low-fat diet. Fat accumulation (and associated ultra-structural changes) occurred despite an enriched diet, supplemented with vitamins, minerals, and choline [4].

FIGURE 9-4.

Effect on total hepatic lipids of five types of liquid diets fed to rats for 24 days. Isocaloric substitution of fat with ethanol resulted in striking hepatic fat accumulation. This accumulation did not result from carbohydrate depletion because isocaloric replacement with fat (instead of alcohol) had no such effect. Similarly, mere depletion in carbohydrates (hypocaloric diets) did not result in fat accumulation [4].

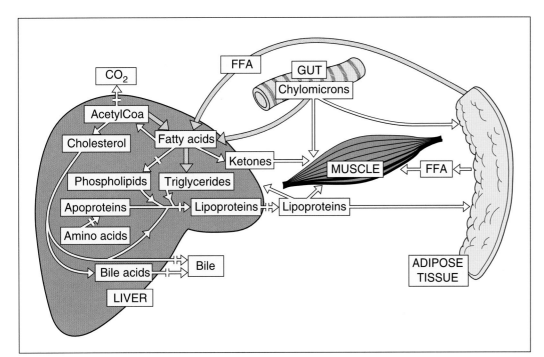

FIGURE 9-6.

Possible mechanisms of fatty liver production through either increases (*shaded arrows*) or decreases (*open arrows*) of lipid transport and metabolism [1]. FFA—free fatty acids.

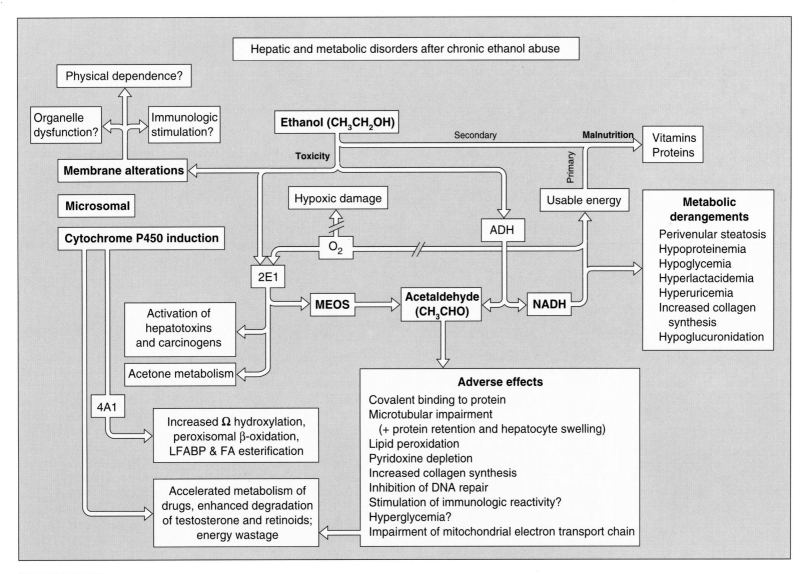

FIGURE 9-7.

Hepatic and metabolic disorders after chronic ethanol abuse. Malnutrition, whether primary or secondary, has been differentiated from direct toxicity. The latter has been attributed, in part, to redox changes or effects secondary to microsomal induction, acetaldehyde, direct membrane alternations, or hypoxia [5]. ADH—alcohol dehydrogenase; FA—fatty acid; LFABP—liver fatty acid binding protein; MEOS—microsomal ethanol-oxidizing system; NADH—reduced nicotinamide-adenine dinucleotide.

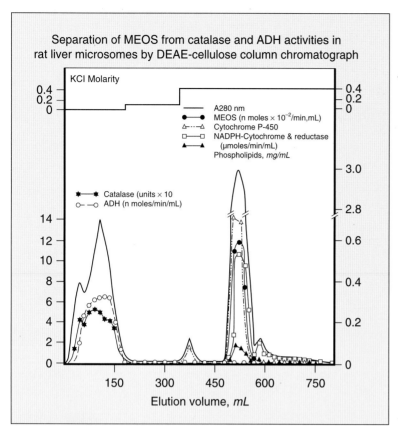

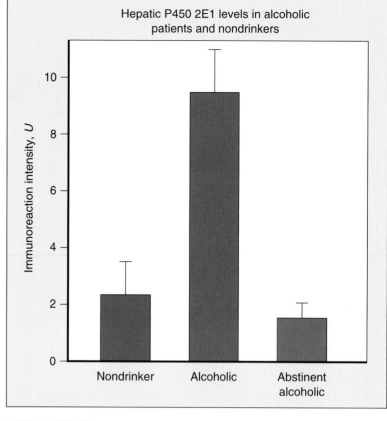

FIGURE 9-8.

Separation of microsomal ethanol-oxidizing system (MEOS) from catalase and alcohol dehydrogenase (ADH) activities in rat liver microsomes by diethylaminoethanol (DEAE)-cellulose column chromatography. A preparation was obtained that is clearly devoid of ADH and catalase but contains cytochrome P450 and oxidizes ethanol. NADPH—reduced nicotinamide-adenine-dinucleotide phosphate. (*Modified from* Teschke *et al.* [6]; with permission.)

FIGURE 9-9.

Hepatic P450 2E1 levels in alcoholics and nondrinkers illustrating the striking 2E1 induction, a key biochemical difference between heavy and moderate drinkers (or abstainers). P450 2E1 was quantitated by scanning of western blots of percutaneous liver biopsies, using anti-2E1 antibodies. By contrast with microsomal ethanol-oxidizing systems, no induction of liver alcohol dehydrogenase has been reported after high alcohol consumption (not shown). (*Data from* Tsutsumi [7]; with permission.)

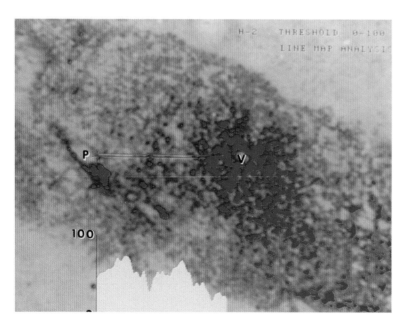

FIGURE 9-10.

Image analysis of 2E1 messenger RNA (mRNA) and complementary DNA (cDNA) hybrids in a human liver section. After in situ hybridization with a 2E1 cDNA, the liver specimen (from a control subject) was subjected to computerized image analysis to quantitate 2E1 mRNA and cDNA hybridization signals and to determine the mRNA signal density gradient in the hepatic acinus. The perivenular location of 2E1 mRNA was associated with a corresponding selective perivenular preponderance of the 2E1 protein (not shown) [7]. Area measurements were made on the red portions of the section, which represented acinar regions positive for 2E1 mRNA transcripts. Hybridization signal densities within the narrow red rectangle overlaid between a portal and terminal hepatic venule (*V*) were measured along the width by horizontal scanning. The actual computer drawn line map corresponding to this scan spanning the portal triad (*P*) to *V* area is illustrated in white below the section. The 2E1 mRNA hybridization signal intensity has been plotted inversely on the Y axis, where *100* denotes no specific signal and *0* denotes the most intense signal [8].

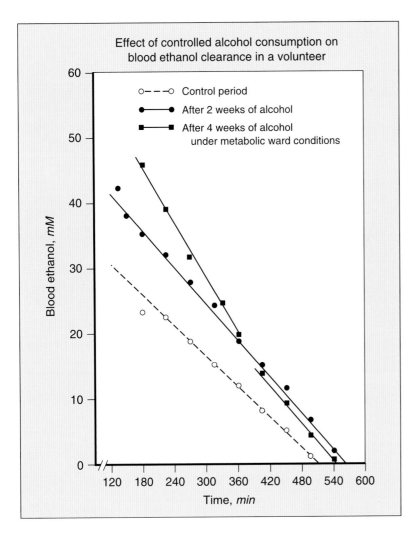

Effect of controlled alcohol consumption on blood ethanol clearance in a volunteer

Blood ethanol, *mM*

- ○ – – ○ Control period
- ●——● After 2 weeks of alcohol
- ■——■ After 4 weeks of alcohol under metabolic ward conditions

Time, *min*

FIGURE 9-11.

Effect of chronic alcohol consumption on blood ethanol elimination curves in a human volunteer. After a period of abstinence (6 weeks), a clearance test was done with a dose of ethanol of 1.0 g/kg. Next, the subject was given 2 to 4 g/kg ethanol per day (divided in six doses) over 4 weeks. Clearance tests were repeated with 1.3 g/kg of alcohol after 2 weeks and 1.5 g/kg after 4 weeks. The progressive acceleration in clearance occurred primarily at the higher blood alcohol levels, consistent with the relatively high kilometers of microsomal ethanol-oxidizing systems (MEOS) for ethanol and the selective induction of MEOS activity upon chronic ethanol consumption. This study illustrates the metabolic tolerance to ethanol that develops in the chronic drinker [9].

INTERACTIONS OF ETHANOL WITH OTHER DRUGS, HEPATOTOXIC AGENTS, AND VITAMINS

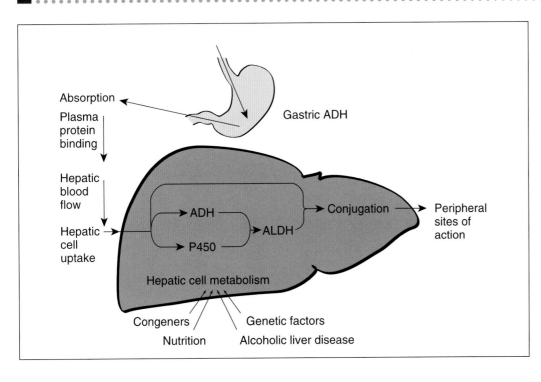

Absorption

Plasma protein binding

Hepatic blood flow

Hepatic cell uptake

Gastric ADH

ADH

P450

ALDH

Conjugation

Peripheral sites of action

Hepatic cell metabolism

Congeners

Nutrition

Genetic factors

Alcoholic liver disease

FIGURE 9-12.

Schematic illustration of some of the sites of ethanol-drug interactions. Metabolic interactions may affect conjugation, microsomal cytochrome P450–dependent pathways (P450), alcohol dehydrogenase (ADH), and acetaldehyde dehydrogenase (ALDH) [10].

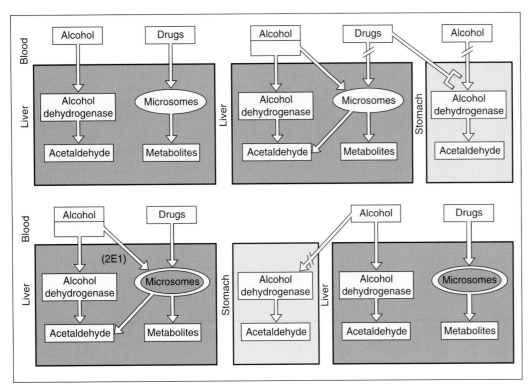

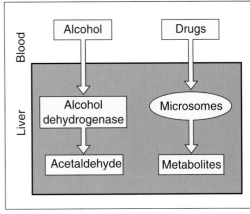

FIGURE 9-14.

Hepatic metabolism of alcohol by alcohol dehydrogenase and drugs by microsomes.

FIGURE 9-13.

Schematic representation of hepatic ethanol-drug interactions involving the alcohol dehydrogenase pathway (in liver and stomach) and the hepatic microsomes (*See* Figs. 9-14 to 9-17) [3].

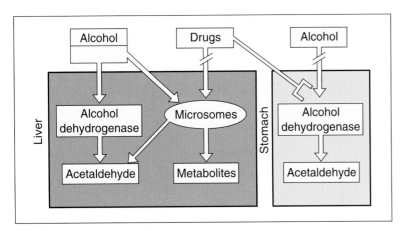

FIGURE 9-15.

Inhibition of hepatic microsomal drug metabolism in the presence of high concentrations of ethanol, in part through competition for a common microsomal detoxification process and inhibition of gastric ethanol metabolism by drugs.

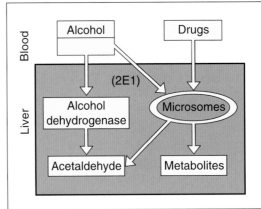

FIGURE 9-16.

Microsomal induction after chronic alcohol consumption and its contribution to accelerated hepatic metabolism of ethanol at high blood levels.

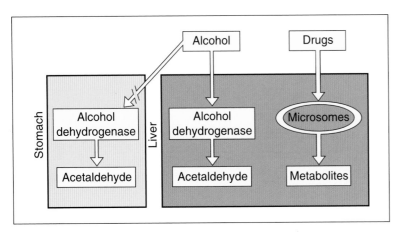

FIGURE 9-17.

Decreased gastric alcohol dehydrogenase activity and gastric ethanol metabolism after chronic alcohol abuse, as well as increased hepatic drug metabolism and xenobiotic activation because of the persisting microsomal induction after withdrawal from chronic alcohol consumption.

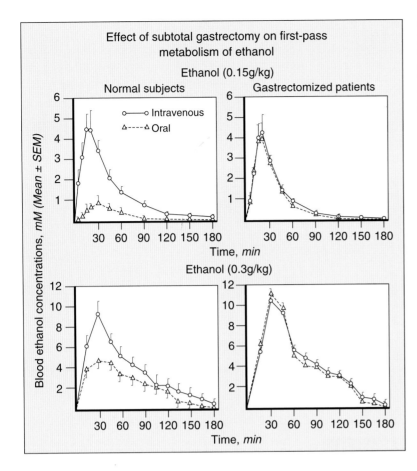

FIGURE 9-18.

First-pass metabolism of ethanol and its abolition by gastrectomy. At two different doses of ethanol, blood levels were lowered when the same amount was given orally rather than intravenously (first-pass metabolism). No such effect was seen in gastrectomized subjects [11].

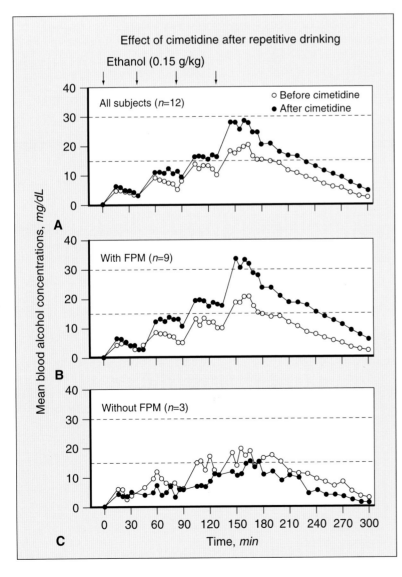

FIGURE 9-19.

Effect of cimetidine (400 mg twice a day for 7 days) on blood alcohol levels after oral consumption of four small doses of ethanol (150 mg/kg) at 45-minute intervals in all twelve subjects studied (**A**), in the nine subjects with substantial first-pass metabolism (FPM) (**B**), and the three subjects with minimal FPM of alcohol before treatment with the drug (**C**). In individuals with FPM, cimetidine resulted in a significant increase in blood-alcohol levels that stayed above the threshold for impairment of psychomotor functions (15 mg/dL) or judgment (30 mg/dL). In some subjects, blood alcohol levels exceeded 50 to 80 mg/dL, the legal threshold for driving in many countries and some states in the United States [12].

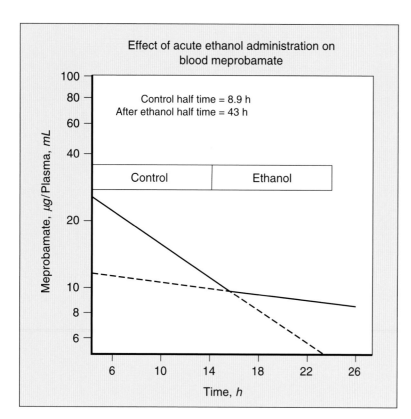

FIGURE 9-20.

Effect of acute ethanol intoxication on disappearance of meproba-mate from the blood in a volunteer subject given meprobamate, 12 to 15 mg/kg orally. Fourteen hours later, 1 g/kg of ethanol was given and followed by 24 g every 2 hours. *Solid lines* are plotted from experimental points; *dashed lines* are extrapolated [1].

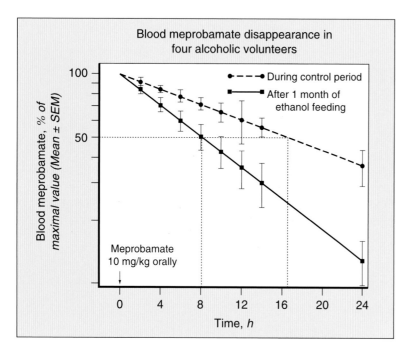

FIGURE 9-21.

Effect of chronic ethanol consumption on clearance of meproba-mate from blood. Four alcoholic volunteers were tested before and after 1 month of ethanol ingestion which resulted in a striking acceleration of meprobamate disappearance; half-lives are shown by the *dotted lines* on x and y axis [13].

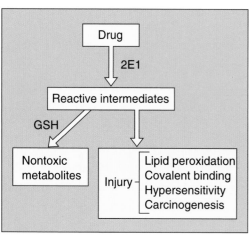

FIGURE 9-22.

Mechanism for enhancement of drug-induced toxicity after chronic ethanol consumption. Whereas microsomal systems usually detoxify xenobiotics, including drugs, on occasion the system backfires and toxic reactive metabolites are produced that cause liver injury unless sufficiently detoxified, for instance by reduced glutathione (GSH). Lack of GSH such as it occurs in nutritional deficiencies or acetaldehyde toxicity (*see* Fig 9-38) will therefore potentiate the toxicity. One example is provided by carbon tetrachloride (*see* Fig. 9-23).

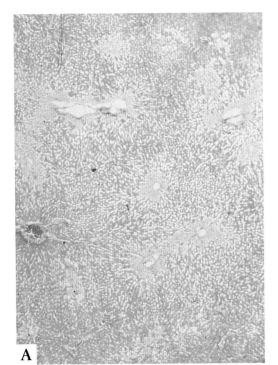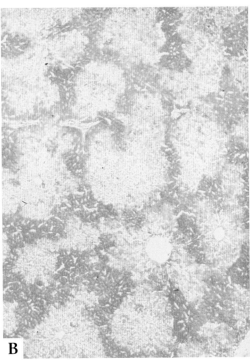

FIGURE 9-23.

Increased carbon tetrachloride (CCl$_4$) hepatotoxicity. **A**, Liver histology (hematoxylin and eosin stain) of a rat given a single dose of CCl$_4$; **B**, littermate given the same dose but after 3 weeks of alcohol consumption, illustrating the striking potentiation of the perivenular hepatotoxicity. (*Data from* Hasumura *et al.* [14]; with permission.)

TABLE 9-2. VULNERABILITY OF THE ALCOHOLIC PATIENT TO HEPATOTOXIC AGENTS

Industrial solvents	Carcinogens
Anesthetics	Vitamins
Drugs	Ethanol
Analgesics	

TABLE 9-2.

Because of the activation by 2E1 of many xenobiotics to hepatotoxic agents and carcinogens, and also because of the spill over of the induction of 2E1 to that of other microsomal systems, alcoholic patients develop an increased vulnerability to a variety of xenobiotics, including drugs such as sedatives, tranquilizers, hypoglycemic agents, anticoagulants, and vitamins.

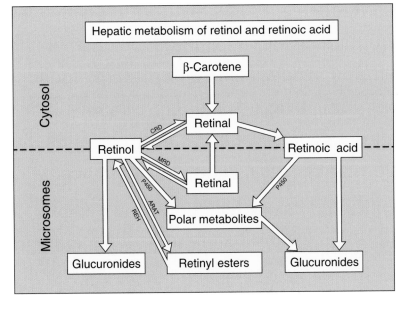

FIGURE 9-24.

Schematic representation of the role of cytosolic and microsomal systems in the hepatic metabolism of retinol. Microsomal degradation is induced after chronic alcohol consumption [15]. ARAT—acyl-CoA:retinol acyltransferase; CRD—cytosolic retinol dehydrogenase; MRD—microsomal retinol dehydrogenase; REH—retinyl ester hydrolase.

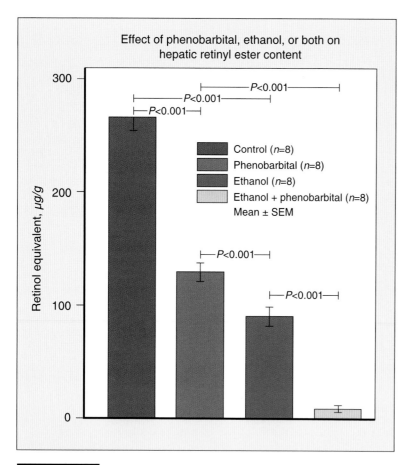

FIGURE 9-25.

Effect of phenobarbital, ethanol, or both on hepatic retinyl ester content. Both drugs resulted in a significant depletion of hepatic retinyl ester. The combination of phenobarbital with ethanol produced a most striking depletion, resulting in negligible hepatic retinyl ester levels. Similar effects were observed with a combination of ethanol and butylated hydroxytoluene [16].

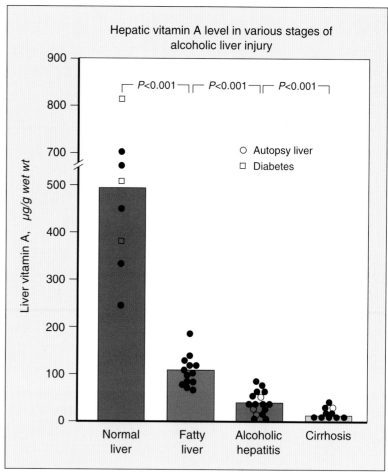

FIGURE 9-26.

Hepatic vitamin A levels in subjects with normal livers and various stages of alcoholic liver injury. Already at the early fatty liver stage and in the absence of manifestation of malnutrition and maldigestion, severe hepatic vitamin A depletion was present [17].

FIGURE 9-27.

Potentiation of hepatotoxicity of ethanol by vitamin A. A combination of ethanol and vitamin A supplementation resulted in the appearance of giant mitochondria (*red areas*) visible by light microscopy. No such lesions were seen with the same amount of either ethanol alone or vitamin A alone (hematoxylin and eosin, magnification × 1000). (*From* Leo *et al.* [18]; with permission.)

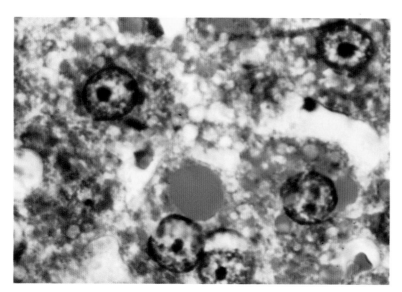

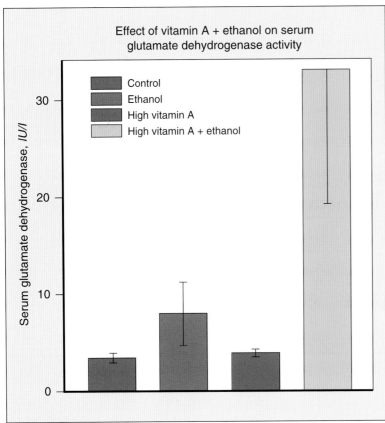

FIGURE 9-28.

Effect of vitamin A and ethanol on serum glutamate dehydrogenase activity. The structural lesions of the mitochondria (*see* Fig. 9-27) had its biochemical counterpart, namely a striking potentiation of the leakage, into the blood stream of the mitochondrial enzyme glutamic dehydrogenase. (*Data from* Leo and Lieber [19]; with permission.)

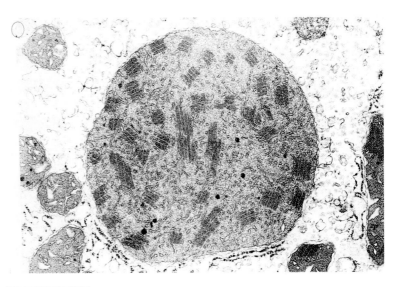

FIGURE 9-29.

Electron micrograph of a liver biopsy of an alcoholic patient supplemented with vitamin A (10,000 IU/d for 4 months) showing giant mitochondria (adjacent to normal-sized organelles) with severe disorganization of the inner cristae and containing a very dense matrix with multiple fine filamentous or crystalloid-like structures [15]. (Uranyl acetate and osmium staining, magnification × 17,000.)

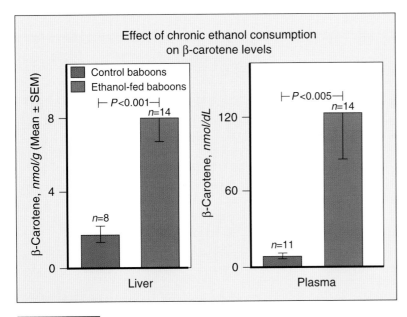

FIGURE 9-30.

Effect of chronic ethanol consumption on β-carotene levels. A survey of a baboon colony fed liquid diets (with or without ethanol) and a daily carrot (200 g corresponding to 30 mg β-carotene) revealed that the liver and plasma β-carotene levels, measured by high-pressure liquid chromatography, were significantly higher in ethanol-fed animals than in pair-fed controls [20].

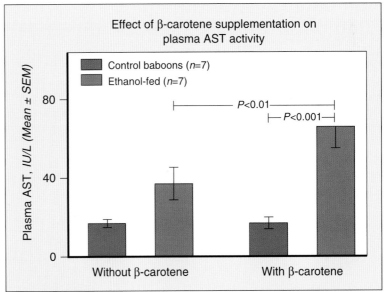

FIGURE 9-31.

Effect of β-carotene supplementation on plasma aspartate aminotransferase (AST) levels in baboons. A striking increase in plasma AST activity was observed when alcohol was combined with β-carotene supplementation [20].

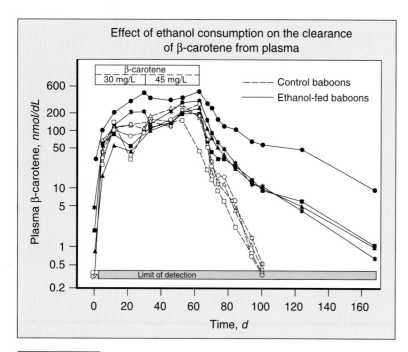

FIGURE 9-32.

Effect of ethanol consumption on the clearance of β-carotene from plasma in baboons. Ethanol slowed the clearance of β-carotene upon cessation of the supplementation [20].

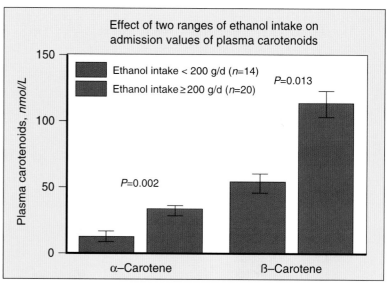

FIGURE 9-33.

Effect of two ranges of ethanol intake on admission values of plasma carotenoids in alcoholics. Contrary to expectation, those drinking most heavily had the lowest plasma carotenoids. (*Data from* Ahmed *et al.* [21]; with permission.)

TOXIC EFFECTS OF ACETALDEHYDE

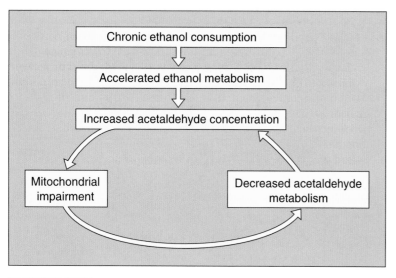

FIGURE 9-34.

Possible relationship between ethanol consumption, altered acetaldehyde levels, and mitochondrial impairment through a "vicious cycle." (*Modified from* Lieber [1]; with permission.)

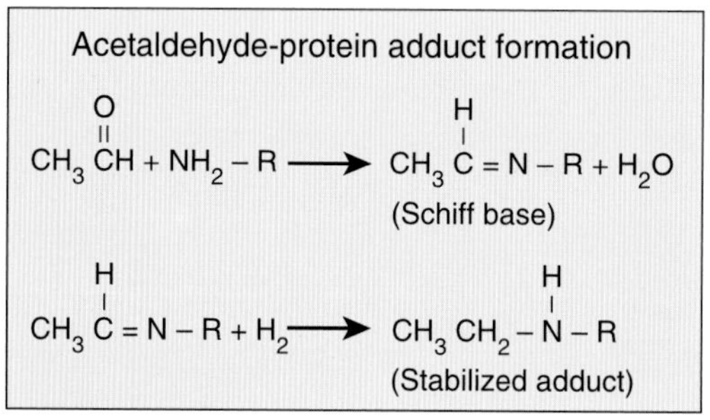

Acetaldehyde-protein adduct formation

$$CH_3 \overset{O}{\overset{\|}{C}}H + NH_2 - R \longrightarrow CH_3 \overset{H}{\overset{|}{C}} = N - R + H_2O$$
(Schiff base)

$$CH_3 \overset{H}{\overset{|}{C}} = N - R + H_2 \longrightarrow CH_3 \overset{H}{\overset{|}{C}}H_2 - \overset{|}{N} - R$$
(Stabilized adduct)

FIGURE 9-35.

Adduct formation between acetaldehyde and proteins. Acetaldehyde readily reacts with other compounds, for instance through formation of Schiff bases that can be stabilized by reducing compounds.

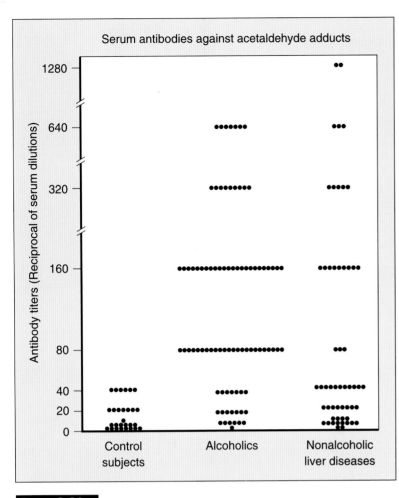

FIGURE 9-36.

Serum antibody titers against acetaldehyde adducts in healthy control subjects, alcoholics, and patients with nonalcoholic liver diseases. The difference was significant when we compared alcoholic patients with control subjects ($P<0.0001$), nonalcoholic patients with control subjects ($P<0.0005$), and alcoholic with nonalcoholic patients ($P<0.001$) (x^2 tests) [22].

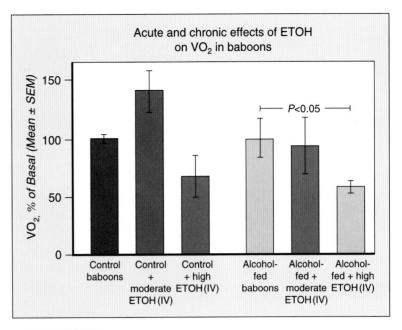

FIGURE 9-37.

Acute and chronic effects of ethanol (ETOH) on flow-independent hepatic tissue oxygen consumption (VO_2) in baboons. Acutely, ETOH increased VO_2, but at higher dosage or in animals fed ETOH chronically, this effect disappeared and decreased oxygen consumption prevailed. IV—intravenous. (*Data from* Lieber *et al.* [23]; with permission.)

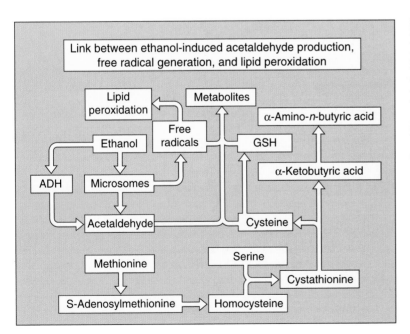

FIGURE 9-38.

Hypothetical link between accelerated acetaldehyde production, increased free radical generation by the "induced" microsomes, enhanced lipid peroxidation, and increased α-amino-n-butyric acid production. This scheme illustrates how reduced glutathione (GSH) depletion (secondary to increased acetaldehyde and free radical generation by the ethanol-induced microsomes) exacerbates liver injury (*ie*, lipid peroxidation) and how GSH repletion can be promoted by supplying precursors (*ie*, S-adenosylmethionine) [3]. ADH—alcohol dehydrogenase.

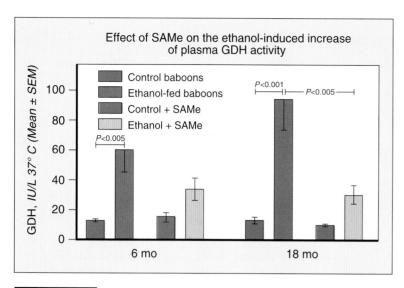

FIGURE 9-39.

Effect of S-adenosylmethionine (SAMe) on the ethanol-induced increase of plasma glutamic dehydrogenase activity (GDH). SAMe clearly attenuates this parameter of ethanol-induced liver injury. (*Data from* Lieber *et al.* [24]; with permission.)

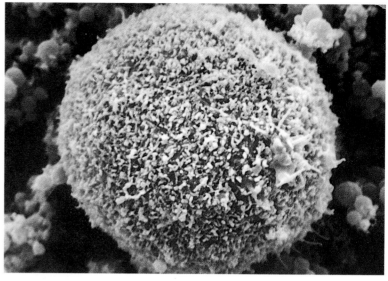

FIGURE 9-40.

Scanning electron micrograph of isolated hepatocytes. Typical hepatocyte from control rat showing abundant microvilli uniformly covering the cell surface [25].

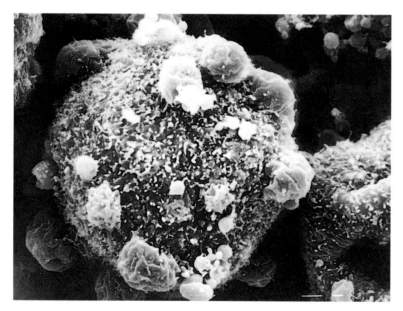

FIGURE 9-41.

Scanning electron micrograph of isolated hepatocytes. Hepatocyte from a ethanol-fed rat showing the appearance of blebs on the cell surface with a diminished number of microvilli [25].

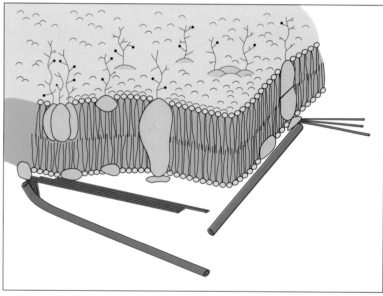

FIGURE 9-42.

Schematic representation of membranes as bilayer of phospholipids, which represents the "backbone" of the membrane. (*Adapted from* Singer and Nicholson [26]; with permission.)

FIGURE 9-43.

Formula of dilinoleoylphosphatidylcholine, the main compound of the polyenylphosphatidylcholine used in Figure 9-44.

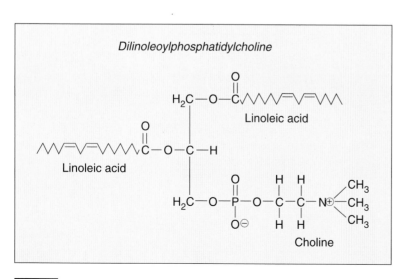

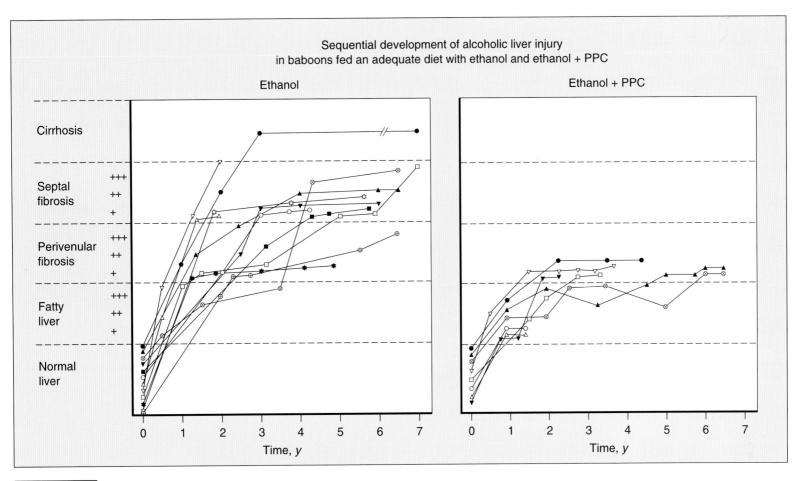

Sequential development of alcoholic liver injury
in baboons fed an adequate diet with ethanol and ethanol + PPC

FIGURE 9-44.

Sequential development of alcoholic liver injury in baboons fed ethanol with normal (*left*) or dilinoleoylphosphatidylcholine (PPC)-enriched diet (*right*). Liver morphology in animals pair-fed controls diets and administered PPC without alcohol remained normal (not shown) [2].

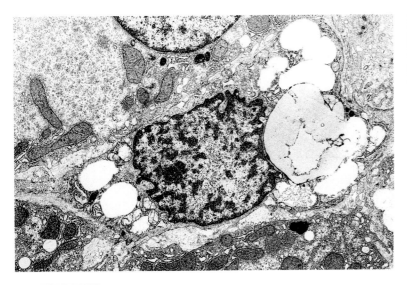

FIGURE 9-45.

Lipocyte from a patient with fatty liver. The lipocyte contains lipid droplets of variable sizes with a total lipid volume density of more than 20% of the cell. The rough endoplasmic reticulum is randomly distributed in the cytoplasm as short narrowed cisternae. The Golgi apparatus is relatively inconspicuous. Collagen fibers are present in the extracellular space. (*Modified from* Lieber [1]; with permission.)

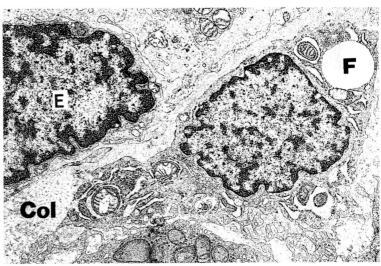

FIGURE 9-46.

Transitional cell in the Disse space in a cirrhotic liver. The cell contains a small lipid droplet (*F*) with a total lipid volume density of less than 20% of the cell volume. The rough endoplasmic reticulum appears conspicuous. Note that the cell profile appears smaller compared with that of the lipocyte in Figure 9-45. In the extracellular space, an abundant amount of collagen fibers is present. An endothelial cell nucleus (*E*) is shown [1].

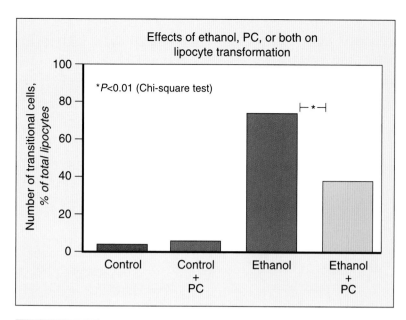

FIGURE 9-47.

Effects of ethanol, phosphatidylcholine (PC), or both on lipocyte transformation. PC resulted in a significant attenuation of the ethanol-induced increase in transitional cells. (*Data from* Lieber *et al.* [2]; with permission.)

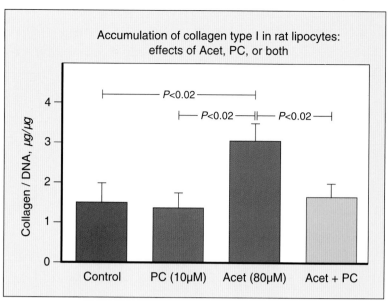

FIGURE 9-48.

Accumulation of collagen type I in rat lipocytes: effects of acetaldehyde (Acet), phosphatidylcholine (PC), or both. PC prevented the Acet-mediated collagen increase [27].

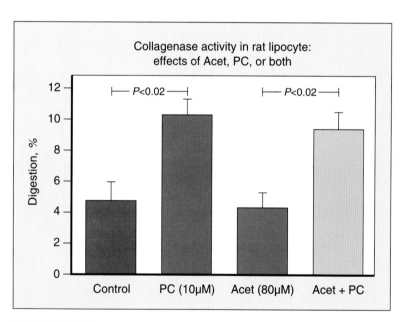

FIGURE 9-49.

Collagenase activity in rat lipocytes: effects of acetaldehyde (Acet), phosphatidylcholine (PC), or both. Polyunsaturated lecithin stimulated collagenase activity in cultured lipocytes, a most likely mechanism for the prevention of the Acet-mediated hepatic collagen accumulation [27].

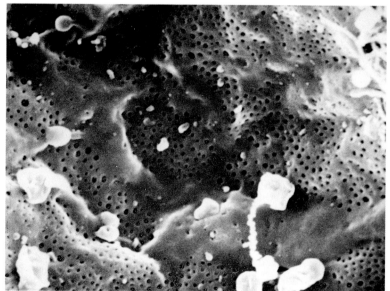

FIGURE 9-50.

Scanning electron micrograph of the luminal surface of the hepatic sinusoidal endothelium of a control baboon. Luminal view of cytoplasmic extension showing fenestrations arranged in clusters [28].

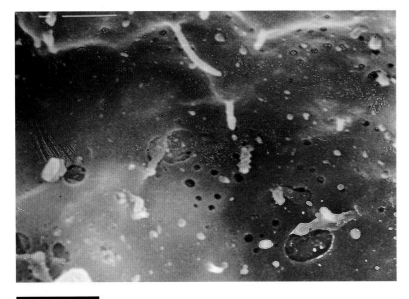

FIGURE 9-51.

Scanning electron micrograph of the luminal surface of the hepatic sinusoidal endothelium of an alcohol-fed baboon. Distinctly fewer fenestration in the endothelium exist here than in control baboons (*see* Fig. 9-50) [28].

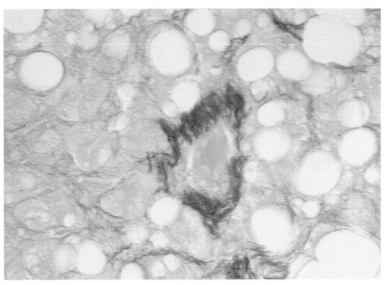

FIGURE 9-52.

Sirius red stain (original magnification × 250) of a liver biopsy from a patient with alcoholic fatty liver without evidence of alcoholic hepatitis. Note the fibrous rim around the terminal hepatic venule (perivenular fibrosis). Some fibrous strands surround the adjacent sinusoids and hepatocytes (perisinusoidal and pericellular fibrosis). (*Courtesy of* F. Paronetto, Bronx, NY)

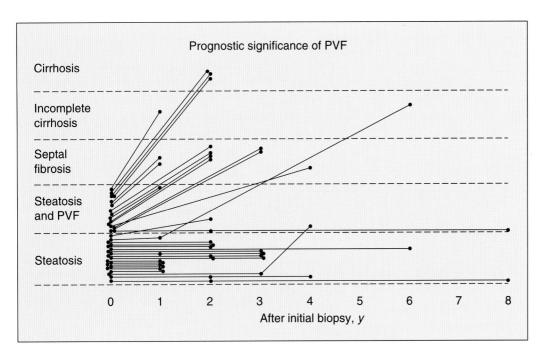

FIGURE 9-53.

Progression of fibrosis in alcoholic patients without hepatitis followed up to 8 years after initial biopsy. Presence of perivenular fibrosis (PVF) on the initial biopsy specimen was a harbinger of rapid development of fibrosis to more severe stages, including cirrhosis [29].

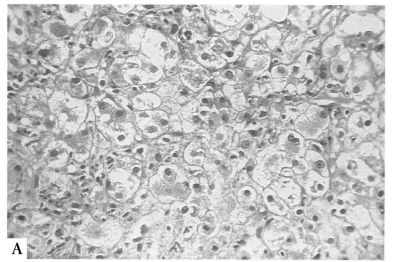

A

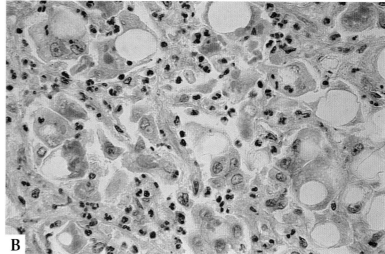

B

FIGURE 9-54.

Major features found on liver biopsy from a patient with alcoholic hepatitis include marked variation in cell size, evidence of cell necrosis, and variable inflammation with a mixture of polymorphonuclear and mononuclear cells. There is evidence of variable sinusoidal compression. Pericellular fibrosis is an important feature. In many patients, eosinophilic inclusions (Mallory bodies) are found. The Mallory bodies represent masses of intermediate filaments. Often the most intense alcoholic-induced injury is in Zone III (centrilobular). **A**, Masson trichrome stain. **B**, Hematoxylin and eosin stain.

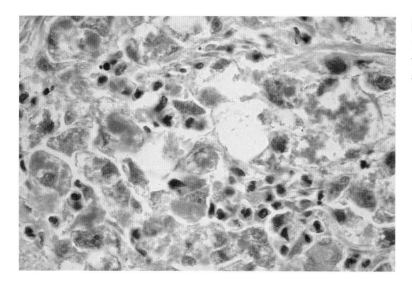

FIGURE 9-55.

Liver biopsy from a patient with active alcoholic hepatitis replete with Mallory bodies (alcoholic hyaline). Hematoxylin and eosin stain. (*Courtesy of* Z. Goodman, Washington, D.C.)

TABLE 9-3. TREATMENT

Nutrition	Steroids
Antioxidants (Vitamin E)	Colchicine
S-adenosylmethionine	Propylthiouracil
Polyunsaturated lecithin	Transplantation
Anticytokines	Abstinence

TABLE 9-3.

Therapeutic modalities in alcoholic liver disease. In addition to correction of nutritional deficiencies (when present), therapy with some "supernutrients" may be contemplated (such as S-adenosylmethionine). Other treatments are still experimental except for abstinence and, in some limited groups, steroids (for severe alcoholic hepatitis) and transplantation.

TABLE 9-4. ALCOHOLIC HEPATITIS: CORTICOSTEROID TREATMENT

INDICATIONS
Spontaneous encephalopathy

4.6 (PT-control) + serum bilirubin > 32

CONTRAINDICATIONS
Active gastrointestinal bleeding

Active infection

PREDNISOLONE
40 mg/d (4wk), 20 mg/d (1 wk), 10 mg/d (1 wk)

TABLE 9-4.

In patients with severe alcoholic liver disease, as indicated by spontaneous encephalopathy or elevated protime and bilirubin (elevated Maddrey's discriminant function), corticosteroid treatment has been shown to be useful [30].

REFERENCES AND RECOMMENDED READING

1. Lieber CS: *Medical and Nutritional Complications of Alcoholism: Mechanisms and Management.* New York: Plenum Press; 1992:579.

2. Lieber CS, Robins SJ, Li J, *et al.*: Phosphatidylcholine protects against fibrosis and cirrhosis in the baboon. *Gastroenterology* 1994, 06:152–159.

3. Lieber CS: Alcohol and the liver: 1994 update. *Gastroenterology* 1994, 106:1085–1105.

4. Lieber CS: Chronic alcoholic hepatic injury in experimental animals and man: Biochemical pathways and nutritional factors. *Fed Proc* 1967, 26:1443–1448.

5. Lieber CS: The metabolism of alcohol and its implications for the pathogenesis of disease. In *Ethanol and The Gastrointestinal Tract: Mechanisms in Disease* Edited by Preedy VR, Watson RR. Boca Raton: CRC Press; (in press).

6. Teschke R, Hasumura Y, Joly J, *et al.*: Microsomal ethanol-oxidizing system (MEOS): Purification and properties of a rat liver system free of catalase and alcohol dehydrogenase. *Biochem Biophys Res Commun* 1972, 49:1187–1193.

7. Tsutsumi M, Lasker JM, Shimizu M, *et al.*: The intralobular distribution of ethanol-inducible P450IIE1 in rat and human liver. *Hepatology* 1989, 10:437–446.

8. Takahashi T, Lasker JM, Rosman AS, Lieber CS: Induction of cytochrome P4502E1 in human liver by ethanol is due to a corresponding increase in encoding RNA. *Hepatology* 1993, 17:236–245.

9. Salaspuro MP, Lieber CS: Non-uniformity of blood ethanol elimination: Its exaggeration after chronic consumption. *Ann Clin Res* 1978, 10:294–297.

10. Lieber CS: GI pharmacology and therapeutics: Alcohol liver disease. In *Gastrointestinal Pharmacology and Therapeutics.* Edited by McCallum RW, Friedman G, Jacobson ED. New York: Raven Press, (in press).

11. Caballeria J, Frezza M, Hernandez-Munoz R, *et al.*: The gastric origin of the first pass metabolism of ethanol in man: effect of gastrectomy. *Gastroenterology* 1989, 97:1205–1209.

12. Gupta AM, Baraona E, Lieber CS: Potentiation of the cimetidine-induced increase in blood alcohol levels after repeated small ethanol doses. *Alcoholism: Clin Exp Res* 1994, 18:420.

13. Misra PS, Lefevre A, Ishii H, *et al.*: Increase of ethanol, meprobamate and pentobarbital metabolism after chronic ethanol administration in man and in rats. *Am J Med* 1971, 51:346–351.

14. Hasumura Y, Teschke R, Lieber CS: Increased carbon tetrachloride hepatotoxicity, and its mechanism, after chronic ethanol consumption. *Gastroenterology* 1974, 66:415–422.

15. Leo MA, Lieber CS: Hypervitaminosis A: A liver lover's lament. *Hepatology* 1988, 8:412–417.

16. Leo MA, Lowe N, Lieber CS: Potentiation of ethanol-induced hepatic vitamin A depletion by phenobarbital and butylated hydroxytoluene. *J Nutr* 1987, 117:70–76.

17. Leo MA, Lieber CS: Hepatic vitamin A depletion in alcoholic liver injury. *N Engl J Med* 1982, 307:597–601.

18. Leo MA, Arai M, Sato M, Lieber CS: Hepatotoxicity of vitamin A and ethanol in the rat. *Gastroenterology* 1982, 82:194–205.

19. Leo MA, Lieber CS: Hepatic fibrosis after long term administration of ethanol and moderate vitamin A supplementation in the rat. *Hepatology* 1983, 3:1–11.

20. Leo MA, Kim CI, Lowe N, Lieber CS: Interaction of ethanol with beta-carotene: Delayed blood clearance and enhanced hepatotoxicity. *Hepatology* 1992, 15:883–891.

21. Ahmed S, Leo MA, Lieber CS: Interactions between alcohol and β-carotene in patients with alcoholic liver disease. *Am J Clin Nutr* 1994, 60:430–436.

22. Hoerner M, Behrens UJ, Worner TM, *et al.*: The role of alcoholism and liver disease in the appearance of serum antibodies against acetaldehyde adducts. *Hepatology* 1988, 8:569–574.

23. Lieber CS, Baraona E, Hernandez-Munoz R, *et al.*: Impaired oxygen utilization: A new mechanism for the hepatotoxicity of ethanol in sub-human primates. *J Clin Invest* 1989, 83:1682–1690.

24. Lieber CS, Casini A, DeCarli LM, *et al.*: S-adenosyl-L-methionine attenuates alcohol-induced liver injury in the baboon. *Hepatology* 1990, 11:165–172.

25. Yamada S, Mak KM, Lieber CS: Chronic ethanol consumption alters rat liver plasma membranes and potentiates release of alkaline phosphatase. *Gastroenterology* 1985, 88:1799–1806.

26. Singer SJ, Nicholson GL: The fluid mosaic model of the structure of cell membranes. *Science* 1972, 175:720–730.

27. Li J-J, Kim C-I, Leo MA, *et al.*: Polyunsaturated lecithin prevents acetaldehyde-mediated hepatic collagen accumulation by stimulating collagenase activity in cultured lipocytes. *Hepatology* 1992, 15:373–381.

28. Mak KM, Lieber CS: Alterations in endothelial fenestration in liver sinusoids of baboons fed alcohol: A scanning electron microscopic study. *Hepatology* 1984, 4:386–391.

29. Worner TM, Lieber CS: Perivenular fibrosis as precursor lesion of cirrhosis. *JAMA* 1985, 254:627–630.

30. Ramond MU, Poynard T, Rueff B: A randomized trial of prednisone in patienta with severe alcoholic hepatitis. *N Engl J Med* 1992, 326:507–512.

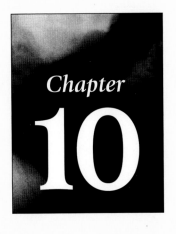

Chapter 10

Cirrhosis: Ascites and Spontaneous Bacterial Peritonitis

FLORENCE WONG

LAURENCE BLENDIS

Abnormalities in renal sodium handling and disturbed volume status are common complications of liver cirrhosis and can contribute to the development of ascites in these patients. The pathogenesis of this impaired renal sodium and water excretion remains controversial.

In this chapter, the pathogenesis and clinical aspects of cirrhotic ascites is discussed. In addition, one of the most important complications of chronic ascites in patients with advanced liver disease, spontaneous bacterial peritonitis, is reviewed with regard to pathogenesis, diagnosis, and therapy.

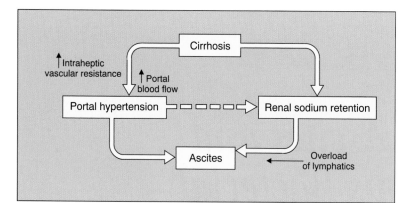

FIGURE 10-1.

Changes occur in cardiovascular and renal physiology in patients with cirrhosis, which encourage renal sodium and water retention. Increased intrahepatic vascular resistance to portal venous outflow, together with an increased inflow into the portal vein from splanchnic and splenic hyperemia, results in portal hypertension. This portal hypertension increases the hydrostatic pressure in the sinusoidal bed. When hepatic lymphatic drainage can no longer accommodate the excess fluid that leaves from the sinusoids, ascites develops.

■ ASCITES

Pathophysiology of ascites formation

Afferent mechanisms of renal sodium retention in cirrhosis

PERIPHERAL ARTERIAL VASODILATATION HYPOTHESIS

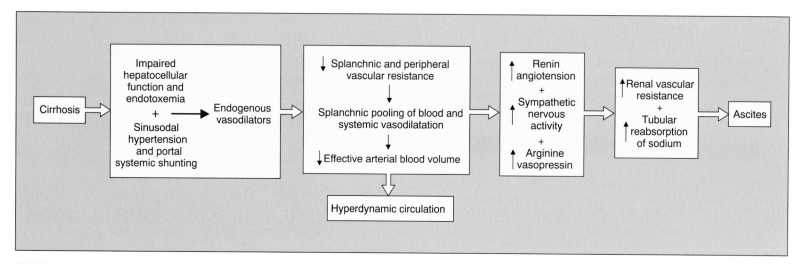

FIGURE 10-2.

One of several theories proposed to explain the pathogenesis of renal sodium and water retention in cirrhosis is the *Peripheral Arterial Vasodilatation Hypothesis*. Profound hemodynamic changes complicate the clinical course of chronic liver disease. There are openings of arteriovenous shunts and splanchnic and peripheral arteriolar vasodilatation. These openings result in lowered arterial blood pressure and systemic vascular resistance, leading to a reduction in the effective arterial blood volume and a hyperdynamic circulation. These changes, in turn, activate neurohumoral pressor systems, promoting renal sodium and water retention in an attempt to restore the effective arterial blood volume and maintain blood pressure. When increased renal sodium reabsorption cannot compensate for the arterial vasodilatation, arterial underfilling occurs. Then the cascade of further activation of various neurohumoral pressor systems begins, leading to increased renal sodium retention and ultimately, formation of ascites.

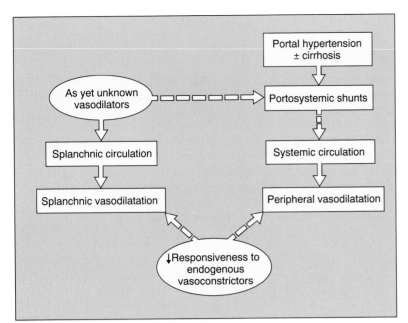

FIGURE 10-3.

Early studies indicate this systemic vasodilatation may partly result from refractoriness of the cardiovascular system to the elevated levels of as yet unknown endogenous vasoactive compounds. The presence of increased amounts of endogenous vasodilators, however, originating from the splanchnic circulation and gaining access into the systemic circulation through portosystemic shunts, has also been postulated, but the nature of the vasodilators remains speculative.

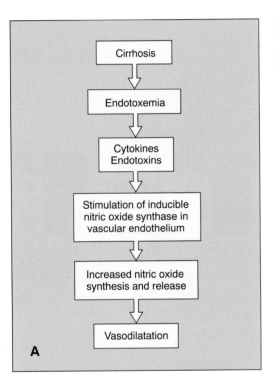

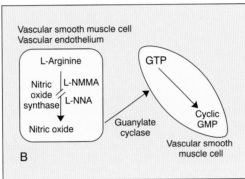

FIGURE 10-4.

A, The most recently proposed vasodilator is nitric oxide or endothelial-derived relaxing factor. Chronic endotoxemia that is associated with cirrhosis may stimulate synthesis and release of nitric oxide; although it more likely results from shear stress on the endothelium secondary to portal hypertension. **B,** Nitric oxide released from the endothelium stimulates the enzyme guanylate cyclase in the myocytes, leading to the production of cyclic guanosine monophosphate in the vascular smooth muscle cell, resulting in smooth muscle cell relaxation and vasodilatation. However, recent studies in animal models examining the role of nitric oxide as a vasodilator have yielded conflicting results. Therefore, the role of nitric oxide remains controversial. GMP—guanosine monophosphate; GTP—guanosine triphosphate; L-NMMA—N^G-monomethyl-L-arginine; L-NNA—N^G-nitro-L-arginine. (*Adapted from* Stark and Szurszewski [1]; with permission.)

TABLE 10-1. PUTATIVE VASODILATORS

Glucagon
Prostaglandins
Insulin
GABA
Substance P
VIP
Bile acids

TABLE 10-1.

Several other putative vasodilators have also been proposed. Glucagon is a vasodilator and its plasma concentration increases in rats with portal hypertension. Glucagon also increases azygous blood flow in patients with cirrhosis. Prostaglandins I_2 and E_2 have vasodilatory actions. Prostanoids are released into the portal vein in patients with liver disease. Increased urinary prostanoids have also been found in cirrhosis; the administration of indomethacin has resulted in worsening of renal hemodynamics, indicating the dependence of the kidneys on these vasodilatory prostaglandins in these patients. Insulin has both vasodilatory and antinatriuretic effects in normal subjects. Hyperinsulinemia in cirrhosis is well documented, although the link between the hyperinsulinemia and vasodilatation has not been formally assessed in these patients. γ-Aminobutyric acid (GABA) is a potent neuroinhibitor. In advanced liver disease, its hepatic clearance may be reduced and thus cause vasodilatation. Other putative vasodilators include substance P, vasoactive intestinal peptide (VIP), and bile acids. None of these have been definitely proven to be responsible for systemic vasodilatation.

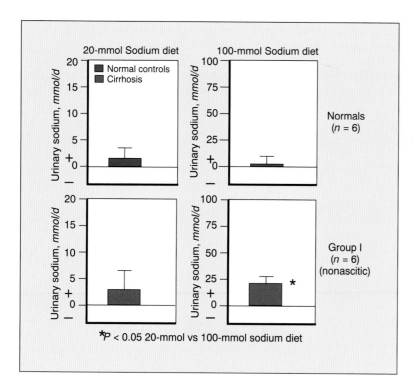

FIGURE 10-5.

More recent human data in pre- and early ascites have not, however, conformed to the Peripheral Arterial Vasodilatation Hypothesis. Evidence is now accumulating that these patients are retaining sodium and showing expanded volume before *underfilling,* which is secondary to systemic vasodilatation as proposed by the Peripheral Arterial Vasodilatation Hypothesis. When assessed with sodium balance studies, preascitic patients clearly demonstrate sodium retention compared with control subjects who were placed on a 100-mmol sodium per day diet. (*Adapted from* Warner *et al.* [2]; with permission.)

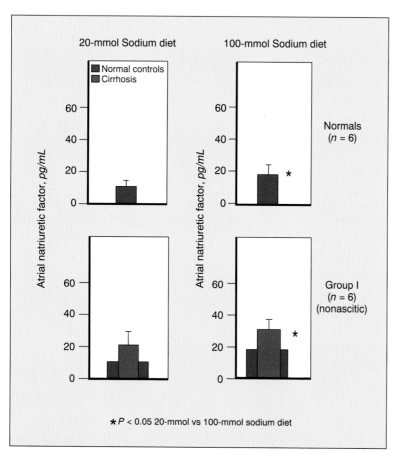

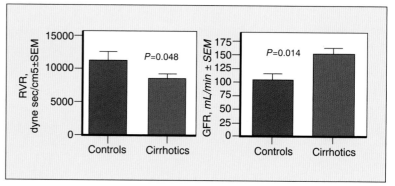

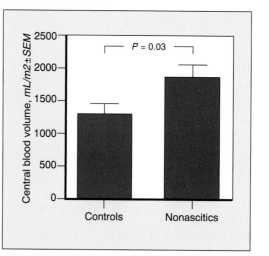

FIGURE 10-6.

Other findings that support intravascular volume expansion, rather than underfilling, of the circulatory volume in preascitic cirrhotic patients include 1) elevated levels of plasma atrial natriuretic factor indicating atrial stretch (**A**), 2) glomerular hyperfiltration and increased renal plasma flow (**B**), increased central blood volume (**C**), and normal or suppressed plasma renin activity, plasma

(Continued on next page)

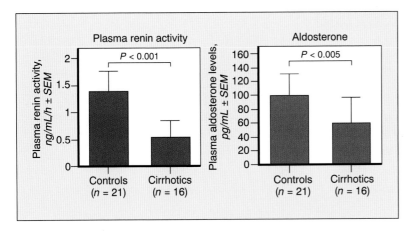

FIGURE 10-6. (CONTINUED)

aldosterone, and norepinephrine levels, indicating an adequately filled arterial volume (**D**). GFR—glomerular filtration rate; RVR—renal vascular resistance. (**A**, *Adapted from* Warner *et al.* [2]; with permission.) (**B**, *Adapted from* Wong *et al.* [3]; with permission.) (**C**, *Adapted from* Wong *et al.* [4]; with permission.) (**D**, *Adapted from* Bernardi *et al.* [5]; with permission.)

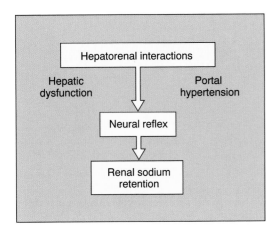

FIGURE 10-7.

The findings in Figure 10-6 all suggest an abnormality in sodium handling leading to sodium retention before onset of systemic vasodilatation and underfilling of the intravascular space. The next obvious question is "could the renal sodium retention be caused by some other abnormalities associated with cirrhosis?" It is feasible that hepatorenal interaction initiates renal sodium retention, and as cirrhosis progresses, splanchnic and peripheral vasodilatation contribute to, and may perpetuate, it (as described by the concept of Peripheral Arterial Vasodilatation Hypothesis). The hepatorenal interaction is as yet undefined. It is possible that hepatic dysfunction may either directly contribute to the sodium retention or play a permissive role in concert with sinusoidal portal hypertension, perhaps through some neurogenic pathway, to promote renal sodium retention in cirrhosis. The following experimental evidence is supportive of each one of these mechanisms being involved in the sodium retention.

SINUSOIDAL PORTAL HYPERTENSION

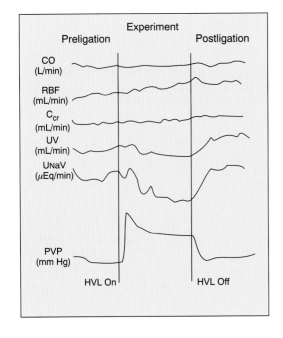

FIGURE 10-8.

In an acute animal model, production of sinusoidal portal hypertension by a ligature around the hepatic vein, with renal blood flow maintained constant with canine plasma, is associated with sodium retention. However, the same ligature around the portal vein, yielding the same height of portal hypertension at the presinusoidal level, does not produce renal sodium retention, suggesting that sinusoidal rather than presinusoidal portal hypertension is necessary for the development of sodium retention. C_{CR}—creatinine clearance; CO—cardiac output; HVL—hepatic vein ligation; PVP—portal venous pressure; RBF—renal blood flow; UNaV—urinary sodium excretion; UV—urinary volume. (*Adapted from* Campbell *et al.* [6]; with permission.)

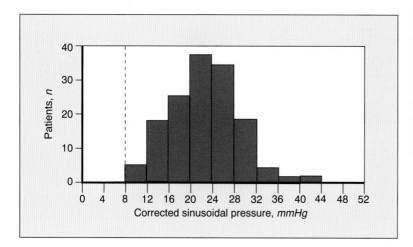

FIGURE 10-9.

It has also been shown that, in a cohort of cirrhotic patients, there is a critical level of sinusoidal portal hypertension of 8 mm Hg below which ascites does not occur. The recent introduction of the transjugular intrahepatic portosystemic stent shunt to reduce sinusoidal portal pressure, leading to the disappearance of ascites, also supports the important role of sinusoidal portal hypertension in the pathogenesis of sodium retention in cirrhosis. (*Adapted from* Morali *et al.* [7]; with permission.)

HEPATIC DYSFUNCTION

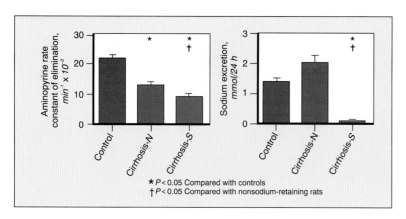

FIGURE 10-10.

Sinusoidal portal hypertension, however, is not the sole factor responsible for renal sodium retention in cirrhosis. In carbon tetrachloride–induced cirrhosis in the rat, the onset of renal sodium retention has been demonstrated to be related to a critical level of hepatic dysfunction as measured by the aminopyrine breath test, suggesting that hepatic dysfunction may also play a role in the pathogenesis of renal sodium retention. N—nonsodium-retaining rats; S—sodium-retaining rats. (*Adapted from* Wensing *et al.* [8]; with permission.)

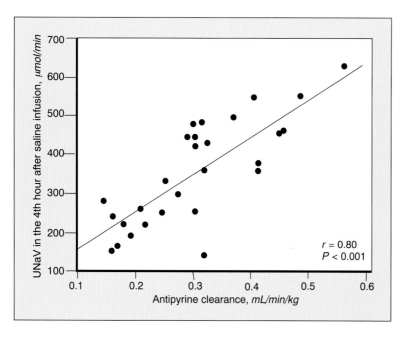

FIGURE 10-11.

A more recent study confirms a correlation between the ability of a group of preascitic cirrhotic patients to handle an intravenous saline load and antipyrine clearance, a measure of the functional hepatocellular mass, thus further strengthening the association between hepatic dysfunction and sodium retention. UNaV— urinary sodium excretion. (*Adapted from* Wong *et al.* [9]; with permission.)

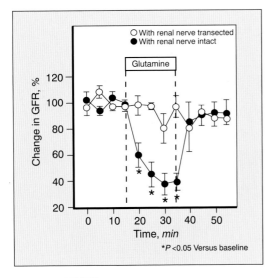

FIGURE 10-12.

Whether sinusoidal portal hypertension or hepatic dysfunction initiates the signal for renal sodium retention, it appears that a hepatorenal neural reflex is involved in causing renal sodium retention. Glutamine induces hepatocellular swelling. When it is infused into the superior mesenteric vein in rats, the glomerular filtration rate (GFR) is promptly reduced. This reduction is abolished when the renal nerve is transected, thus suggesting a neural link between the liver and the kidney. (*Adapted from* Lang *et al*. [10]; with permission.)

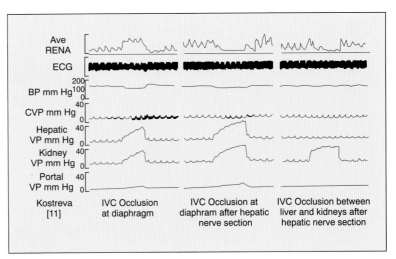

FIGURE 10-13.

In another experimental dog model, occlusion of the inferior vena cava (IVC) leading to sinusoidal portal hypertension results in increased hepatic and renal sympathetic nervous activities. Hepatic nerve section abolishes the increase in renal sympathetic nervous activities. It is therefore possible that hepatic dysfunction may either directly contribute to the sodium retention or play a permissive role in concert with sinusoidal portal hypertension, perhaps through some neurogenic pathway, to promote renal sodium retention in cirrhosis. Ave RENA—average renal sympathetic efferent nerve activity; BP—blood pressure; CVP—central VP; ECG—electrocardiograph; VP—venous pressure. (*Adapted from* Kostreva *et al*. [11]; with permission.)

Efferent mechanisms of renal sodium retention in cirrhosis

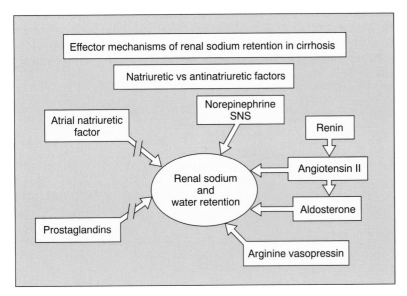

FIGURE 10-14.

Whatever the pathogenetic process is in initiating renal sodium and water retention in cirrhosis, the efferent mechanisms involved in effecting the sodium retention are multifactorial. The predominance of either natriuretic or antinatriuretic factors will ultimately decide if the patient will remain in sodium balance or retain sodium. SNS—sympathetic nervous system. (*From* Wong and Blendis [12]; with permission.)

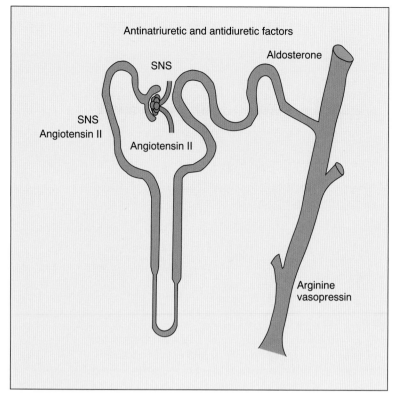

FIGURE 10-15.

The antinatriuretic, antidiuretic factors include an activated sympathetic nervous system (SNS), increased renin-angiotensin-aldosterone levels, as well as elevated arginine vasopressin concentrations. Chronic SNS stimulation in cirrhosis is well documented. It affects both renal hemodynamics as well as renal tubular function. An increase in renal SNS activity leads to an increase in renal vascular resistance, located predominantly at the level of the afferent arteriole, and a decrease in glomerular filtration rate and renal blood flow. An increase in α-adrenergic tone also results in increased proximal tubular reabsorption of sodium, and an increase in β-adrenergic tone results in increased renin excretion. Increased renin production is caused mainly by increased secretion by the kidney. This increased renin production is the result of increased renal sympathetic activity, directly stimulating renin release from the juxtaglomerular apparatus, as well as because of impaired renal perfusion secondary to both decreased renal perfusion pressure and increased afferent arteriolar tone. Increased renin secretion leads to increased production of angiotensin II, which then increases renal vascular resistance by preferentially increasing efferent arteriolar tone, thereby decreasing renal blood flow and increasing glomerular filtration rate. Angiotensin II increases proximal tubular reabsorption of sodium independent of renal hemodynamic changes. It also stimulates secretion of aldosterone from the adrenal cortex, which in turn stimulates the reabsorption of sodium at the distal renal tubule, promoting more avid sodium retention. There is nonosmotic hypersecretion of arginine vasopressin in response to volume receptor activation by the systemic and splanchnic vasodilatation. This action impairs water excretion in the collecting tubule.

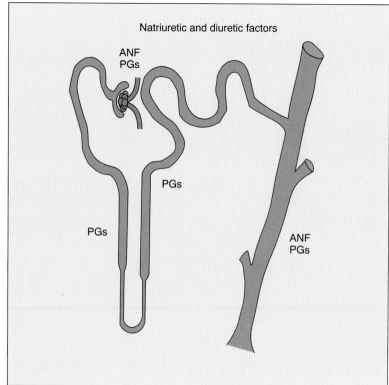

FIGURE 10-16.

The natriuretic, diuretic factors include elevated atrial natriuretic factor (ANF) concentrations as well as increased production of renal prostaglandins. ANF is both a vasodilatory as well as a natriuretic hormone and increased secretion is stimulated by atrial stretch. It increases the glomerular filtration rate by afferent vasodilatation and efferent vasoconstriction. ANF increases natriuresis independent of its renal hemodynamic effects by directly inhibiting sodium reabsorption in the inner medullary collecting duct. Renal prostaglandins are autocoids that decrease renal vascular tone, preferentially dilating the afferent arteriole in the presence of pressor agents such as norepinephrine and angiotensin II. They also promote a natriuresis by altering chloride transport and hence sodium reabsorption in the medullary segment of the thick ascending limb of the loop of Henle and inducing a diuresis by reducing the tonicity of the renal medullary interstitium as well as by inhibiting the effects of arginine vasopressin on the collecting tubule. PG—prostaglandin.

Factors localizing fluid retention to the peritoneal space

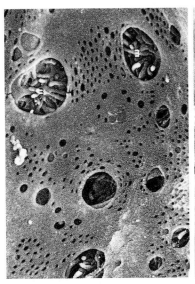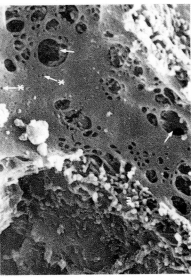

FIGURE 10-17.

The hepatic sinusoidal bed is a specialized capillary bed. The sinusoidal endothelium, with its fenestrae and lack of a basement membrane, is freely permeable to albumin; therefore no trans-sinusoidal oncotic pressure gradient can develop to retain fluid in the intravascular space.

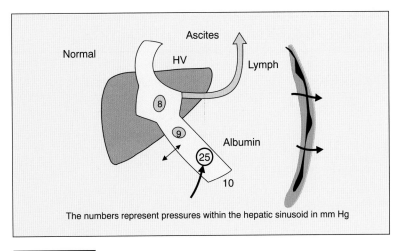

FIGURE 10-18.

The hepatic sinusoidal bed is normally a low pressure venous bed resulting from high presinusoidal resistance in the hepatic arterioles. Sinusoidal hydrostatic pressure is therefore very low. There is minimal pressure gradient from the portal venous end to the hepatic venous end of the sinusoidal bed. Interstitial fluid that escapes from the sinusoids into the hepatic parenchyma is drained away by hepatic lymphatics and very little escapes through the liver capsule into the peritoneal cavity. HV—hepatic vein.

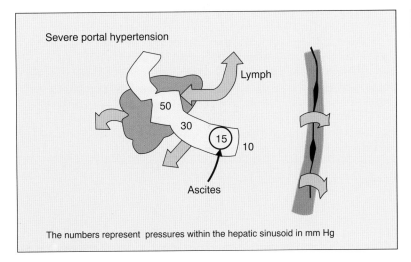

FIGURE 10-19.

When cirrhosis develops, there is a hepatic venous outflow block, leading to sinusoidal portal hypertension. Sinusoidal hydrostatic pressure increases markedly, which favors transudation of fluid into the interstitial space. There remains no oncotic pressure gradient across the sinusoids caused by free passage of albumin through the sinusoidal fenestrae. Regional hepatic lymphatics become tortuous and dilated and increase their drainage capacity as much as 20-fold. Fluid begins to escape through the liver capsule into the peritoneal cavity as ascites. Once sequestered within the peritoneal cavity, ascitic fluid can be reabsorbed by the peritoneal lymphatics at a maximal rate of 900 mL/d. When hepatic lymph production exceeds the drainage capacities of the hepatic and peritoneal lymphatics, ascites will accumulate.

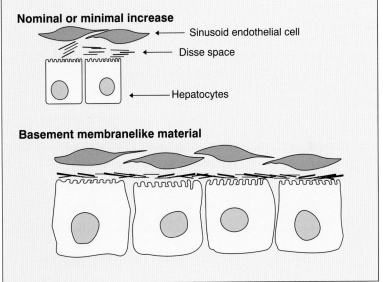

FIGURE 10-20.

In the later stage of cirrhosis, a basement membranelike material that *capillarises* the sinusoid is laid down. This membrane reduces the sinusoidal permeability; an oncotic pressure gradient develops between the hepatic interstitial space and the sinusoidal lumen. The development of this oncotic pressure gradient acts to counterbalance the hydrostatic pressure gradient, thereby decreasing hepatic lymph production. Accumulation of ascitic fluid in the peritoneal cavity also leads to a rise of the intra-abdominal pressure. This pressure is transmitted back to the hepatic parenchyma and results in a rise in interstitial pressure, counteracting further fluid loss. At this stage of cirrhosis, however, these compensatory mechanisms are no longer adequate to eliminate ascites. (*Adapted from* Orrego *et al.* [13]; with permission.)

TABLE 10-2. HEPATORENAL INTERACTION

No ascites	Responsive ascites	Unresponsive ascites	Hepatorenal syndrome
ANF-normal or ↑	ANF compensation fails	ANF compensation fails	ANF ↓
Compensated sodium handling	ANF responsiveness maintained	ANF responsiveness fails	PRA, Aldo ↑↑↑
PRA, Aldo-normal or ↓	PRA, Aldo ↑	PRA, Aldo ↑↑	Renal PGs ↓
Renal PGs-normal or ↑	Renal PGs ↑	Renal PGs ↑↑	Renal vasoconstriction ↑
Renal vasodilatation	Renal vasoconstriction	Renal vasoconstriction	Systemic vasodilatation ↑
Systemic vasodilatation	Systemic vasodilatation	Systemic vasodilatation	Precipitating factors:
			Jaundice
			Sepsis
			Hemorrhage
			Volume disturbance
			Nephrotoxic drugs

TABLE 10-2.

In the natural history of cirrhosis, the patient passes through many stages of renal sodium handling. Before the clinical appearance of ascites or at the preascites stage of cirrhosis, patients already have a tendency to retain sodium. This abnormality is subtle but can be readily demonstrated when these patients are challenged by a sodium load. Intravascular volume expands, associated with renal sodium retention. These preascitic cirrhotic patients remain in sodium balance, presumably as a result of the natriuretic effect of elevated antinatriuretic factor (ANF) levels, unopposed by normal or low levels of antinatriuretic forces. As the cirrhotic disease progresses, sodium and water retention also become more severe. Ascites develops when local factors preferentially localize the excess fluid into the peritoneal cavity. In early ascites, diuretic-induced increased delivery of sodium to the distal nephron enables the increased ANF secretion to facilitate the necessary increase in sodium excretion. Later, systemic arterial vasodilatation develops. Activation of pressor systems as a result of relative arterial under-filling not only promotes further renal sodium and water retention but also stimulates renal vasoconstriction. Increased activities of the renin angiotensin and the sympathetic nervous systems therefore blunt the natriuretic response to diuretics and elevated ANF levels. These changes also stimulate renal prostaglandin (PG) secretion, thereby maintaining the integrity of renal function and the patient remains diuretic responsive. When the increased prostaglandin secretion cannot overcome the vasoconstrictive and antinatriuretic forces, refractory ascites ensues. Finally, prostaglandin secretion fails, and the unopposed vasoconstrictive influences lead to marked sodium retention and ultimately hepatorenal syndrome. Aldo—aldosterone; PRA—plasma renin activity. (*Adapted from* Wong and Blendis [14]; with permission.)

Clinical features and consequences of ascites

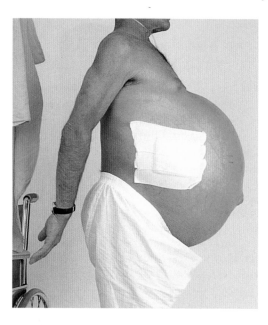

FIGURE 10-21.

Ascites often develops insidiously over the course of months and the patient presents with abdominal distension. Ascites may develop suddenly if there is a precipitating cause such as infection, an alcoholic binge, development of a hepatoma, or thrombosis of the hepatic vein. Once ascites becomes clinically obvious, the patient usually is ill with moderate muscle wasting. The umbilicus is everted. Pedal edema is common, partly related to the hypoalbuminemia and partly related to the pressure on the inferior vena cava by the abdominal fluid.

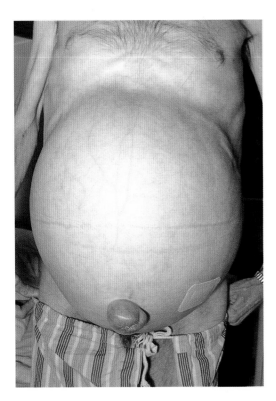

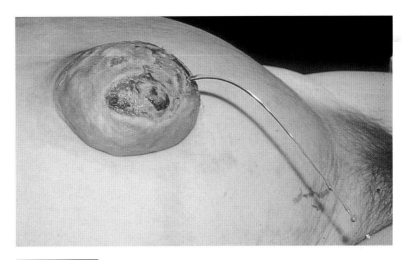

FIGURE 10-22.

Increased intra-abdominal pressure favors development of hernias in the umbilicus, the inguinal regions, and through abdominal incisions. Pressure from the ascites-filled hernial sacs may cause considerable discomfort.

FIGURE 10-23.

Occasionally, tense ascites can lead to rupture of an umbilical hernia, thereby predisposing the patient to the potentially fatal complication of bacterial peritonitis. We recommend, therefore, prophylactic repair of umbilical hernias after removal of the ascites. This repair is usually associated with a low mortality rate. Rupture of an umbilical hernia requires wide-spectrum antibiotics, as well as surgical repair. The morality rate, however, is high.

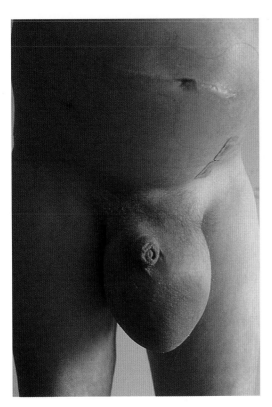

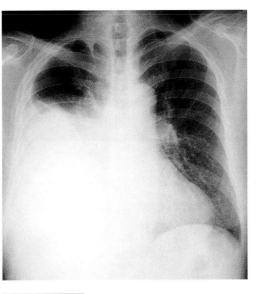

FIGURE 10-24.

Frequently ascitic fluid can track down to the scrotum, causing scrotal and penile edema. Scrotal edema can be mistaken for a hydrocele. Treatments include bed rest with the foot of the bed raised, scrotal support bandages, and diuretics to reduce the ascites. Drainage of the scrotal edema is not recommended, because it often results in a permanent fistula.

FIGURE 10-25.

Pleural effusion is present in about 6% of patients with ascites and usually is on the right side. This effusion is the result of a defect in the diaphragm that allows the ascitic fluid to pass up into the pleural cavity. In contrast, a left-sided pleural effusion in an ascitic patient may indicate pulmonary pathology. Occasionally, a pleural effusion can be seen in the absence of ascites caused by the negative intrathoracic pressure drawing up the ascitic fluid through the diaphragmatic defect into the pleural cavity. Thoracentesis is followed by rapid refilling of the pleural cavity because of the negative intrathoracic pressure, and control of the pleural effusion can only be achieved with the control of ascites.

Diagnosis of ascites

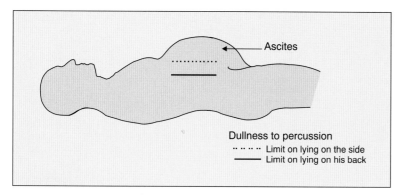

FIGURE 10-26.

The earliest sign of ascites present in the abdominal cavity is bulging of the flanks. There is at least 2 L of fluid in the abdominal cavity when dullness to percussion in the flank is detected. The presence of fluid in the abdominal cavity can be confirmed by the shifting of the percussion dullness when the patient changes position. A fluid thrill usually means much more free fluid, with the fluid under tension.

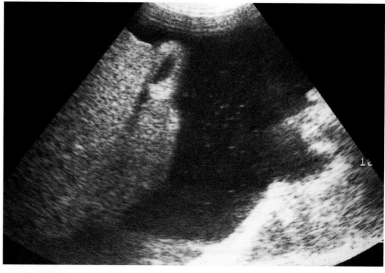

FIGURE 10-27.

Less than 2 L of peritoneal fluid is difficult to detect clinically. Abdominal ultrasound is useful in defining small amounts of ascites, and therefore this investigation is the standard criterion for the detection of ascites. Ascitic fluid is shown as a space around a shrunken cirrhotic liver. The ultrasonographer can add a suitable surface marker to aid the clinician who is about to perform diagnostic abdominal paracentesis.

TABLE 10-3. PARACENTESIS IS REQUIRED

At first presentation

Alteration of the patient's clinical state

Sudden increase in ascites

Worsening of hepatic encephalopathy

Presence of fever

TABLE 10-3.

Diagnostic paracentesis should be performed at first presentation no matter how obvious the cause of the ascites or when there is alteration of the patient's clinical state, such as a sudden increase in the amount of ascitic fluid, worsening of encephalopathy, or presence of fever, in order to rule out other complications such as spontaneous bacterial peritonitis and hepatocellular carcinoma.

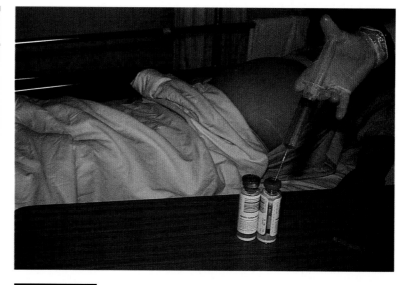

FIGURE 10-28.

Direct inoculation of at least 10 mL of ascitic fluid into two blood culture bottles at the bedside, one for aerobic and one for anaerobic organisms, is important as this process increases the positive culture yield should bacterial peritonitis be present. Further samples should be sent separately for biochemical analysis and cell count.

TABLE 10-4. ASCITIC FLUID ANALYSIS

Polymorphonuclear count
> 250/µL is diagnostic of spontaneous bacterial peritonitis
Ascitic fluid albumin concentration
Serum-ascitic fluid albumin gradient > 11 g/L is suggestive of cirrhotic, rather than malignant, ascites

TABLE 10-4.

Ascitic fluid analysis should include a total polymorphonuclear count and albumin concentration. A serum-ascitic fluid albumin gradient of greater than 11 g/L represents cirrhotic rather than malignant ascites. A high-protein content may be associated with Budd-Chiari syndrome or pancreatic ascites. A total polymorphonuclear count of greater than 250/µL is diagnostic of spontaneous bacterial peritonitis.

Differential diagnosis of ascites

TABLE 10-5. DIFFERENTIAL DIAGNOSIS OF ASCITES

Cirrhosis	Constrictive pericarditis
Hepatoma	Nephrotic syndrome
Tuberculous peritonitis in the malnourished alcoholic	Pancreatitis
Peritoneal carcinomatosis	Malignant chylous ascites, especially lymphoma
Right-sided cardiac failure	

TABLE 10-5.

Many causes of noncirrhotic ascites exist. Hepatic venous obstruction or Budd-Chiari syndrome must be considered, especially if the protein count of the ascitic fluid is high. Severe right-sided heart failure or constrictive pericarditis is usually clinically obvious and can be confirmed with the characteristic echocardiographic findings. A chest radiograph will also demonstrate the changes of right heart failure or calcification of the pericardium as causes of constrictive pericarditis. Similarly, nephrotic syndrome as a cause of ascites can be easily diagnosed by the presence of generalized edema and proteinuria. Tuberculous ascites should be suspected in the severely malnourished alcoholic cirrhotic. The patient is usually febrile, but fever may be absent in half of the patients. The leukocyte count of the ascitic fluid is usually, but not always, elevated. These leukocytes are usually lymphocytes, but sometimes can be polymorphs. The protein content of the ascitic fluid is usually greater than 3.5 g/L. The ascitic fluid should be stained for acid-fast bacilli, but the smears are rarely positive. Positive culture is found in only half the patients. Malignant ascites is often blood stained and the protein count is high. Cytology of the ascitic fluid is often negative. Chylous ascites suggests metastatic cancer, predominantly lymphoma. Pancreatic ascites can complicate acute pancreatitis but is rarely gross. A high-ascitic amylase level of greater than 1000 U/L is diagnostic of pancreatic ascites.

Treatment of ascites

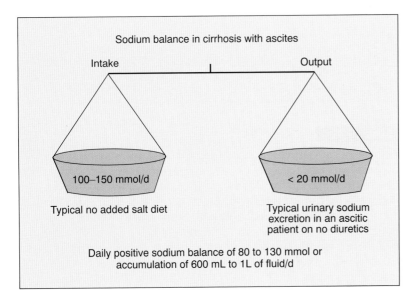

Sodium balance in cirrhosis with ascites

Intake — Output

100–150 mmol/d — < 20 mmol/d

Typical no added salt diet — Typical urinary sodium excretion in an ascitic patient on no diuretics

Daily positive sodium balance of 80 to 130 mmol or accumulation of 600 mL to 1L of fluid/d

FIGURE 10-29.

Although bed rest will result in a redistribution of body fluid, sodium and fluid restriction is required to mobilize the ascites. Typically, an ascitic patient receiving no diuretics excretes less than 20 mmol of sodium per day. An ascitic patient consuming a typical *no added salt* diet containing approximately 100 to 150 mmol of sodium per day would result in the patient having a positive sodium balance of up to 130 mmol/d or the accumulation of up to 1 L of fluid per day. A negative sodium balance is better achieved by reducing dietary sodium intake. A 20 mmol of sodium per day diet, though unpalatable, is necessary in patients with refractory ascites. In most other patients, however, restriction to 40 mmol of sodium per day should be adequate.

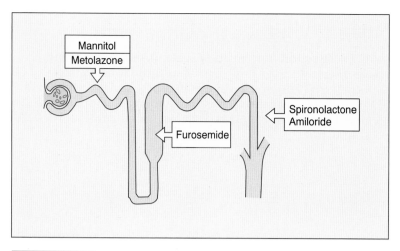

FIGURE 10-30.

Diuretic therapy is usually required in addition to sodium and fluid restriction to control ascites. The aim of diuretic therapy is to block the various renal sodium-retaining mechanisms and thereby increase urinary sodium excretion. Distal diuretics (*eg*, spironolactone, triamterene, amiloride) are relatively weak. The half-life of spironolactone in patients with end-stage cirrhosis is between 10 to 35 hours because of impaired metabolism. There is a lag phase of 2 to 4 days before the onset of action and up to 7 days for offset of action when therapy is discontinued. Therefore, dosages of spironolactone should not be adjusted more often than once every 7 days. Amiloride is preferred because its onset and offset of action are not as long. Loop diuretics are very powerful. They can increase urinary sodium excretion as much as 300%. The onset of action of furosemide is within 30 minutes after oral administration, with a peak effect within 1 to 2 hours and most of the natriuretic activity completed within 3 to 4 hours. The dose-response curve of furosemide is sigmoidal. After a maximal response is reached, administration of higher doses does not produce a further natriuretic response. Diuretics that act on the proximal renal tubule are very potent. They should not be used without careful monitoring because severe intravascular volume depletion leading to renal dysfunction is a common complication. They are generally not recommended as outpatient therapy.

TABLE 10-6. DIURETICS USED IN ASCITES

Type of diuretic	Name	Side effects
Distal	Spironolactone	Gynecomastia
		Hyperkalemia
		Renal tubular acidosis
	Amiloride	Hyperkalemia
	Triamterene	
Loop	Furosemide	Hyponatremia
	Ethacrynic acid	Hypokalemia
		Azotemia
Proximal	Metolazone	Hyponatremia
		Hypokalemia
		Azotemia

TABLE 10-6.

Diuretic therapy, especially furosemide, must be balanced against the frequency of occurrence of complications. Intravascular hypovolemia, leading to azotemia and metabolic alkalosis, occurs in 20% of ascitic patients treated with diuretics. Hyponatremia is the result of drug-induced natriuresis and renal impairment to excrete free water. Hyperkalemia and hypokalemia are common, depending on the class of diuretic used. Diuretics can also induce hepatic encephalopathy, mainly through hypovolemia and impaired cerebral perfusion. The kidney is a very important source of ammonia, and diuretics increase the production of ammonia in the renal vein. Other troublesome side effects of spironolactone include painful gynecomastia, decreased libido, and impotence. Chronic treatment with diuretics can also cause muscle cramps in the lower extremities.

Refractory ascites

TABLE 10-7. REFRACTORY ASCITES

Prolonged history of ascites unresponsive to 400 mg of spironolactone or 30 mg of amiloride plus up to 120 mg of furosemide daily for 2 weeks

Patients who cannot tolerate diuretics because of side effects are also regarded as diuretic resistant

TABLE 10-7.

Refractory, or resistant, ascites is defined as a prolonged history of ascites unresponsive to 400 mg of spironolactone or 30 mg of amiloride plus up to 120 mg of furosemide daily for 2 weeks. Patients who cannot tolerate diuretics because of their side effects are also regarded as diuretic resistant. Some 5% to 10% of ascitic patients admitted to hospital for treatment of ascites have refractory ascites. It is worthwhile to perform a sodium balance study on these patients while they are under strict dietary sodium and fluid control in hospital. Some of these patients are not truly diuretic resistant, rather, their noncompliance when treated as outpatients accounts for the lack of response. Demonstration of weight loss in hospital when under strict dietary control can sometimes bring the message home. There are various treatment options for refractory ascites.

TABLE 10-8. COMPLICATIONS DURING THE FIRST HOSPITAL STAY IN PATIENTS FROM GROUP 1 (TREATED WITH PARACENTESIS) AND GROUP 2 (TREATED WITH DIURETICS)

	GROUP 1 (*n* = 58)	GROUP 2 (*n* = 59)	*P*
Patients with complications	10	36	< 0.001
Hyponatremia	3	18	< 0.001
Encephalopathy	6	17	< 0.002
Renal impairment	2	16	< 0.001
Hyperkalemia	1	7	NS
Gastrointestinal bleeding	2	6	NS
Peritonitis	0	4	NS
Bacteremia	2	0	NS
Others	0	4*	NS

* Two patients with possible infections, one patient with respiratory failure, and one patient with strangulated hernia. NS—not significant.

TABLE 10-8.

Repeated large volume paracentesis (4 to 6 L/d) together with intravenous albumin infusion has been shown in a randomized controlled trial to be safer and more effective in eliminating ascites than standard diuretics. Furthermore, the incidence of systemic and renal hemodynamic disturbance, hyponatremia, hepatic encephalopathy, and renal impairment was much lower in the patients treated with paracentesis than in those treated with diuretics. The duration of patient hospital stay was also shorter.

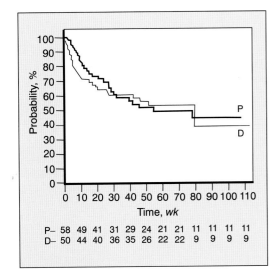

FIGURE 10-31.

In contrast to Table 10-8, there was no difference in the rate of hospital readmission, probability of survival, and cause of death in this study. P—paracentesis; D—diuretics. (*Adapted from* Gines *et al.* [15]; with permission.)

TABLE 10-9. PATIENTS DEVELOPING COMPLICATIONS DURING THE FIRST HOSPITAL STAY IN GROUP 1 AND GROUP 2 AND TYPES OF COMPLICATIONS*

	GROUP 1 (*n* = 52)	GROUP 2 (*n* = 53)	*P*
Patients with complications	6	16	NS
Hyponatremia and/or renal impairment	0	9	< 0.01
Hyponatremia and/or renal impairment plus other complications	1	2	NS
Other complications	8	5	NS
Number of complications	13	23	NS
Hyponatremia	1	9	< 0.01
Renal impairment	0	6	< 0.05
Encephalopathy	6	3	NS
Gastrointestinal hemorrhage	2	1	NS
Severe infection	4†	4‡	NS

* Group 1 equals paracentesis plus intravenous albumin; group 2 equals paracentesis without intravenous albumin. † Three patients with bacteremia and one patient with pneumonia. ‡ Two patients with bacteremia and two patients with peritonitis. NS—not significant.

TABLE 10-9.

The next question is "should cirrhotic patients with tense ascites be treated with repeated large volume paracentesis with or without intravenous albumin infusion?" In a trial from Barcelona [16], paracentesis plus intravenous albumin was shown not to induce any significant changes in renal function tests, plasma renin activity, or plasma aldosterone levels. However, repeated large volume paracenteses without volume expansion resulted in significant hyponatremia, increases in plasma renin activity and aldosterone concentrations, as well as impairment of renal function. (*Adapted from* Gines *et al.* [16]; with permission.)

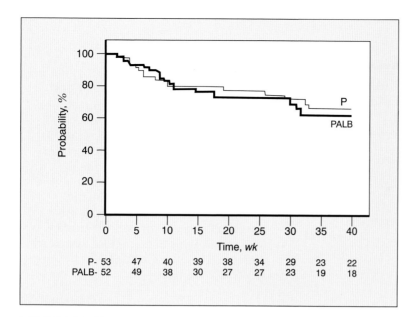

Figure 10-32.

Once again, there was no difference in the probability of survival between the patients whose ascites was treated with paracentesis together with albumin (PALB) and those without albumin infusion (P).

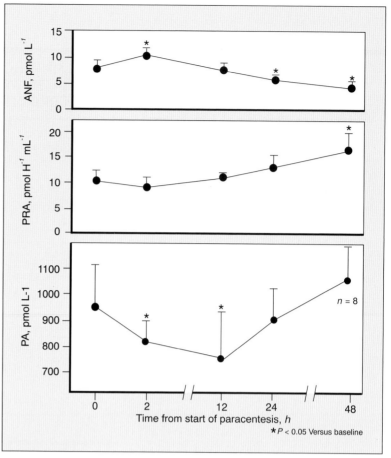

Figure 10-33.

More recently, a single large volume paracentesis with albumin infusion has been demonstrated to have no significant deleterious effect on systemic hemodynamics and renal function. Single total paracentesis without albumin infusion, however, is associated with the same complications as repeated paracentesis without albumin infusion. The atrial natriuretic factor (ANF) decreased and plasma renin activity (PRA) and plasma aldosterone (PA) levels increase significantly indicating intravascular volume depletion. Patients treated with paracentesis still require dietary sodium restriction and diuretic therapy to prevent the reaccumulation of ascites. (*Adapted from* Panos *et al.* [17]; with permission.)

Peritoneovenous (LeVeen) shunt

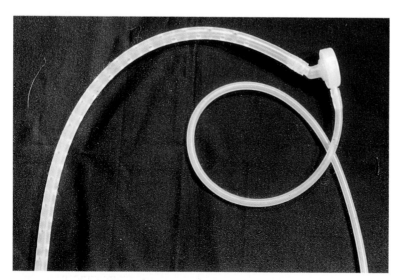

Figure 10-34.

A peritoneovenous shunt is a device consisting of a perforated intra-abdominal tube connected through a one-way pressure sensitive valve to a silicone tube, which traverses the subcutaneous tissue up to the neck, where it enters the internal jugular vein.

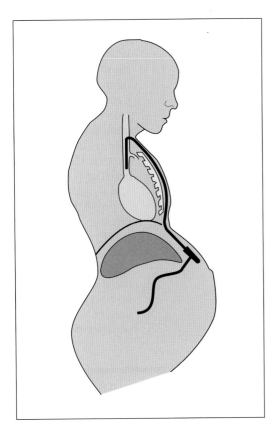

FIGURE 10-35.

The lower end of the LeVeen shunt is in the peritoneal cavity. The tip of the intravenous end is located in the superior vena cava. The shunt allows one-way passage of the ascitic fluid back into the systemic circulation. Flow in the shunt is maintained if there is a 3- to 5-cm H_2O pressure gradient between the abdominal cavity and the superior vena cava. A fall in the gradient will cause the valve to close, thus preventing blood from flowing back into the tubing.

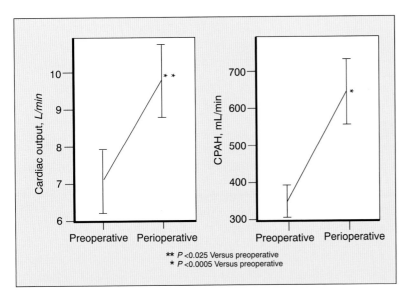

** $P < 0.025$ Versus preoperative
* $P < 0.0005$ Versus preoperative

FIGURE 10-36.

A, Infusion of ascitic fluid into systemic circulation is associated with many physiologic changes. Circulating blood volume increases. Cardiac output and renal plasma flow, as measured by para-amino-hippurate clearance (CPAH), increase. Because arterial pressure does not increase, there is a concomitant reduction in systemic vascular resistance. **B,** Plasma atrial natriuretic factor concentrations increase and, together with the suppression of plasma renin activity (PRA), plasma aldosterone, and norepinephrine concentrations, result in a significant natriuresis and diuresis in most patients. (*Adapted from* Blendis *et al.* [18]; with permission.)

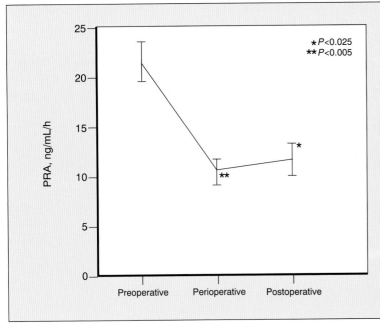

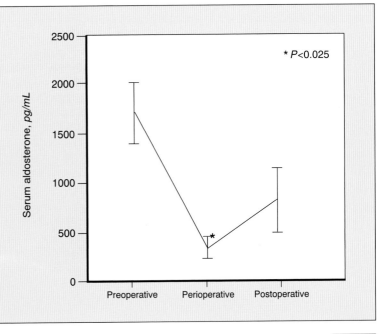

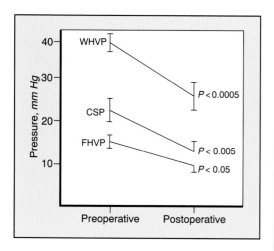

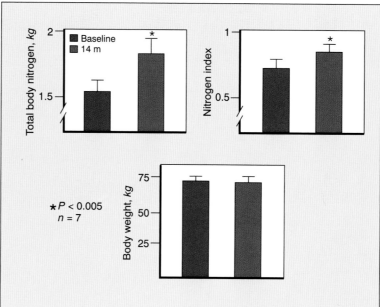

FIGURE 10-37.

When followed up for longer periods, those patients with a successful peritoneovenous shunt demonstrate a significant reduction in their corrected sinusoidal pressure (CSP) (**A**) and a significant improvement in nitrogen balance (**B**). FHVP—free hepatic venous pressure; WHVP—wedged hepatic venous pressure. (*Adapted from* Blendis *et al.* [19]; with permission.)

TABLE 10-10. PERITONEOVENOUS SHUNTING

EARLY COMPLICATIONS

Technical	Kinking/dislodgement
Cardiopulmonary	Pulmonary edema
Coagulopathy	Disseminated intravascular coagulation
Infection	
Esophageal variceal rupture	

TABLE 10-10.

Despite these positive effects of a peritoneovenous shunt, a number of both early and late complications exist. Immediate postoperative complications include acute pulmonary edema caused by sudden volume overload. Other early problems include technical problems such as kinking and dislodgement of the shunt, which will require its immediate removal. Shunt infection, if it occurs, is usually caused by *Staphylococcus aureus*. Prophylactic antibiotics have reduced its incidence. Disseminated intravascular coagulation used to follow almost every case of shunt insertion. Disseminated intravascular coagulation is thought to be caused by the infusion of activated coagulation factors from the ascitic fluid into the systemic circulation. Surgeons now routinely remove ascitic fluid and replace it with normal saline to reduce its occurrence. Rapid expansion of the plasma volume is associated with an acute increase in portal pressure and increases the risk of variceal hemorrhage. This complication can be prevented by removing most of the ascitic fluid at operation.

TABLE 10-11. PERITONEOVENOUS SHUNT

LATE COMPLICATIONS

Shunt obstruction	Mesenteric fibrosis
Superior vena cava syndrome	Small bowel obstruction
Recurrent bacteremia	

TABLE 10-11.

Shunt obstruction is the most common complication during follow-up. This complication is usually the result of fibrin deposition within the shunt. Occasionally, shunt obstruction may also be caused by thrombosis of the venous limb of the prosthesis. Superior vena cava syndrome is much less common. Recurrent bacteremia indicates colonization of the shunt or endocarditis, and the shunt should be removed. Finally, mesenteric fibrosis and small bowel obstruction have been reported in a small percentage of patients with peritoneovenous shunt. Shunt obstruction is not associated with the recurrence of ascites in a small proportion of patients. If ascites reaccumulates and renal function deteriorates, however, a new shunt should be inserted.

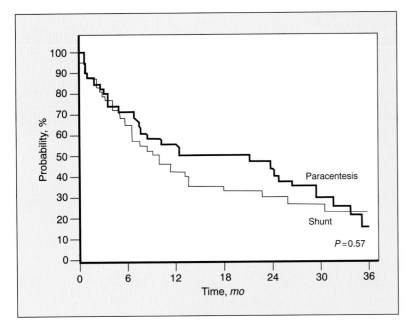

FIGURE 10-38.

Although peritoneovenous shunt can improve systemic hemodynamics and sodium homeostasis, its beneficial effects are usually
short lived because of the high incidence of obstruction. Morbidity
and survival correlate with the degree of hepatic dysfunction.
Recent multicenter randomized control trials did not show it to
be superior to either routine medical therapy or repeated paracentesis in terms of hospital readmission rate or survival. (*Adapted
from* Gines *et al.* [20]; with permission.)

TABLE 10-12. PVS

SELECTION CRITERIA	RELATIVE CONTRAINDICATIONS
Serum bilirubin < 60 μmol/L	Previous abdominal surgery
Prothrombin time < 4 seconds prolonged	Spontaneous bacterial peritonitis
Platelet count > 50 X 10⁶/L	Large esophageal varices

TABLE 10-12.

Peritoneovenous shunt (PVS) should be restricted to be used in
patients with refractory ascites and preserved hepatic function.
Initial studies by LeVeen [21] indicated that patients with high
postoperative mortality were those with deep jaundice and those
who had a severe coagulopathy with an elevated prothrombin
time and thrombocytopenia. The criteria listed in the table for
patient selection for PVS are recommended for improved long-
term shunt function and survival.

Transjugular intrahepatic portosystemic stent shunt

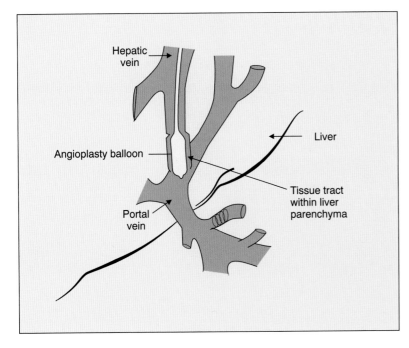

FIGURE 10-39.

Transjugular intrahepatic portosystemic stent shunt has been used
as an alternative treatment for patients with variceal bleeding who
have failed sclerotherapy. It was observed that patients who had
concomitant ascites either had reduction or disappearance of their
ascites. The very first transjugular intrahepatic portosystemic shunt
was a venous shunt in the liver parenchyma between the portal
and hepatic veins. It was initially devised to decompress the portal
system as a treatment for esophageal varices. The major complication with the tissue shunt was shunt occlusion. (*Adapted from*
Gordon *et al.* [22]; with permission.)

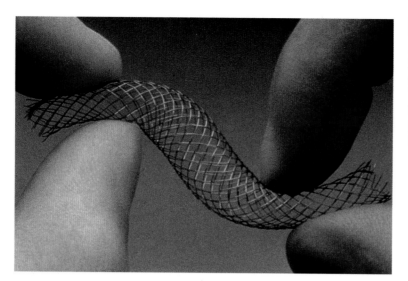

FIGURE 10-40.

More recently, an expandable flexible metal shunt prosthesis, originally designed for strictures of the biliary tract, has been used. This stent has proven to be successful in maintaining shunt patency. The stent is, however, comparatively short and often cannot span the total distance between the portal vein and the extrahepatic portion of the hepatic vein. This results in residual hepatic vein narrowing, requiring an additional one or two stents in series.

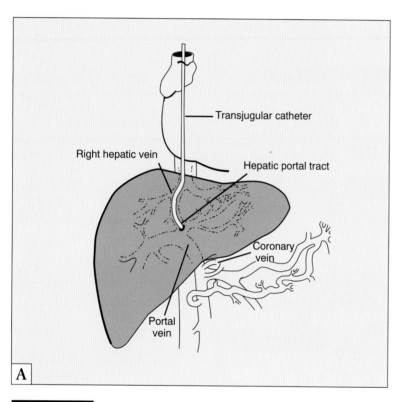

Transjugular catheter

Right hepatic vein

Hepatic portal tract

Coronary vein

Portal vein

A

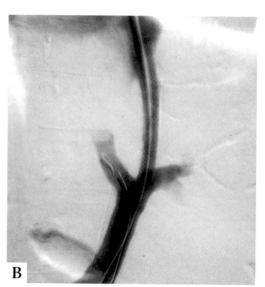

B

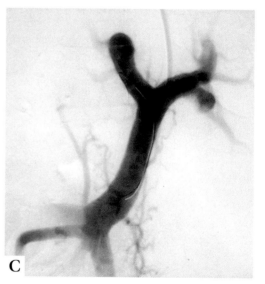

C

FIGURE 10-41.

A, The right hepatic vein is cannulated using the transjugular approach. Under fluoroscopic guidance, a needle is then passed through the cannula to puncture the liver, aiming at a main branch of the portal vein. Once the needle is in the portal vein, the cannula is advanced over the needle. **B,** Results of a portal venogram confirm that the portal vein has been entered. The cannula is then replaced with an angioplasty balloon. The intrahepatic tract is dilated. **C,** The angioplasty catheter is then replaced with the stent, which is then deployed in the intrahepatic tract. A repeat venogram confirms the patency of the shunt.

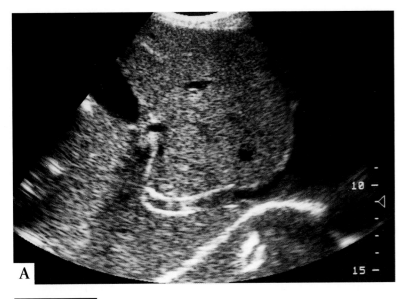

FIGURE 10-42.

Subsequent assessment of shunt patency can be performed using Doppler ultrasound. **A,** The metal stent appears as a bright echogenic object on ultrasound. **B,** Doppler measurement of shunt flow velocity of greater than 100 cm/s confirms shunt patency. Shunt obstruction can be managed by balloon dilatation of the shunt. If this procedure is not successful, a new stent can be inserted parallel to the original stent. It is recommended that shunt patency assessment be performed immediately after insertion, at 1 month, and thereafter every 3 months.

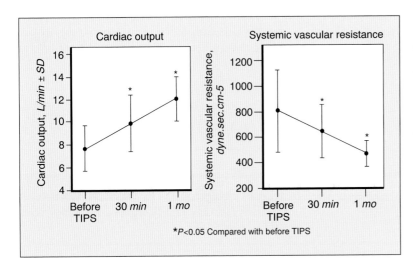

FIGURE 10-43.

As with peritoneovenous shunt, successful placement of transjugular intrahepatic portosystemic stent shunt (TIPS) is associated with profound hemodynamic changes. Corrected sinusoidal pressure falls significantly; there is also exacerbation of the hyperdynamic circulation. Cardiac output increases significantly and significant systemic vasodilatation occurs immediately following TIPS. These changes become more pronounced at 1 month after TIPS. (*Adapted from* Azoulay *et al.* [23]; with permission.)

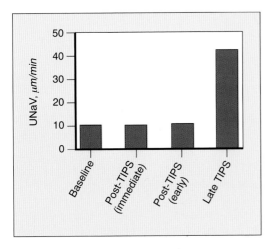

FIGURE 10-44.

Unlike peritoneovenous shunt, natriuresis is delayed. Evidence exists that further activation of the sympathetic nervous system, counteracting the falling levels of plasma renin activity and aldosterone, may be responsible for the lack of natriuresis immediately after insertion of the transjugular intrahepatic portosystemic stent shunt (TIPS). Natriuresis can be expected when plasma renin activity and aldosterone levels decrease significantly to within normal range as well as reduction of sympathetic nervous activity towards the baseline levels. UNaV—urinary sodium extraction.

TABLE 10-13. COMPLICATIONS OF TIPS

Shunt stenosis/occlusion
Hepatic encephalopathy
Worsening of renal function in those with prior renal dysfunction
Reappearance of ascites in noncompliant patients
Shunt hemolysis

TABLE 10-13.

Complications of transjugular intrahepatic portosystemic stent shunt (TIPS) include shunt occlusion, which can be easily detected by Doppler ultrasound, and hepatic encephalopathy. Encephalopathy is significant in 30% of patients, and the risk is higher in those with a prior history of spontaneous encephalopathy and those older than 60 years. Encephalopathy improves with time and can be controlled with lactulose. Moderate renal impairment before TIPS (creatinine levels greater than 250 μmol/L) can lead to worsening of renal function and may even precipitate renal failure. This failure is thought to be caused by further renal vasoconstriction associated with the markedly activated sympathetic activity immediately after TIPS. In addition, these patients are exquisitely sensitive to the renal damaging effects of the radiographic dye. The presence of a metal prosthesis within the liver also predisposes these patients to hemolysis, and increased bilirubin levels has frequently been observed in patients following TIPS. Dietary sodium restriction is mandatory after TIPS to prevent reappearance of ascites.

TABLE 10-14. TIPS–PATIENT SELECTION

ABSOLUTE CONTRAINDICATIONS	RELATIVE CONTRAINDICATIONS
Hepatic encephalopathy	Dental sepsis
Cardiac disease	Spontaneous bacterial peritonitis
Renal dysfunction	
Noncompliance with sodium and fluid restrictions	Hepatocellular carcinoma

TABLE 10-14.

Patient selection is very important. Transjugular intrahepatic portosystemic stent shunt (TIPS) is generally not recommended if the patient has a prior history of spontaneous hepatic encephalopathy, cardiac or renal disease, and noncompliance with dietary sodium and fluid restriction. Dental and other foci of sepsis and bacterial peritonitis have to be treated before TIPS insertion, because infection of the shunt will be very difficult to eradicate. Similarly, patients with previous spontaneous bacterial peritonitis must remain on prophylactic antibiotic therapy, such as norfloxacin, for life. The presence of a hepatocellular carcinoma is also a relative contraindication. If, however, the prognosis is longer than 6 months and the patient does not have any other contraindications, then TIPS should be used as a treatment for refractory ascites. In the suitable patient, TIPS can significantly improve quality of life.

Liver transplantation

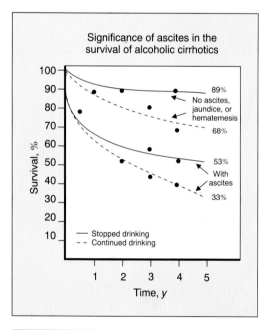

FIGURE 10-45.

Development of ascites in patients with cirrhosis is associated with a poor prognosis. In a study by Powell and Klatskin [24] in a cohort of alcoholic cirrhotic patients, the 5-year survival rate was reported as only 53% after ascites developed; this rate fell to 33% in those who continued to drink. After ascites has become refractory, probability of survival falls to 50% at 2 years (see Fig. 10-30). Therefore, refractory ascites has increasingly become an indication for liver transplantation, however, shortage of resources has made this an option possible for only a few selected patients. (*Adapted from* Powell and Klatskin [24]; with permission.)

TABLE 10-15. POOR PROGNOSTIC INDICATORS OF SURVIVAL IN CIRRHOTIC PATIENTS WITH ASCITES

Mean arterial pressure	≤ 82 mm Hg
Urinary sodium excretion	< 1.5 mEq/d
Glomerular filtration rate	≤ 50 mL/min
Plasma norepinephrine	> 570 pg/mL
Nutritional status	Poor
Hepatomegaly	Present
Serum albumin	≤ 28 g/L

TABLE 10-15.

Various studies have assessed the prognostic value of predictors of survival in cirrhotic patients with ascites. Llach *et al.* [25] found seven independent prognostic indicators that include mean arterial pressure, urinary sodium excretion, glomerular filtration rate, plasma norepinephrine, nutritional status, hepatomegaly, and serum albumin. These findings indicate that parameters of systemic hemodynamics, renal and hepatic function, and nutritional status should be considered in the selection of patients for liver transplantation. (*Adapted from* Llach *et al.* [25]; with permission.)

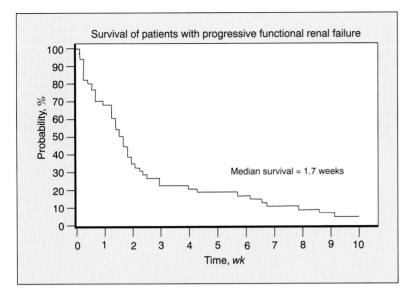

Figure 10-46.

A, Liver transplantation should be performed before there is any significant deterioration of renal function, because after hepatorenal syndrome has developed, the median period of survival is only 1.7 weeks. **B**, Furthermore, probability of survival after liver transplantation in cirrhotic patients with ascites is significantly lower in those with preoperative functional renal failure. In fact, earlier studies using multivariate analyses of etiology, liver, and renal function tests found that the worst prognostic indicator for posttransplant morbidity and mortality was an elevated serum creatinine level. (**A**, *Adapted from* Gines *et al.* [26]; with permission.) (**B**, *Adapted from* Forns *et al.* [27]; with permission.)

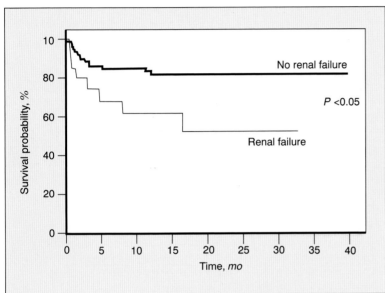

SPONTANEOUS BACTERIAL PERITONITIS

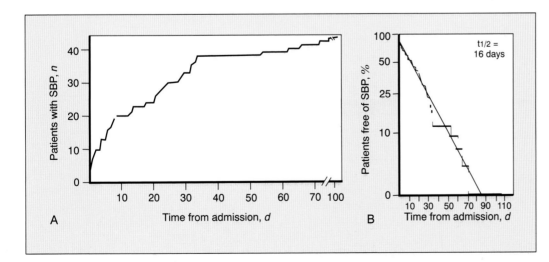

Figure 10-47.

A and **B**, Spontaneous bacterial peritonitis (SBP) is a clinical syndrome in which ascites becomes infected in the absence of a recognizable cause of peritonitis. Over the past decade, the apparent increase in incidence may be caused by greater recognition. Routine paracentesis has documented a 10% to 27% prevalence of SBP at the time of hospital admission for patients with ascites.

Pathogenesis

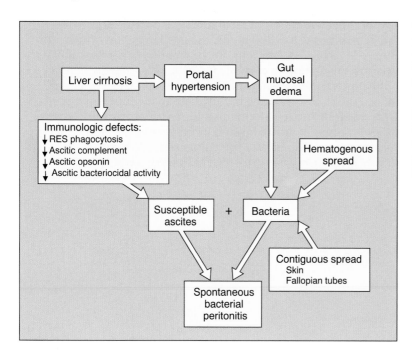

FIGURE 10-48.

Recent publications suggest that spontaneous bacterial peritonitis is the result of translocation of bacteria across the gastrointestinal epithelium into the lymphatics and then into the peritoneal cavity with seeding of susceptible ascites. Decompensated, and especially jaundiced, cirrhotic patients have impaired reticuloendothelial function with reduced phagocytic activity, low ascitic fluid protein concentration, and low ascitic opsonin activity, all of which predispose the patient to spontaneous infection within the ascites. RES—reticuloendothelial system.

Clinical features

TABLE 10-16. SPONTANEOUS BACTERIAL PERITONITIS

CLINICAL FEATURES

Significant fever	Worsening encephalopathy
Chills	Worsening of ascites
Abdominal pain	Hypotension
Abdominal tenderness	Asymptomatic
Reduced bowel sounds	

TABLE 10-16.

The clinical features of spontaneous bacterial peritonitis are quite variable and the diagnosis requires a high index of suspicion. These features can range from the classical picture of fever, chills, generalized abdominal pain, and absent bowel sound to one of a totally asymptomatic patient. Frequently, patients only present with worsening of liver function or hepatic encephalopathy. (*From* Hoefs and Runyon [28]; with permission.)

Diagnosis

TABLE 10-17. SBP

DIAGNOSIS

Standard criterion–PMN cell count > 250/µL

Culture negative neutrocytic ascites = SBP

TABLE 10-17.

The diagnosis of spontaneous bacterial peritonitis (SBP) is made by paracentesis. The standard criterion is the ascitic polymorphonuclear (PMN) cell count. A PMN cell count of greater than 250/µL is diagnostic. This PMN cell count has a sensitivity of 84%, a specificity of 93%, and a diagnostic accuracy of 90%. A variant of SBP known as culture-negative neutrocytic ascites occurs in patients who have suspected SBP but with negative culture of their ascitic fluid and an ascitic fluid PMN cell count of greater than 250 cells/µL. These cases carry the same unfavorable prognosis as culture positive SBP.

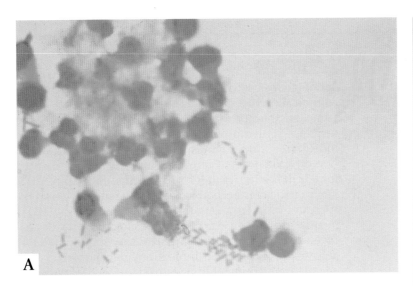
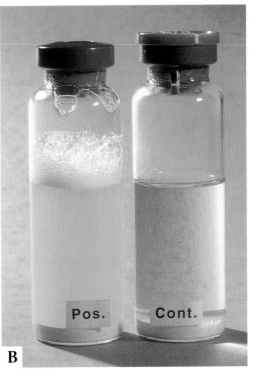

FIGURE 10-49.

A, Gram stains of ascitic fluid are only positive in 10% to 50% of infected patients. **B,** Cultures may take up to 48 hours to become positive. The percentage of possibility is maximized by injection of 10 mL of ascitic fluid directly into blood culture bottles at the bedside.

Organisms isolated

TABLE 10-18. SBP

ORGANISMS ISOLATED

GRAM-NEGATIVE BACILLI (70%)	ANAEROBES (5%)	GRAM-POSITIVE ORGANISMS (25%)
E. coli	Bacteroides	Streptococcus viridans
Klebsiella	Clostridia	Group D Streptococcus
C. freundii	Lactobacillus	S. pneumoniae
Proteus		S. aureus
Enterobacter		

TABLE 10-18.

Many cases of spontaneous bacterial peritonitis (SBP) are caused by microorganisms of intestinal origin. Nonenteric organisms are only responsible for 20% of episodes of SBP. Gram-negative bacilli overall account for 70% of all patients, with *Escherichia coli* as the most common pathogen isolated, being found in 50% of patients. Other gram-negative organisms include *Klebsiella* species, *Citrobacter freundii*, *Proteus*, and *Enterobacter*. Gram-positive organisms are responsible for 25% of cases and include *Streptococcus pneumoniae*, *Streptococcus viridans*, group D *Streptococci*, and *Staphylococcus aureus*. Anaerobic organisms are uncommon causes of SBP because the oxygen tension in the ascitic fluid is too high for their survival. Among these, *Bacteroides* species appear to be more common than other anaerobes. A small percentage of cases are polymicrobial, and every effort should be made to look for an underlying cause of the infection in such cases.

Treatment

TABLE 10-19. TREATMENT FOR SBP

Cefotaxime	Less nephrotoxic
	Broad spectrum
	2 g, 8 hourly
Cefoxitine	Enterococcal cover
	1 g, 6 to 8 hourly
Aztreonam	500 mg, 8 hourly
Amoxicillin-clavulanic acid	1 g amoxicillin & 200 mg clavulanic acid, 6 hourly

Do not use aminoglycosides because they can precipitate renal failure

Do not wait for culture results

Prompt treatment reduces mortality

TABLE 10-19.

Spontaneous bacterial peritonitis (SBP) is a severe infective complication of ascites. If untreated, it has a mortality rate of 50%. Therefore antibiotic therapy should be given immediately after a diagnostic polymorphonuclear count is available without waiting for culture results. Cefotaxime, a new broad-spectrum third generation cephalosporin, is now recognized as the treatment of choice for SBP. It is effective in 85% of patients, and the incidence of nephrotoxicity is negligible with the therapeutic doses used. Its spectrum includes most organisms responsible for SBP. The recommended dose is 2 g every 8 hours. Cefoxitine provides good cover for enterococcal infections, whereas newer antibiotics including amoxicillin-clavulanic combinations and aztreonam are also adequate. The number of patients in the studies assessing the efficacy of these antibiotics is, however, small. Aminoglycosides should never be used in cirrhotic patients, because the risk of nephrotoxicity is high and the development of nephrotoxicity is not related to serum concentrations. The ascitic fluid polymorphonuclear count should decrease rapidly once treatment is given, returning to normal within 48 hours, together with a parallel clinical improvement.

TABLE 10-20. TREATMENT OF SBP

| | CEFOTAXIME | | |
	5-DAY COURSE	P	10-DAY COURSE
Patients, n	43	NS	47
Days of hospitalization	31 ± 38	NS	50 ± 68
Recurrence of infection	5	NS	6
Hospital mortality	14	NS	20
Drug and administration costs/patient	259 ± 34	< 0.0001	486 ± 117

TABLE 10-20.

Recently, two studies have demonstrated that 5 days of cefotaxime is an adequate course of therapy. The mortality and recurrence rates were similar to those receiving 10 days of therapy. The cost of this treatment can therefore be significantly reduced by shortening the hospital stay. NS—not significant. (*Adapted from* Runyon *et al.* [29]; with permission.)

Secondary versus spontaneous bacterial peritonitis

TABLE 10-21. SECONDARY VERSUS SPONTANEOUS BACTERIAL PERITONITIS

	SECONDARY BACTERIAL PERITONITIS	SPONTANEOUS BACTERIAL PERITONITIS
Organisms	Multiple	Single
Ascitic protein count	> 1 g/dL	< 1 g/dL
Ascitic glucose concentrations	< 50 mg/dL	Approximate simultaneous serum value
Response to treatment		
(1) Polymorphonuclear cell count	Continues to rise despite treatment	Falls exponentially
(2) Ascitic culture	Remains positive	Rapidly becomes sterile

TABLE 10-21.

Secondary bacterial peritonitis should be considered as a differential diagnosis if the following features are present 1) multiple organisms are grown from the ascitic fluid, 2) ascitic fluid protein concentration greater than 1 g/dL, and 3) polymorphonuclear count remains high despite appropriate antibiotic therapy. In such cases, radiographic examinations are required to exclude perforation of the gastrointestinal tract.

TABLE 10-22. SPONTANEOUS BACTERIAL PERITONITIS

PREDICTORS OF INFECTION RESOLUTION

Band neutrophil in the leukocyte count

Blood urea nitrogen

Serum aspartate aminotransferase

Hospital- versus community-acquired infection

TABLE 10-22.

In a study that includes 213 consecutive episodes of spontaneous bacterial peritonitis in 185 cirrhotic patients, a multivariate analysis identified four independent predictors of infection resolution. These predictors include band neutrophils in the leukocyte count, blood urea nitrogen, serum aspartate amino transferase, and hospital- versus community-acquired infection. (*Adapted from* Toledo *et al.* [30]; with permission.)

Recurrence

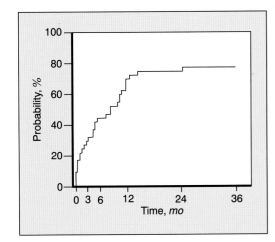

FIGURE 10-50.

A, Because the underlying predisposing factors remain unchanged despite adequate antibiotic therapy, spontaneous bacterial peritonitis recurs frequently in cirrhotic patients. The probability of recurrence has been estimated to be 43% at 6 months, 69% at 1 year, and 74% at 2 years. **B,** Three parameters have been identified as predictors for spontaneous bacterial peritonitis recurrence. These are serum bilirubin levels of greater than 4 mg/dL, a prothrombin time of less than or equal to 45% of control, and an ascitic fluid protein concentration of less than or equal to 1 g/dL. (*Adapted from* Tito *et al.* [31]; with permission.)

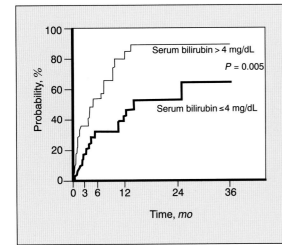

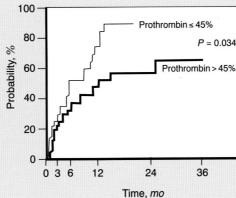

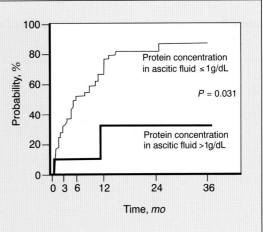

Prophylaxis

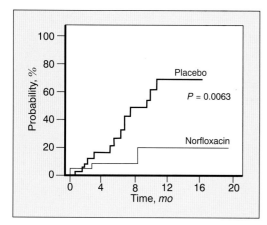

FIGURE 10-51.

Various therapeutic modalities have been tried to reduce the risk of recurrence. Diuretic therapy has been shown to increase ascitic protein content and opsonin activity but not to influence outcome. Selective intestinal decontamination to eliminate aerobic gram-negative bacilli with oral nonabsorbable antibiotics has proved to be effective in reducing the recurrence of spontaneous bacterial peritonitis. Norfloxacin (400 mg daily) has been shown to be significantly better than placebo to reduce the incidence of recurrence of spontaneous bacterial peritonitis. It is the drug of choice, because it has the advantages of rarely causing bacterial resistance and of having a low incidence of side effects when administered long term. (*Adapted from* Gines *et al.* [32]; with permission.)

Prognosis

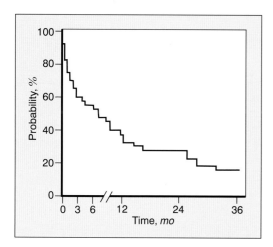

FIGURE 10-52.

Despite successful treatment of spontaneous bacterial peritonitis, the underlying predisposing factors including liver dysfunction and portal hypertension remain unchanged, and therefore the prognosis of these patients remains poor. The cumulative survival rate has been reported to be less than 20% at 2.5 years. (*Adapted from* Tito *et al.* [31]; with permission.).

TABLE 10-23. SBP

PREDICTORS OF SURVIVAL

Blood urea nitrogen

Serum aspartate aminotransferase

Hospital- versus community-acquired infection

Age

Pugh score

Ileus

TABLE 10-23.

Independent predictors of survival after a first episode of spontaneous bacterial peritonitis (SBP) are blood urea nitrogen, serum aspartate aminotransferase, hospital- versus community-acquired infection, age, Pugh score, and paralytic ileus. Despite improved treatment and decreased SBP recurrence rates with prophylactic antibiotics, no change in mortality has yet been demonstrated. All patients who have experienced one episode of SBP should be considered for liver transplantation. (*Adapted from* Toledo *et al.* [30]; with permission.)

REFERENCES AND RECOMMENDED READING

1. Stark ME, Szurszewski JH: Role of nitric oxide in gastrointestinal and hepatic function and disease. *Gastroenterology* 1992, 103:1928–1949.

2. Warner LC, Campbell PJ, Morali G, *et al.*: The response of atrial natriuretic factor (ANF) and sodium excretion to dietary sodium challenge in cirrhotic patients. *Hepatology* 1990, 12:460–466.

3. Wong F, Massie D, Colman J, Dudley F: Glomerular hyperfiltration in patients with well compensated alcoholic cirrhosis. *Gastroenterology* 1993, 104:884–889.

4. Wong F, Liu P, Tobe S, *et al.*: Central blood volume in cirrhosis: Measurement by radionuclide angiography. *Hepatology* 1994, 19:312–321.

5. Bernardi M, Trevisani F, Santini C, *et al.*: Aldosterone related blood volume expansion in cirrhosis before and during the early phase of ascites formation. *Gut* 1983, 24:761–766.

6. Campbell V, Greig P, Cranford J, *et al.*: A comparision of acute reversible pre and post-sinusoidal portal hypertension on salt and water retention in the dog. *Hepatology* 1982, 2:54–58.

7. Morali G, Sniderman K, Deitel KM, *et al.*: Is sinusoidal portal hypertension a necessary factor for the development of hepatic ascites. *J Hepatology* 1992, 16:249–250.

8. Wensing G, Sabra R, Branch R: Renal and systemic hemodynamics in experimental cirrhosis in rats: Relation to hepatic function. *Hepatology* 1990, 12:13–19.

9. Wong F, Massie D, Hsu P, Dudley F: The renal response to a saline load in well compensated alcoholic cirrhosis. *Hepatology* 1994, 20:873–881.

10. Lang F, Tschernko E, Schulze E, *et al.*: Hepatorenal reflex regulating kidney function. *Hepatology* 1991, 14:590–594.

11. Kostreva DR, Castana A, Kampine JP: Reflex effects of hepatic baroreceptors on renal and cardiac sympathetic nerve activity. *Am J Physiol* 1980, 238:R390–R394.

12. Wong F, Blendis L: Transjugular intrahepatic portosystemic shunt for refractory ascites: Tipping the sodium balance. *Hepatology* 1995, in press.

13. Orrego H, Medline A, Blendis LM, *et al.*: Collagenisation of the Disse space in alcoholic liver disease. *Gut* 1979, 20:673–679.

14. Wong F, Blendis L: Foreward. Hepatorenal disorders. *Semin Liver Dis* 1994, 14:1–3.

15. Gines P, Arroyo V, Quintero E, *et al.*: Comparison of paracentesis and diuretics in the treatment of cirrhosis with tense ascites. Result of a randomized study. *Gastroenterology* 1987, 93:234–241.

16. Gines P, Tito L, Arroyo V, *et al.*: Randomized comparative study of paracentesis with and without intravenous albumin in cirrhosis. *Gastroenterology* 1988, 94:1493–1502.

17. Panos M, Moore K, Vlavianos P, *et al.*: Single total paracentesis for tense ascites: Sequential hemodynamic changes and right atrial size. *Hepatology* 1990, 11:662–667.

18. Blendis LM, Greig PD, Langer B, *et al.*: The renal and hemodynamic effects of the peritoneovenous shunt for intractable hepatic ascites. *Gastroenterology* 1979, 77:250–257.

19. Blendis LM, Harrison J, Russell DM, *et al.*: Effects of peritoneovenous shunting on body composition. *Gastroenterology* 1986, 90:127–134.

20. Gines P, Arroyo V, Vargas V, *et al.*: Paracentesis with intravenous infusion of albumin as compared with peritoneovenous shunting in cirrhosis with refractory ascites. *N Engl J Med* 1991, 325:829–835.

21. LeVeen H: The LeVeen Shunt. *Ann Rev Med* 1985, 36:453–469.

22. Gordon JD, Colapinto RF, Abecassis M, *et al.*: A non-operative approach to life threatening variceal bleeding. *Can J Surg* 1987, 30:45–49.

23. Azoulay D, Castaing D, Dennison A, *et al.*: Transjugular intrahepatic portosystemic shunt worsens the hyperdynamic circulatory state of the cirrhotic patients. Preliminary report of a prospective study. *Hepatology* 1994, 19:129–134.

24. Powell WJ, Klatskin G: Duration of survival in patients with Laennec's cirrhosis. Influence of alcohol withdrawal, and possible effects of recent changes in general management of the disease. *Am J Med* 1968, 44:406–420.

25. Llach J, Gines P, Arroyo V, *et al.*: Prognostic value of arterial pressure, endogenous vasoactive systems, and renal function in cirrhotic patients admitted to the hospital for the treatment of ascites. *Gastroterology* 1988, 94:482–487.

26. Gines A, Escorsell A, Gines P, *et al.*: Incidence, predictive factors and prognosis of the hepatorenal syndrome in cirrhosis with ascites. *Gastroenterology* 1993, 105:229–236.

27. Forns X, Gines A, Gines P, Arroyo V: Management of ascites and renal failure in cirrhosis. *Semin Liver Dis* 1994, 14:82–96.

28. Hoefs JC, Runyon BA: Spontaneous bacterial peritonitis. *Dis Mon* 1985, 31:1–48.

29. Runyon BA, McHutchinson JG, Antillon MR, *et al.*: Short-course versus long-course antibiotic treatment of spontaneous bacterial peritonitis. A randomised controlled study. *Gastroenterology* 1991, 100:1737–1742.

30. Toledo C, Salmeron J-M, Rimola A, *et al.*: Spontaneous bacterial peritonitis in cirrhosis: Predictive factors of infection, resolution and survival in patients treated with cefotaxime. *Hepatology* 1993, 17:251–257.

31. Tito L, Rimola A, Gines P, *et al.*: Recurrence of spontaneous bacterial peritonitis in cirrhosis, frequency and predictive factors. *Hepatology* 1988, 8:27–31.

32. Gines P, Rimola A, Planas R, *et al.*: Norfloxacin prevents spontaneous bacterial peritonitis recurrence in cirrhosis. Results of a double-blind placebo controlled trial. *Hepatology* 1990, 12:716–724.

Chapter 11

Bleeding Varices and Hepatic Encephalopathy

HAROLD O. CONN

The illustrations reproduced here have been collected over a career of more than 40 years that was devoted primarily to the clinical management and investigation of hepatic diseases. These images are related predominantly to disorders of portal hypertension. Most of the color illustrations were generously given to me by friends who are also practicing clinical investigators. They were offered as gifts for my own personal enjoyment and edification. I am nearing the end of that career and have chosen to share these images with interested colleagues, especially the readers of *Gastroenterology and Hepatology: The Comprehensive Visual Reference*. Most of the black-and-white illustrations have been published in articles in the medical literature, the authors and publishers of which have given permission for reproduction. Some of them are original diagrams created for specific purposes and some were carefully selected for their content and style. I acknowledge the gracious generosity of the donors and thank them personally and in behalf of the editors, publishers, and readers of this volume.

The invitation to prepare this chapter by such a fine, meticulous cadre of colleagues has given me the opportunity to exhibit this collection in an optimal format. I take great pleasure and pride in having these images published in this volume.

■ HEMORRHAGE FROM ESOPHAGEAL VARICES

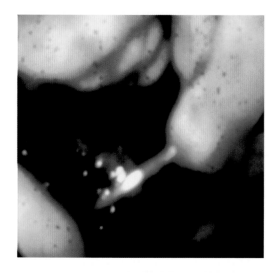

FIGURE 11-1.

Active hemorrhage from an esophageal varix. Pressure within esophageal varices averages almost 30 mm Hg in cirrhotic patients. Coughing, straining, defecation, or lifting may increase variceal pressure to arterial pressure levels. Indeed, bleeding at such high pressures may give rise to arterial jets, as shown in this remarkable endoscopic photograph. Needless to say, large volumes of blood can quickly be lost from such lesions. (*Courtesy of* N. Currey, Rancho Mirage, CA)

Endoscopic prognostic findings

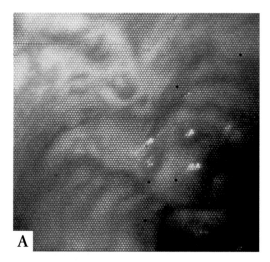
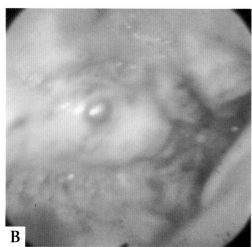
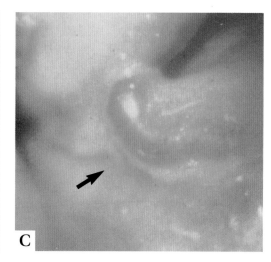

A
B
C

FIGURE 11-2.

Endoscopic red markings on esophageal varices. Beppu and co-workers [1] discovered a series of endoscopic lesions—cherry red spots (**A**), hemocystic spots (**B**), and red wale markings (**C**)—that are indicative of increased risk of rupture of the varices. Red spots are the most common, the hemocystic spots are larger versions of the red spots, and red wales appear to have the worst prognosis.

These lesions represent localized dilatations on the surface of esophageal varices that may be related to the ebb and flow of blood in esophageal varices that are associated with the respiratory cycle (*see* Figs. 11-3 and 11-4). (**A**, *Courtesy of* A. Dagradi, Los Angeles, CA) (**B** and **C**, *Courtesy of* K. Beppu, Los Angeles, CA)

Esophageal variceal blood flow

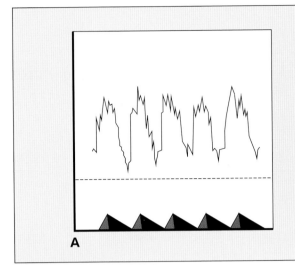
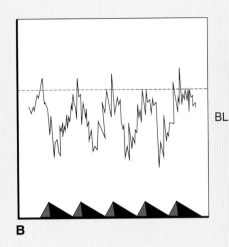
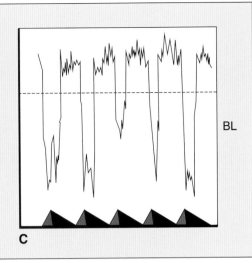

Figure 11-3.

Variable direction of blood flow in esophageal varices. During investigations of endoscopic sclerotherapy using a radiopaque sclerosant, McCormack and coworkers [2] noted that the direction of blood flow in the varices was usually, but not always, cephalad. Occasionally, it was both cephalad and caudad at the same time. Doppler recordings of variceal blood flow show blood flowing cephalad (upward, *ie, above the dotted line*) with increased velocity during inspiration (*open portion of the triangle*) in some of the varices of all the patients studied (**A**), blood flowing caudad (downward, *ie, below the dotted line*) in other locations in the varices of about half the patients (**B**), and blood flowing in one direction during inspiration and in the opposite direction during expiration (*solid portion of the triangle*) (**C**). (*From* McCormack *et al.* [2]; with permission.)

Tidal basin hypothesis of variceal blood flow

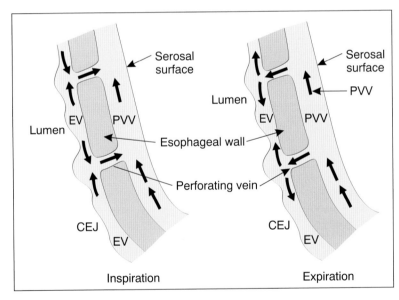

Figure 11-4.

The *Tidal Basin* hypothesis of esophageal varices. McCormack and co-workers [2] explained these findings in terms of the peculiar vascular anatomy of the esophagus as follows. Submucosal esophageal varices are connected to subserosal, paraesophageal vessels by a series of small perforating or communicating veins that penetrate the muscles of the esophageal wall (*pink areas*) [3]. The blood flow in these perforating vessels reverses direction with each inspiration and expiration. Thus, the submucosal varices tend to dilate and flow caudad during inspiration and to collapse and flow cephalad during expiration [2,3]. Blood flow into and out of the varices is trapped in an endless cycle that converts the varices into a tidal basin, which is characterized by perpetual turbulence. The turbulence creates lateral pressure, which results in dilation of the involved vessels, just as it does distal to a vascular constriction (poststenotic dilation). This phenomenon may cause the varices to become the dilated, thin-walled protuberances that resemble clusters of grapes rather than linear blood-carrying veins (*see* Fig. 11-5). CEJ—cardioesophageal junction; EV—esophageal varices.

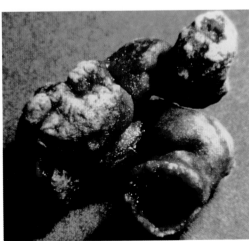

Figure 11-5.

Buteryl-2-cyanoacrylate casts of esophagogastric varices. These irregular, spheroidal varices can be best appreciated by the casts of varices sloughed into the esophagogastric lumen days or weeks after sclerotherapy using polymeric tissue adhesives such as buteryl-2-cyanoacrylate [4]. These spherical sloughs may be greater than 1 cm in diameter. (*Courtesy of* N. Soehendra, Hamburg, German

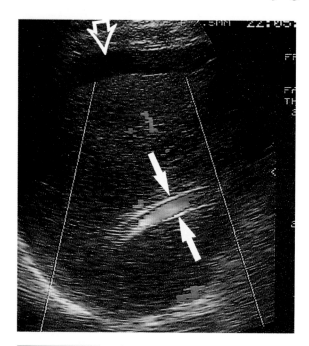

FIGURE 11-6.

Transjugular intrahepatic portosystemic shunt (TIPS). This hepatic Doppler sonogram in a 55-year-old man with alcoholic cirrhosis and portal hypertension shows the position of a patent TIPS [5]. The procedure was performed because of refractory, debilitating ascites. The shunt shows characteristic echogenicity (*solid arrows*) and an intense blue signal caused by shunted blood flow. Ascites (*open arrow*) is present anterior to the liver. After the placement of the shunt, the patient's esophageal varices diminished in size and the ascites began to disappear without further therapy. The patient was awaiting liver transplantation at the time of this ultrasonographic examination. The shunt became occluded 8 months later. (*From* Sadler and Shapiro [5]; with permission.)

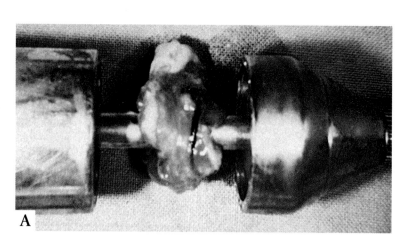

FIGURE 11-7.

Esophageal transection with SPTU Russian staple gun [6]. **A,** The excised esophageal ring surrounds the stem of the staple gun. **B,** Cross-sectional view of the excised ring of esophagus. (*From* Ponce *et al.* [7]; with permission.)

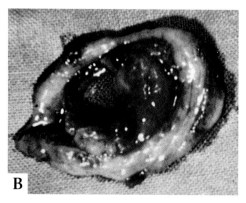

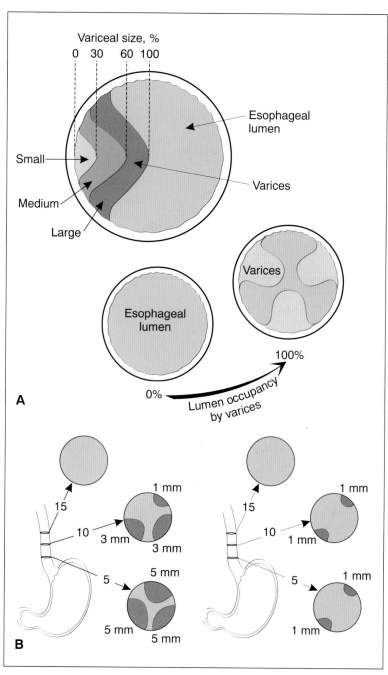

FIGURE 11-8.

Depiction of variceal size and the extent of the esophageal lumen occupied by varices. **A,** Variceal size is expressed as the percentage of the theoretical maximum size, which is defined as the percentage of the radius of the esophagus (100%) when varices bulge to the center of the esophageal lumen and kiss [7]. **B,** Small, medium, and large varices are defined as occupying less than 30%, 30% to 50%, and greater than 50%, respectively, of the luminal area. Lumen occupancy of 0% is defined as a lumen that is free of varices; 100% is defined as a lumen completely occluded by varices. A similar method has been described by Parra and coworkers [8]. (*From* Beppu *et al.* [6]; with permission.)

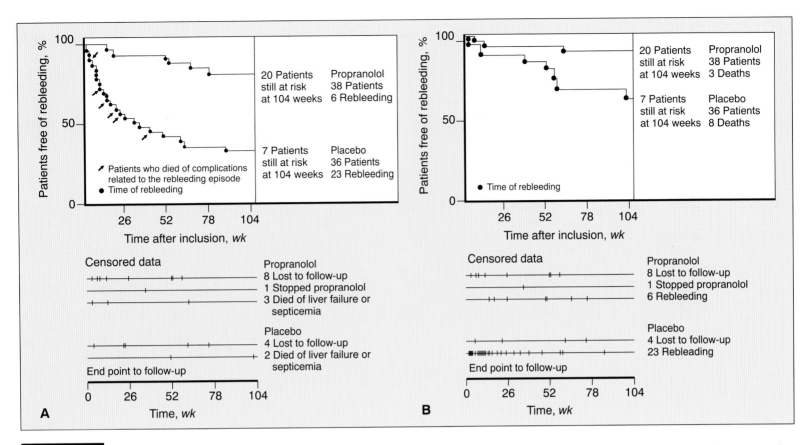

FIGURE 11-9.

Effect of propranolol (or placebo) on recurrent hemorrhage from varices. This randomized clinical trial is the first trial with β-adrenergic blockade (propranolol) in patients who survived variceal hemorrhage. It is a landmark study that opened the era of pharmacologic therapy in portal hypertension [9]. A, The data about cumulative freedom from variceal rebleeding are shown. B, Survival data are given. By virtue of presenting censored data in this manner, readers have the opportunity to examine the data critically. For example, it is possible to calculate the effects of censoring rebleeding episodes in the 23 patients in the placebo group. Whether or not these patients are retained in or excluded from the calculations will affect the significance of the survival calculations [10]. A, The *upper curve* shows the time of rebleeding in the patients in the propranolol group; the *lower curve* shows the time of rebleeding in the placebo group. The *lower portion* of the figure shows the censored data, *ie*, those patients who were lost to follow-up, who stopped taking propranolol, or who died of other causes. Some of the recurrent hemorrhages were from acute gastric erosions (none in the propranolol group and three in the placebo group). B, The *upper curve* shows cumulative survival in the propranolol group, the *lower curve* in the placebo group. (*From* Lebrec *et al.* [9]; with permission.)

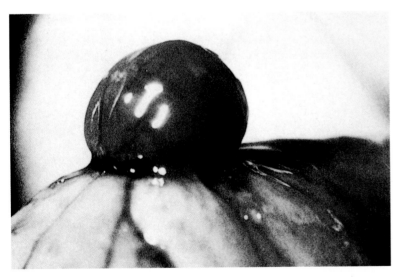

FIGURE 11-10.

Gastric mucosal ligation demonstrating a ligated varix 10 mm in diameter ensnared by the ligating O ring. (*From* Van Steigmann *et al.* [11]; with permission.)

Esophageal ligation versus endoscopic sclerotherapy

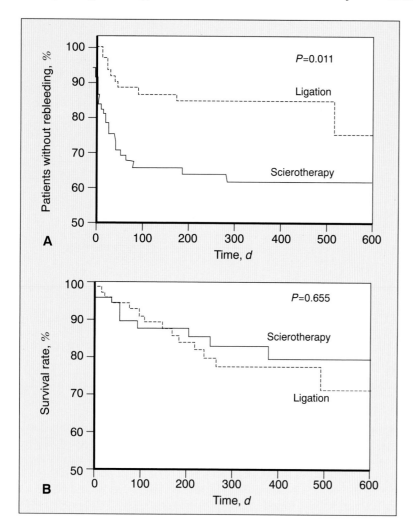

FIGURE 11-11.

Comparison of recurrent bleeding treated with endoscopic sclerotherapy versus endoscopic ligation of varices [12]. **A,** Decrease in recurrent bleeding after initial treatment of variceal bleeding by endoscopic sclerotherapy or endoscopic ligation in patients with cirrhosis. The difference between groups is statistically significant ($P=0.011$). **B,** Cumulative survival rate in patients with cirrhosis and bleeding esophageal varices treated with endoscopic ligation was similar to that in patients treated with endoscopic sclerotherapy. (*From* Hou *et al.* [12]; with permission.)

Emergency portacaval shunts

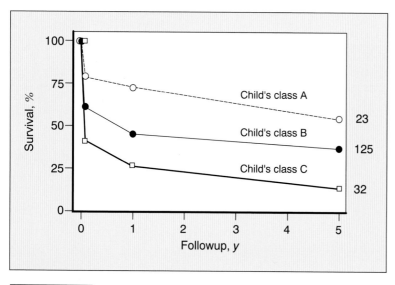

FIGURE 11-12.

Percentage survival after emergency portacaval anastomosis in relation to Child's classification [13]. Almost 70% of the patients were Child's class B; 18% were class C; and 13% were class A. The 30-day operative mortality rate increased progressively and proportionately as Child's classification worsened from A to B to C. Survival was similar thereafter in the three groups. (*Adapted from* Orloff *et al.* [13]; with permission.)

FIGURE 11-13.

Transjugular intrahepatic portosystemic stent shunts. This diagram demonstrates how the stent connects the hepatic vein or one of its branches to the portal vein or one of its branches [14]. (*From* McCormick *et al.* [14]; with permission.)

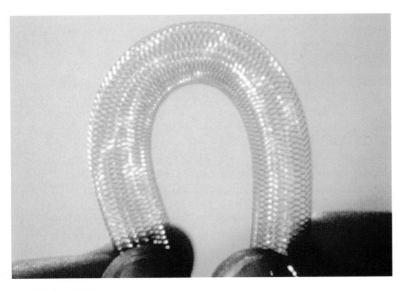

FIGURE 11-14.

Wallstent for transjugular intrahepatic portosystemic stent shunts. A stainless steel mesh stent with a 10-mm diameter is shown. The flexibility of this stent, which is obvious in this photograph, is its greatest virtue. This flexibility permits it to be positioned in sharp curves without significant distortion in shape. (*Courtesy of* A. Florey, Minneapolis, MN)

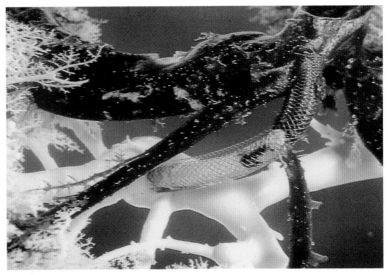

FIGURE 11-15.

Plastic cast of Wallstent transjugular intrahepatic portosystemic stent shunts in situ. This patient's liver had been resected before liver transplantation. The hepatic vein was injected with blue plastic and the portal vein with white plastic. The transected right hepatic vein is seen in the upper right. A long, double-length stent extends from the right hepatic vein to the right portal vein. (*Courtesy of* J.P. Vinel, Toulouse, France)

Azygos blood flow

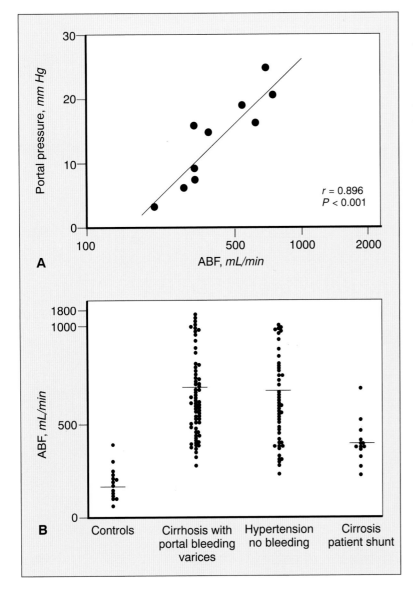

FIGURE 11-16.

Azygos blood flow (ABF). ABF is a gross measure of blood flow through esophageal varices, although it also includes the venous drainage from the posterior intercostal, bronchial, mediastinal, and esophageal veins. Using the thermal dilution method [15], the ABF averages about 175 mL/min in normal individuals. The mean ABF in cirrhotic patients is almost 700 mL/min, indicating that more than 500 mL of blood flow through the esophageal varices each minute [16]. **A,** There is a close correlation between the ABF and the portal venous pressure, *ie*, the hepatic vein pressure gradient. **B,** Based on studies in 100 cirrhotic patients, the ABF averages about 650 mL/min in both those who have and those who have not bled from varices. The ABF is lower in cirrhotic patients with portacaval anastomoses (PCA), indicating that PCA effectively shunts portal venous blood away from the varices. (**A,** *From* Bosch and Groszmann [16]; with permission.) (**B,** *From* Vinel *et al.* [17]; with permission.)

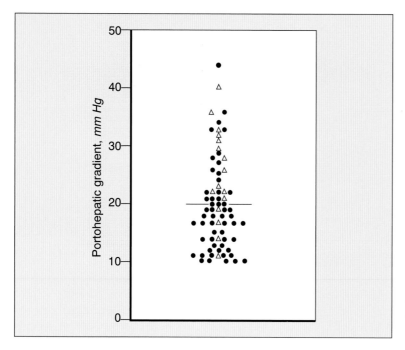

FIGURE 11-17.

FIGURE 11-17.

Portal venous pressure in patients who bled from esophageal varices. The hepatic vein pressure gradient (HVPG), *ie*, the wedged or occluded hepatic venous pressure minus the free hepatic venous pressure, is the *corrected* portal venous pressure. Patients who bled from esophageal varices invariably have a HVPG greater than 12 mm Hg. The pressure tends to be highest at the moment of hemorrhage and to decrease thereafter. This decrement is expected in alcoholic cirrhosis, in which hepatic fatty deposition and inflammation decrease during abstinence after admission to the hospital. Indeed, the HVPG was significantly lower among the 56 patients who survived more than 2 weeks after variceal hemorrhage (mean 26 mm Hg; *closed circles*) than in the 16 patients who died within the first 2 weeks (mean 20 mm Hg; *open triangles*) [17]. The failure to establish a relationship between the height of the HVPG and the risks of variceal hemorrhage and death could represent in part, at best, an artifact of retrospective analysis [18], *ie*, patients with the higher portal venous pressure levels may die before they survive long enough to have their portal venous pressure measured. (*From* Vinel *et al.* [17]; with permission.)

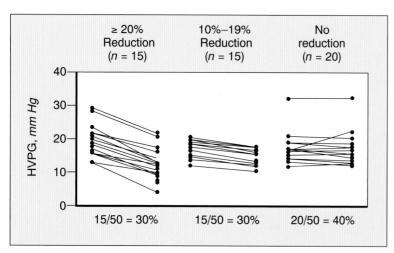

FIGURE 11-18.

Variability of the portal venous pressure to β-adrenergic blockade in cirrhotic patients with portal hypertension. In 50 consecutive cirrhotic patients with esophageal varices and portal hypertension (hepatic vein pressure gradient [HVPG] > 12 mm Hg), oral administration of 40 mg propranolol caused a reduction of 20% or more of basal pressure levels (approximately 4 mm Hg) in 15 patients (30%) [19]. In addition, a decrease of 10% to 19% (2 to 4 mm Hg) was observed in 15 patients (30%) and a decrease of less than 10% (< 2 mm Hg) in 20 patients (40%). The mean basal HVPG in these patients had been approximately 20 mm Hg. Thus, only 60% of patients with portal hypertension showed a significant decrease in portal venous pressure (2 to 6 mm Hg). This investigation indicates that the blind administration of propranolol to cirrhotic patients with esophageal varices will reduce the portal venous pressure significantly (> 3 mm Hg) in only about half the patients. A short therapeutic trial of β-blockade with measurements of the HVPG preceding and following seems indicated before the initiation of β-blockade. (*From* Garcia-Tsao *et al.* [19]; with permission.)

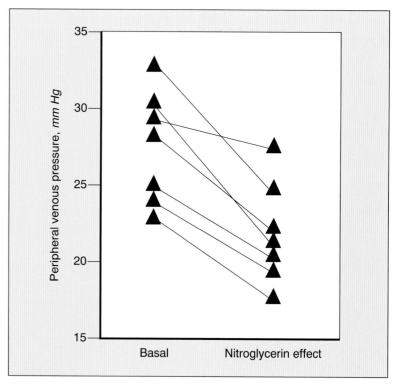

FIGURE 11-19.

The reduction of portal venous pressure by oral nitroglycerin in cirrhotic patients. Nitroglycerin was introduced into the therapy of portal hypertension as an adjunct to intravenous vasopressin [20]. This usage was based on the demonstration that nitroglycerin has an additive effect with vasopressin on portal venous pressure [21]. Because oral nitroglycerin might have greater pharmacologic effects by virtue of its direct delivery to the portal vein, it was administered orally [22]. In all seven cirrhotic patients in whom it was tried, it caused a decrease in portal venous pressure with a mean decrease from 29 to 23 mm Hg. The portal venous pressure was measured using the Chiba (skinny) needle with percutaneous, transhepatic puncture of intrahepatic branches of the portal vein. (*From* Gibson *et al.* [22]; with permission.)

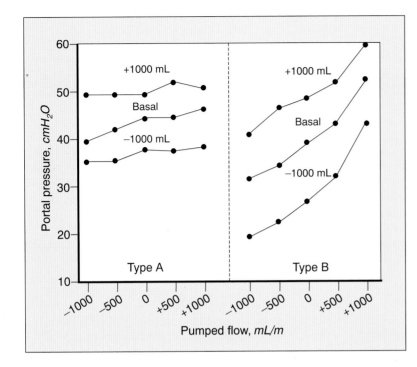

FIGURE 11-20.

The effects of diversion or augmentation of portal venous flow on portal venous pressure in cirrhosis. The interrelationships of plasma volume, portal venous blood flow, portal venous pressure, and hepatic arterial blood flow are complex and poorly understood. In an attempt to elucidate these unknowns, Zimmon and Kessler [23] performed a series of ingenious experiments in cirrhotic and schistosomial patients with portal hypertension. These investigations consisted of decreasing or augmenting portal blood flow, by portal venesection and portal transfusions, respectively. By using an extracorporeal umbilicosaphenous shunt, the investigators were able to demonstrate two types of patient responses. Type A patients tend to compensate and to show relatively little change in portal venous pressure. Type B patients show significant decrements and increments in portal venous pressure with diversion and augmentation, respectively. (*From* Zimmon and Kessler [23]; with permission.)

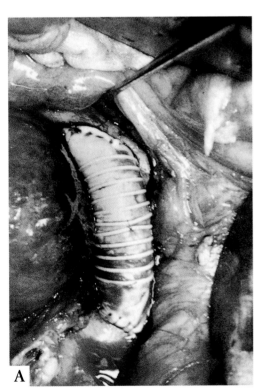

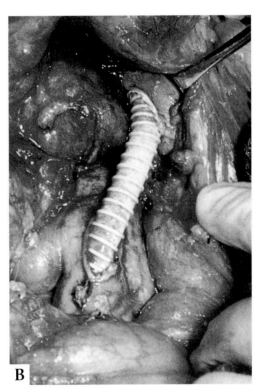

FIGURE 11-21.

Portosystemic anastomoses, usually portacaval, have been the standard method of decompressing the portal venous system since 1945. Difficulties have arisen when the diameter of the shunt is too small or too large. When too small, only partial, inadequate portal decompression is achieved and the shunt tends to clot. When the shunt is too large, portal systemic encephalopathy (PSE) tends to develop. Partial portosystemic anastomosis can be constructed using H grafts to anastomose the portal vein to the inferior vena cava. These photographs show a 16-mm diameter H graft (**A**), which is considered to be a "total" shunt, and an 8-mm diameter H graft (**B**), which is a partial shunt. Controlled trials have shown that total shunts decompress the portal hypertension completely but induce PSE in 43% of the patients [24]. The smaller (8 mm) shunts partially decompress the portal venous system sufficiently to prevent variceal hemorrhage but cause PSE in only 21% of the patients. The ideal size appears to be 10 or 12 mm. (*From* Sarfeh and Rypins [24]; with permission.)

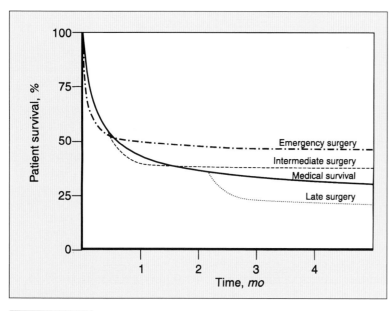

FIGURE 11-22.

Survival after hemorrhage from esophagogastric varices. In a seminal study, Graham and Smith [25] and Smith and Graham [26] constructed a survival curve for patients who had bled from varices. This curve, which starts at the time of hemorrhage, was constructed from a large series of published reports in which the investigators had presented serial survival data. The *solid curve*, which shows the overall survival curve, parallels the curve for the recurrence of hemorrhages from varices in these patients. This curve has several unique characteristics. The initial slope is steepest for the initial interval, whether it represents a day, a week, or a month. It becomes less steep for each succeeding interval until it achieves a steady slope, which approximates the survival rate of these patients before the first episode of hemorrhage.

Several additional curves have been superimposed on the primary curve. Late surgery is the lowest curve (*dotted line*); it represents the probable curve in patients who have a portacaval shunt some months after hemorrhage by which time the patients had regained their prehemorrhage (virginal) survival status. The mortality of the shunt surgery is engrafted on the primary curve. Intermediate surgery (*dashed line*) represents the probable curve as seen in patients operated on a few days to weeks after the acute bleeding episode. There appears to be a small advantage in the survival rate in this subgroup. The survival curve for emergency (immediate) surgery (*alternating dotted and dashed line*) shows a modest survival advantage despite an extremely high-operative (30 day) mortality rate of about 50% [27]. This procedure immediately stops active bleeding and prevents recurrent episodes of variceal bleeding. (*From* Graham and Smith [25]; with permission.)

Postshunt venacaval aneurysm

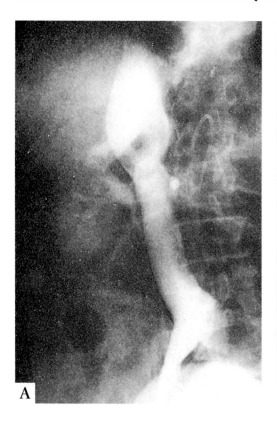

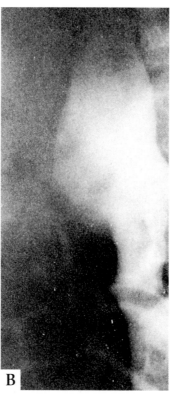

FIGURE 11-23.

Aneurysmal dilation of the inferior vena cava at the site of successful portacaval anastomoses (PCA). The occurrence of post-PCA aneurysmal dilation is a little known phenomenon that is present in the majority of patients with patent PCA [28,29]. These "aneurysms," which apparently result from the turbulence caused by non-laminar blood flow as the portal venous blood joins the inferior vena caval blood, are evident within 1 month of the time the shunt is constructed. These dilations, which are not true aneurysms, tend to persist thereafter as long as the shunt remains patent. In the event of occlusion or stenosis of the shunt, the dilation tends to regress. **A** and **B,** Typical dilations are depicted. These dilations may attain enormous size, reaching 6 cm in both the anteroposterior and transverse diameters, which are approximately three times the diameter of the normal inferior vena cava at that level.

(Continued on next page)

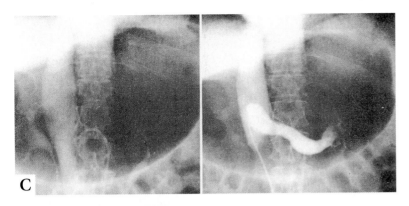

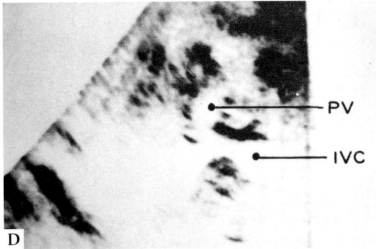

FIGURE 11-23. (CONTINUED)

C, The portal vein entering the dilated inferior vena cava is shown by retrograde injection of contrast medium into the portal vein (portacaval shuntogram). These aneurysms apparently cause no clinical symptoms or signs, although they may cause deformities of the second and third portions of the duodenum by barium contrast examination. They are not visible at autopsy when they are empty of blood but can be confirmed by postmortem recon-struction of the vena cava or by ultrasonographic examination (**D**) [30]. (**A** and **B**, *From* Conn and Rambsy [28]; with permission.) (**C**, *From* Castell and Conn [29]; with permission.) (**D**, *From* Goldberg and Patel [30]; with permission.)

Portal venous devascularization

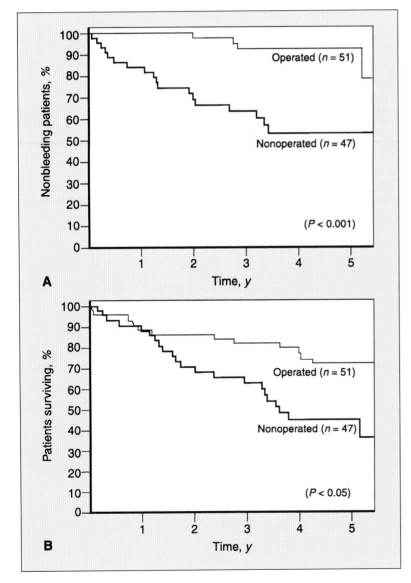

FIGURE 11-24.

Portal devascularization in the prevention of the initial hemor-rhage from esophageal varices. Portal devascularization, the Yamamoto-Sugiura procedure [31], consists of transection and resuturing of the esophagus, ligation of the gastric veins, splenec-tomy, and coronary vein ligation. It is predominantly a Japanese procedure that has not met with popularity in the West. Inokuchi and coworkers [32] performed a randomized controlled trial in almost 100 cirrhotic patients. **A**, Hemorrhage from esophageal varices occurred significantly less commonly in devascularized patients than in unoperated control patients ($P<0.001$). **B**, Cum-ulative survival was significantly better in those patients who had the operations than in those patients who did not ($P<0.05$). This complex procedure performed on Japanese patients appears to be as effective in preventing the initial hemorrhage from varices as prophylactic propranolol in American patients [33], although the patients, the type of cirrhosis, the surgeons, and other factors are different. (*From* Yamamoto *et al.* [31], with permission.)

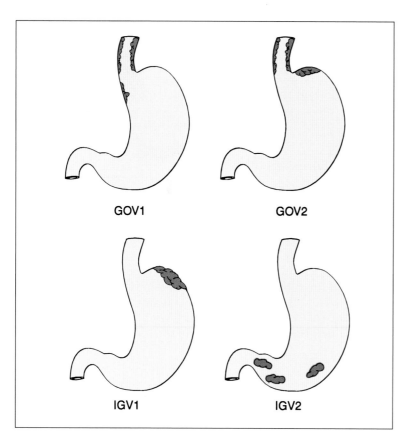

FIGURE 11-25.

GOV1   GOV2

IGV1   IGV2

FIGURE 11-25.

Anatomic distribution of gastroesophageal varices (GOVs). GOVs, which are part of the anatomic constellation of portal hypertensive gastropathy, are poorly understood and defined. Sarin and coworkers [34] in New Delhi have classified GOVs. Those GOVs, which are continuous with esophageal varices, may involve the lesser (GOV1) or the greater curvature (GOV2) of the stomach. Type 1 isolated gastric varices (IGV1), which are not continuous with esophageal varices, are usually found in the fundus of the stomach. Type 2 IVGs (IGV2) may be found anywhere in the stomach and are prone to bleed; type 2 isolated ectopic varices tend not to bleed. Sarin and and coworkers [34] comment about the prevalence and the distribution of these two types of varices and their clinical behavior. (From Sarin *et al.* [34]; with permission.)

■ HEPATIC ENCEPHALOPATHY

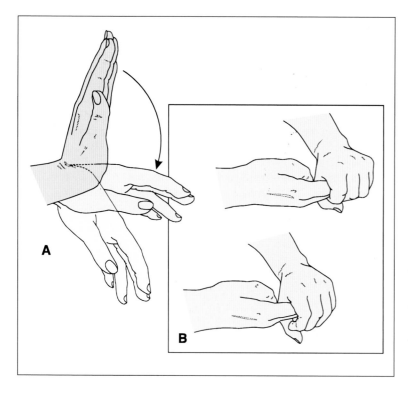

A

B

FIGURE 11-26.

Assessing asterixis: two techniques. Asterixis is a nonspecific neurologic sign that appears to result, at least in part, from dysfunction of the descending reticular system [35]. It may be seen in almost all types of metabolic encephalopathy of both hepatic and nonhepatic origin. **A,** It is defined as a defect of movement that is characterized by an inability to sustain a fixed posture such as holding one's hand in a dorsiflexed position at the wrist. Within 30 seconds, repetitive, irregular, involuntary movements of the hand occur. They appear to be flapping motions, hence its colloquial name *the flapping tremor.* Both the active and opposing muscles are activated. When asterixis is present, transient interruptions in electrical current, which last from 50 to 100 msec, occur. When the current is cut off, the hand falls forward by force of gravity; when the current returns, the position is resumed. Similar abnormalities can be induced in experimental animals by infusion of ammonium salts [36]. **B,** It can be tested for by having the patient squeeze two of the examiner's fingers. When asterixis is present, intermittent relaxation of the squeezing fingers can be felt by the examiner, whose fingers are being squeezed, within 30 seconds. (**A,** *From* Leavitt and Tyler [35]; with permission.) (**B,** *From* Conn and Lieberthal [36]; with permission.)

Mental status

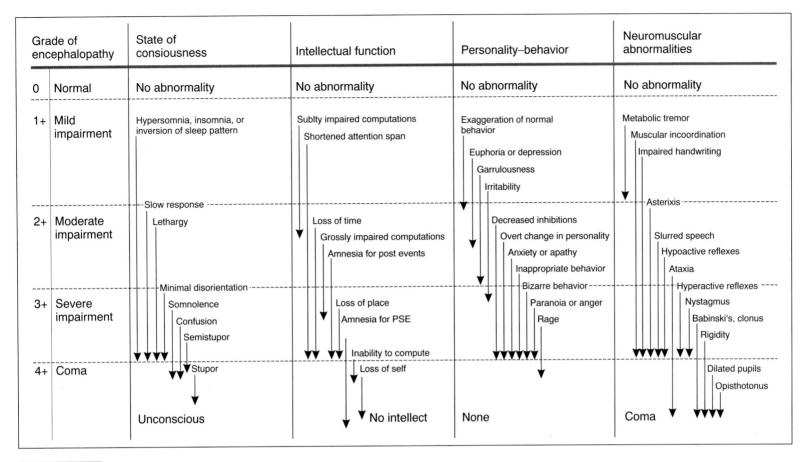

Grade of encephalopathy		State of consiousness	Intellectual function	Personality–behavior	Neuromuscular abnormalities
0	Normal	No abnormality	No abnormality	No abnormality	No abnormality
1+	Mild impairment	Hypersomnia, insomnia, or inversion of sleep pattern	Sublty impaired computations, Shortened attention span	Exaggeration of normal behavior, Euphoria or depression, Garrulousness, Irritability	Metabolic tremor, Muscular incoordination, Impaired handwriting
		Slow response, Lethargy			Asterixis
2+	Moderate impairment		Loss of time, Grossly impaired computations, Amnesia for post events	Decreased inhibitions, Overt change in personality, Anxiety or apathy, Inappropriate behavior	Slurred speech, Hypoactive reflexes, Ataxia
		Minimal disorientation		Bizarre behavior	Hyperactive reflexes
3+	Severe impairment	Somnolence, Confusion, Semistupor	Loss of place, Amnesia for PSE	Paranoia or anger, Rage	Nystagmus, Babinski's, clonus, Rigidity
			Inability to compute		
4+	Coma	Stupor	Loss of self		Dilated pupils, Opisthotonus
		Unconscious	No intellect	None	Coma

FIGURE 11-27.

Clinical spectrum of the disordered mental state in portosystemic encephalopathy (PSE). The grade of PSE is indicated on the *left*. Each of the three components of mental state (state of consciousness, intellectual function, and personality-behavior) plus neuromuscular abnormalities are shown in the four columns. Within each column the grade at which specific abnormalities usually appear is shown by the *tail of the arrow*. The *length of the arrow* indicates the range of grades through which each abnormality may persist. Many features of PSE are not detectable or measurable because testing may require cooperation not possible in comatose patients [36,37]. (*From* Conn and Lieberthal [36]; with permission.)

Pathogenesis

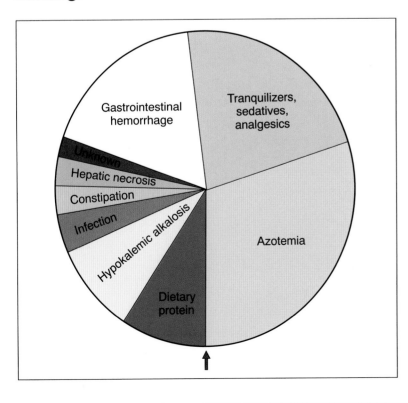

FIGURE 11-28.

Precipitants of hepatic encephalopathy in 100 consecutive patients with hepatic encephalopathy at the West Haven Veterans Administration Hospital, West Haven, Connecticut. The most common precipitant was azotemia, which occurred in one third of the patients [38]. In about half of them the azotemia had been precipitated by diuretic agents such as furosemide. Precipitation of hepatic encephalopathy by tranquilizers, sedatives, or analgesic agents appears to be primarily responsible for induction of impaired mental state in a quarter of the episodes. Ninety-seven episodes had occurred in cirrhotic patients, 13 of whom had portacaval anastomoses. The severity of the encephalopathy tended to be milder in the azotemic and drug-induced patients. Hypokalemic alkalosis, which had been caused by vomiting, diarrhea, or diuretic drugs, was seen in 10% of the patients. Severe encephalopathy occurred in association with gastrointestinal bleeding, infection, or azotemia. (*From* Fessel and Conn [38]; with permission.)

Blood ammonia concentration

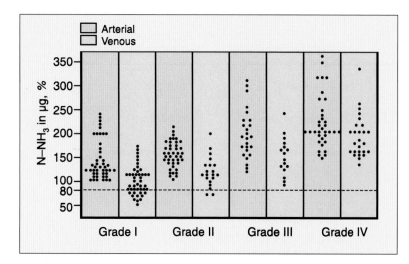

FIGURE 11-29.

Association of blood ammonia concentrations and the grade of hepatic encephalopathy in untreated cirrhotic patients. There is a step-wise progression between the arterial ammonia levels and the degree of portosystemic encephalopathy (PSE) (columns 1, 3, 5, and 7) [39]. There is, however, much overlap in ammonia concentrations between the adjacent grades of PSE. With venous ammonia levels (columns 2, 4, 6, and 8) the same trend is evident, but the degree of overlap is even greater. Arterial ammonia levels correlate much more closely with the degree of hepatic encephalopathy than venous levels. It is not possible to predict these gradients. (*From* Stahl [39]; with permission.)

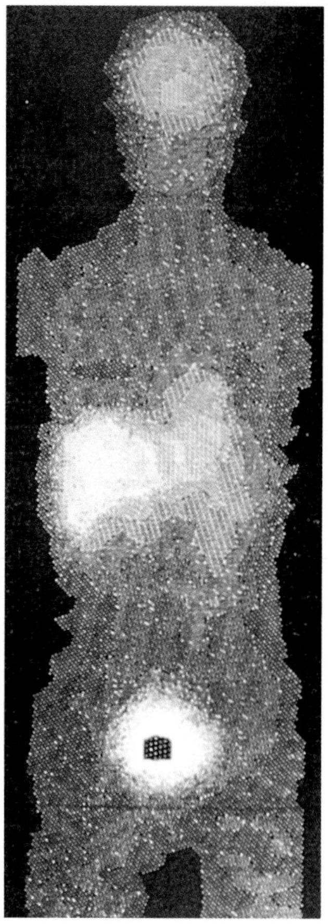

FIGURE 11-30.

A total body scan of a normal subject obtained 20 minutes after an intravenous injection of $^{13}NH_4Cl$ [40]. At this point 7% to 8% of the ammonia had already been converted to urea and had been excreted into the urine where it is visible in the bladder. Similar amounts were found in the liver, in the brain, and in the blood stream. Some 50% of the radioactivity was found in the muscles, which are the primary organs of ammonia removal in the body. The amount of ammonia taken up by the brain was linearly related to the arterial ammonia concentration. (*From* Lockwood *et al.* [40]; with permission.)

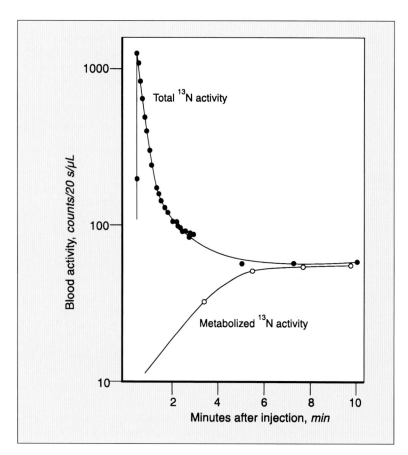

FIGURE 11-31.

The rapidity of ammonia clearance following an intravenous bolus injection of $^{13}NH_4Cl$. Arterial blood samples were withdrawn at the times indicated by *closed circles*. The *open circles* indicate the amount of ^{13}N incorporated into urea. Integration of the curves and subtraction yields the ammonia clearance rate. Clearance was virtually complete within 5 minutes of injection. (*From* Rosenspire *et al.* [41]; with permission.)

Branched-chain amino acid therapy

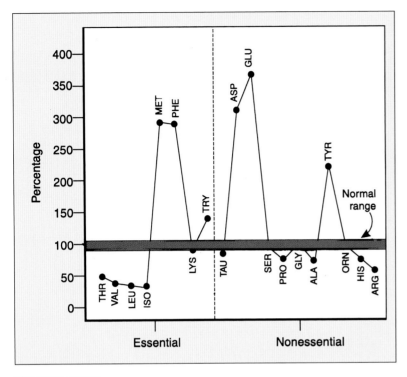

FIGURE 11-32.

The branched-chain amino acid (BCAA)—aromatic amino acid (AAA) hypothesis. The BCAA, *ie*, leucine (LEU), valine (VAL), and isoleucine (ISO), which are metabolized in muscle tissues, exist in parallel to the AAA, *ie*, tyrosine (TYR), phenylalanine (PHE), and tryptophan (TRY), which are metabolized in the liver [42]. These two groups of amino acids compete for transport across the blood brain barrier using the same transport system. In patients with cirrhosis and portal hypertension, the plasma concentrations of the AAAs tend to be increased and those of the BCAAs decreased. Indeed, the molar ratio between the BCAAs and the AAAs, *ie*,

$$\frac{[LEU] + [VAL] + [ISO]}{[TYR] + [PHE]}$$

is usually decreased in cirrhotic patients with hepatic encephalopathy from the normal range of 3.0 to 3.5 to 1.0 to 2.0 [42]. The abnormal ratio is intimately related to the false neurotransmitter hypothesis and to hyperammonemia and is responsible for the therapeutic concept of treating hepatic encephalopathy by administering BCAAs to normalize the BCAA/AAA ratio. Unfortunately, many randomized trials have failed to establish the efficacy of this form of therapy [43], although controversy persists [44].

In this diagram the mean levels of amino acids are depicted as the percentage of normal, which is indicated by the *green zone*. The pattern of decreased VAL, LEU, and ISO and increased PHE and TRY among the essential amino acids is apparent. Among the nonessential amino acids, aspartic acid (ASP), glutamic acid (GLU), and TYR tend to be increased and arginine (ARG) to be decreased. ALA—alanine; GLY—glycine; HIS—histidine; LYS—lysine; MET—methionone; ORN—ornithine; PRO—proline; SER—serine; TAU—tautine; THR—threonine. (*From* Rosen *et al.* [42]; with permission.)

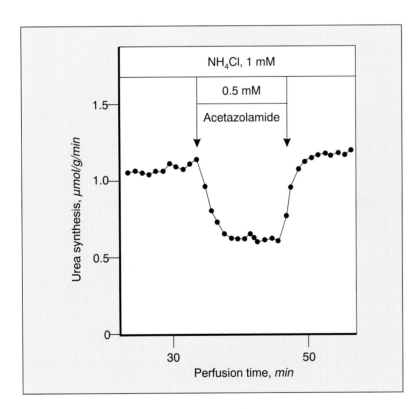

FIGURE 11-33.

Carbonic anhydrase inhibition in the pathogenesis of hyperammonemia and hepatic encephalopathy (HE). Loop diuretic agents such as chlorothiazide and furosemide may induce HE. Hepatic mitochondrial carbonic anhydrase, which is important in the intramitochondrial synthesis of carbamylphosphate, is inhibited by chlorothiazide and acetazolamide, but not by furosemide. It has recently been shown that this effect is associated with inhibition of urea synthesis and is bicarbonate mediated, *ie*, it is not caused by suppression of urea cycle enzymes [45]. In this diagram the effect of acetazolamide (Diamox R$_x$; Lederle Laboratories, Wayne, NJ) (0.5 mM) in inhibiting urea synthesis from ammonium chloride in the isolated, perfused rat liver is shown. (*From* Haussinger *et al.* [45]; with permission.)

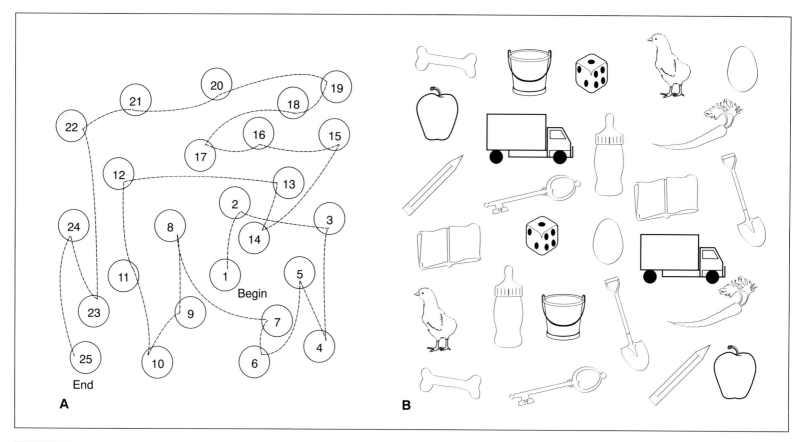

Number Connection Test (NCT). **A**, The NCT is a simple, rapid, inexpensive method of semiquanitatively estimating the severity of hepatic (or other types of) encephalopathy [46]. The patient is asked to connect a series of consecutively numbered circles in numeric order as rapidly as possible. The time in seconds, usually 15 to 60, required to complete this task represents the test time. A series of equally difficult patterns is used to prevent the patient from learning the pathway. These different patterns permit the patient to be studied serially and avoid learning effects which may diminish the precision of the test. The NCT can be incorporated into a Portal Systemic Encephalopathy Index (PSE I), which permits semiquantitative assessment of a variety of aspects of the many faceted syndrome of hepatic encephalopathy [47]. This test has stimulated the creation of a number of other simple psychometric tests. **B**, In this panel, the Familiar Figure Connection Test, pairs of simple figures can be connected by lines. The time it takes the patient to complete this task in seconds is the test time. This particular test appears to be useful in pediatric patients or in those who are illiterate or unfamiliar with Arabic numbers. (*Courtesy of* J. Lagarriga and M. Uribe, Mexico City, Mexico)

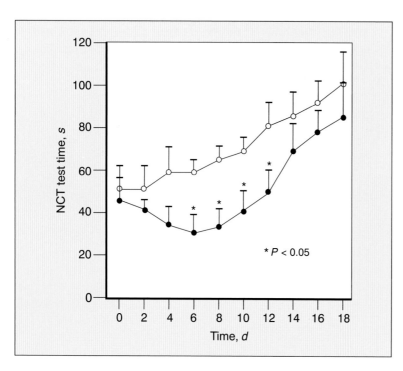

Use of the Number Connection Test (NCT) in testing hepatic encephalopathy. Effect of subtle variations in serum potassium concentration. Hypokalemia, which is often associated with metabolic alkalosis, is a common precipitant of hepatic encephalopathy in susceptible cirrhotic patients [48]. It has recently been shown that the psychometric status of cirrhotic patients with very mild hepatic encephalopahty (grade 1) is affected by minor changes in serum potassium concentration [49]. Patients whose serum potassium concentration was maintained near the upper range of normal (5.4 or 5.5 mEq/L) performed the NCT significantly more rapidly than those whose serum potassium levels were maintained in the low normal range (3.5 or 3.6 mEq/L). Furthermore, the clinical status of these patients who were maintained near the lower limit of normal was better than those who were in the low normal range. (*From* Zavagli *et al.* [49]; with permission.)

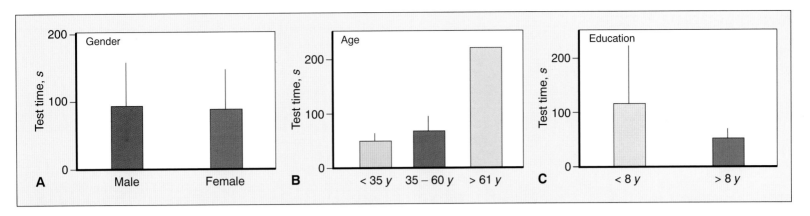

FIGURE 11-36.

Effects of sex, age, and education on the performance of the Number Connection Test (NCT) [50]. Data were obtained in 210 normal subjects. **A**, The mean NCT times in seconds were similar for men and women. **B**, The mean test times were significantly shorter for subjects less than 35 years of age than for those 35 to 60 years of age and for those older than 60 years (*P* < 0.001). **C**, Formal education, which was quantified as years of schooling, was associated with faster performance of the tests, *ie*, shorter mean NCT times in seconds. It is clear that age and education must be controlled for in performing and in interpreting NCT data. (*From* Zeneroli *et al.* [50]; with permission.)

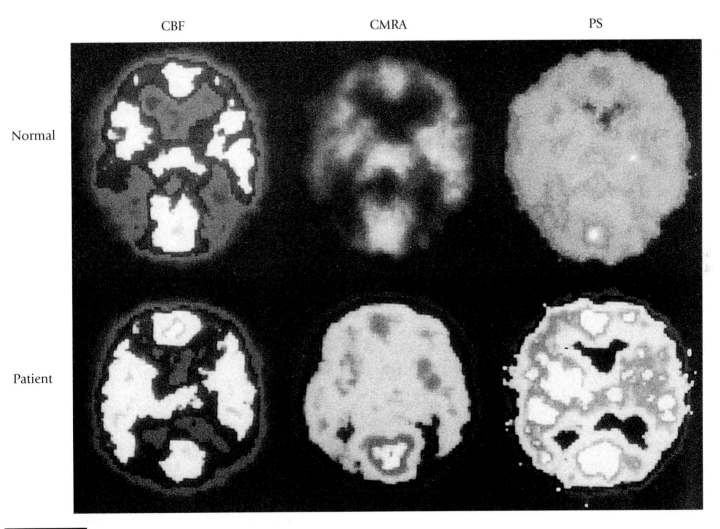

FIGURE 11-37.

Cerebral blood flow (CBF) and cerebral metabolic rate for ammonia (CMRA) using [15]O positron emission tomography [51]. Images are shown for a normal subject (*upper row*) and a patient with mild hepatic encephalopathy and hyperammonemia (*lower row*). CBF showed no significant quantitative differences, although regional variations showed more extensive activity in the temporal regions of the patient compared with those of the normal subject. CMRA was much greater throughout the brain of the encephalo-pathic patient. The permeability surface area product, which is an index of the permeability of the blood brain barrier, shows greater permeability for ammonia in the encephalopathic than in the normal subject (*right column*). The increased permeability surface area product results in the increased brain ammonia concentration, increased encephalopathy, and, indirectly, in increased metabolism of ammonia. (*From* Lockwood [51]; with permission.)

Alzheimer type II cells

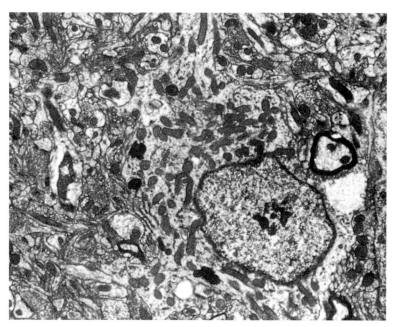

Abnormal astrocytes in hepatic encephalopathy. The clinical syndrome of hepatic encephalopathy is accompanied by the appearance of bizarre astrocytic nuclei [52]. The nuclei of these astrocytes, which are found in the cerebral cortex, putamen, globus pallidus, cerebellum, and other areas, show by light microscopy that their nuclei are larger and appear to have lobular enlargements of the marginal chromatin pattern (Alzheimer type II astrocytes). The severity of the abnormalities parallels the duration and depth of the hepatic encephalopathy. By electron microscopy, this figure shows that patients with chronic hepatic encephalopathy and experimental animals with hyperammonemic coma show marked proliferation of cellular organelles, especially of the mitochondria, which is indicative of increased metabolic activity. The fact that glutamine synthetase is found only in the nuclei of astroglial cells establishes the connection between hyperammonemia and Alzheimer type II astrocytes. Glutamine, the product of ammonia and glutamic acid, is an osmolyte, which when present in high concentration, induces cell swelling and increased intracranial pressure. The electron photomicrograph shown here was taken in a rat with a portacaval shunt, which had been fed an ammoniated resin [53]. (*From* Lockwood [53]; with permission.)

γ-Aminobutyric acid hypothesis

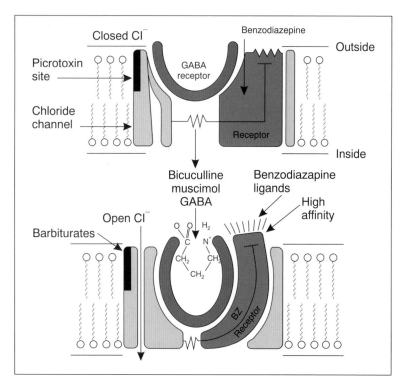

The γ-aminobutyric acid (GABA) hypothesis of the pathogenesis of hepatic encephalopathy. A scientifically sound, experimentally well-documented hypothesis for the pathogenesis of hepatic encephalopathy has been put forward by Jones and Ferenci [54] and supported by many other investigators. Central to this hypothesis is the GABA–benzodiazepine receptor-ionophore complex, which is illustrated here [55]. The finding of benzodiazepine receptor ligands extracted from the brains of patients who died of hepatic encephalopathy [56] and the amelioration induced by flumazenil [57], a benzodiazepine antagonist, support this complex theory. Unfortunately, randomized controlled trials have not confirmed the premise suggested by the authors of the preliminary studies. (*From* Paul *et al.* [55]; with permission.)

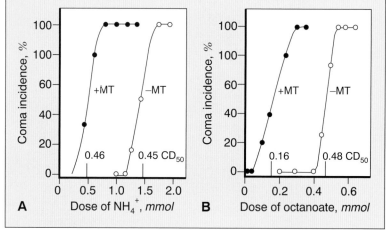

The multifactorial pathogenesis of hepatic encephalopathy. This graph presents data which demonstrate that methanethiol (MT), a mercaptan, enhances the comagenicity of ammonium chloride in rats [58]. *Curves* represent the dosage of ammonium chloride that induces coma in 50% of the exposed animals, *ie*, the coma dose 50 (CD_{50}). **A**, In the absence of MT (-MT) the CD_{50} is 1.45 mM. **B**, When MT is added (+MT), the CD_{50} for ammonium chloride is reduced by a factor of greater than 3. Similar enhancement of the toxicity of ammonium chloride occurs with short-chain fatty acids (SCFA). Furthermore, toxicity of MT can be enhanced by SCFA and vice versa. Similar curves can be constructed for MT with and without SCFA and for SCFA with and without MT (or NH_4Cl) [58]. These relationships, which are well established in experimental animals, have not, of course, been tested in patients. (*From* Zieve *et al.* [58]; with permission.)

Nonabsorbed carbohydrate therapy

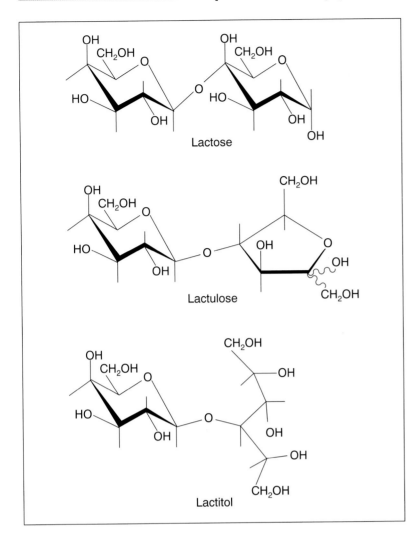

Lactose

Lactulose

Lactitol

FIGURE 11-41.

Lactose, lactulose, and lactitol and their differential therapeutic efficacy in hepatic encephalopathy [59]. The gastrointestinal enzymes are able to split the bond that connects the two monosaccharides (galactose and glucose) of lactose. After cleavage the two monosaccharides are rapidly absorbed and metabolized. Enzymes are unable to cleave the bonds that connect the monosaccharides of lactulose (galactose and fructose) or lactitol (galactose and sorbitol). Formulae are shown to demonstrate the structural similarities and differences of the three disaccharides. These disaccharides are too large to be absorbed and, consequently, pass intact into the lower intestinal tract where bacterial enzymes degrade them to short-chain fatty acids and hydrogen, hydrogen ion, and carbon dioxide. In this environment, ammonia can be corporated directly into bacterial protein [60]. In lactase-deficient patients, lactose cannot be cleaved into its component monosaccharides and acts like lactulose or lactitol. Lactose has been used effectively to treat hepatic encephalopathy in Mexican patients because of their Indian heritage [61]. It should be equally effective in black, Asian, East Indian, Arabic, and Jewish patients, as well as patients from other ethnic groups. In fact, the whole world, except for hyperlactastic northern Europeans, can be considered "lactase-deficient" people, whose hepatic encephalopathy can probably be managed with lactose. (*From* Conn and Bircher [59]; with permission.)

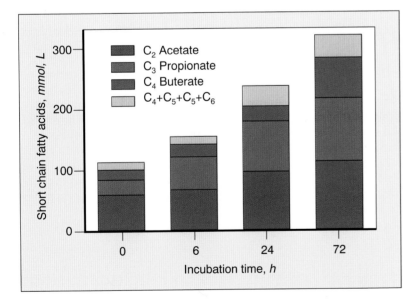

Short chain fatty acids, *mmol, L*

- C_2 Acetate
- C_3 Propionate
- C_4 Buterate
- $C_4+C_5+C_5+C_6$

Incubation time, *h*

FIGURE 11-42.

Effect of lactulose on plasma levels of short-chain fatty acids (SCFAs). Carbohydrates are metabolized to SCFAs, primarily 2-carbon, 3-carbon, and 4-carbon chain length SCFAs (acetate, propionate, and butyrate, respectively.) The comagenicity of the SCFAs increases with carbon-chain length. Acetate is devoid of coma-inducing properties. In the control stool incubation mixture shown, acetate, propionate, and butyrate occur in concentrations of approximately 125, 75, and 50 mM/L, respectively, after 24 hours of incubation. After lactulose is added to the stool incubation mixture, virtually all of the SCFAs exist as acetate [62]. Butyrate and all longer SCFAs are abolished by the lactulose. Thus, lactulose has many actions; it acidifies the intestinal lumen, stimulates cathartic activity, increases the growth of fermentative organisms and suppresses proteolytic bacteria, and stimulates the incorporation of ammonia into bacteria [60]. It also diminishes production of the comagenic SCFAs. (*From* Mortenson *et al.* [62]; with permission.)

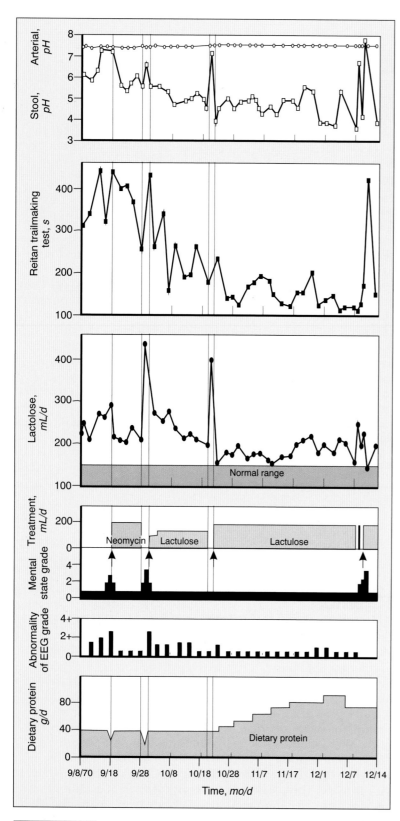

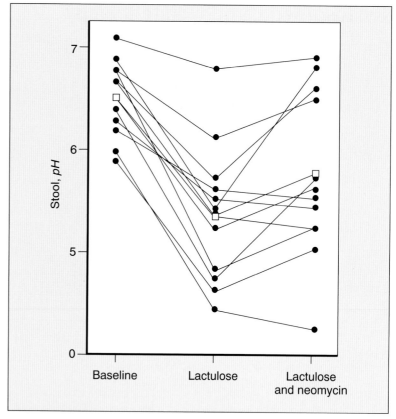

FIGURE 11-44.

Use of lactulose and neomycin in combination in the therapy of hepatic encephalopathy. Occasionally, neither lactulose nor neomycin achieves optimal therapeutic effects in patients with hepatic encephalopathy. In such patients the simultaneous use of both medications may help.

Lactulose requires enteric bacterial activation, which can be confirmed by a reduction in stool pH from its normal value of 7 to less than 6 [60,63]. Neomycin suppresses bacterial activity that may prevent the bacterial activation of lactulose. Furthermore, the antibacterial activity of lactulose is suppressed or eliminated by a reduction in stool pH [64]. Theoretically, the two agents would appear to be mutually antagonistic. In practice, however, they are not. In a group of 12 patients, the stool pH on neomycin alone was 6 or greater in all 12. On lactulose alone the pH was less than 6 in 10 of 12 patients. On neomycin plus lactulose, the stool pH increased to more than 6 in about 25% of the patients, a finding which indicates that lactulose was not being activated by dual therapy. In several patients, the pH remained well below 6, a finding indicative of the therapeutic activity of both agents. In about half the patients, the pH was at intermediate levels, suggesting that lactulose was partially activated and that therapy with both agents in combination was justifiable. (*From* Conn and Lieberthal [63]; with permission.)

FIGURE 11-43.

Effects of neomycin and lactulose in a patient with chronic hepatic encephalopathy [47]. During the basal state, this patient, who was receiving 40 g dietary protein/d, showed gradually worsening hepatic encephalopathy and more abnormal Number Connection Tests (NCT). Neomycin induced improvement in mental state, a decrease in arterial ammonia concentration, and no change in stool pH. When neomycin was stopped, the patient's mental state deteriorated and the blood ammonia level rose sharply. Lactulose quickly restored normal mental state and progressively reduced the arterial ammonia concentration and the NCT time. Cessation of lactulose was promptly followed by relapse. Reinstitution of lactulose resulted in a second remission, which was maintained on lactulose therapy, despite a progressive increase in dietary protein to 100 g/d. EEG—electroencephalograph. (*From* Conn *et al.* [47]; with permission.)

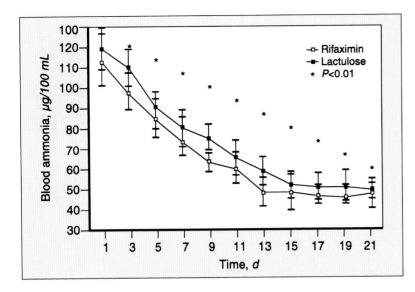

FIGURE 11-45.

Comparative effects of rifaximin and lactulose on hyperammonemic hepatic encephalopathy. Antibiotic therapy with neomycin or related nonabsorbed broad-spectrum antibiotic agents has been a primary form of therapy for hepatic encephalopathy for 20 years. It was frequently toxic, causing renal disease, hearing loss, malabsorption, and other lesions [3]. The recent introduction of rifaximin, a nonabsorbed, nontoxic antibiotic agent, promises to revolutionize the treatment of hepatic encephalopathy [65]. In a randomized comparison of rifaximin (1200 mg/d) and lactulose (40 g/d), the mean venous blood ammonia concentrations were significantly lower in the rifaximin-treated patients than in those who received lactulose in every determination. This figure suggests that rifaximin is at least as effective as lactulose in the management of hyperammonemic hepatic encephalopathy. (*From* Bucci and Palmieri [65]; with permission.)

L-Ornithine-L-aspartate therapy

Chemical structure →

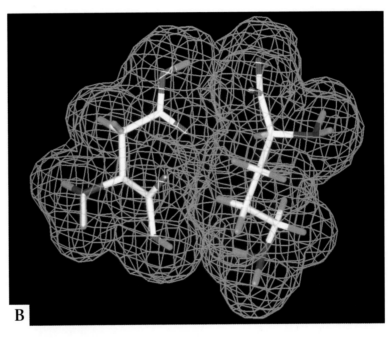

A

FIGURE 11-46.

L-Ornithine-L-aspartate. A new middle-aged therapeutic agent for hepatic encephalopathy. Ornithine-aspartate (OA), the chemical name of which is (S)-2,5-diaminovalerianic acid-(S)-2-amino succinate, has a molecular formula of $C_9H^{19}N3O_6$ and a molecular weight of 265. It is a diamino acid couplet that dissociates in water into its component amino acids [66]. **A,** Conventional chemical structure of OA. **B,** Computer-generated chemical structure of OA. (*Courtesy of* G. Kircheis, Frankfurt, Germany.)

B

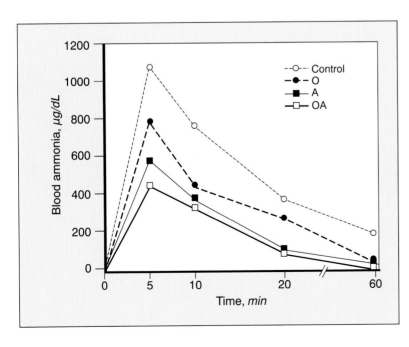

FIGURE 11-47.

Comparative effects of L-ornithine (O), L-aspartate (A), and L-ornithine-L-aspartate (OA) on blood ammonia concentration following ammonium chloride infusion. The control group showed a large sustained hyperammonemia peaking at greater than 1000 µg/dL at the end of the ammonia infusion. When simultaneously treated with an infusion of L-ornithine, the peak ammonia concentration was lower (800 µg/dL). When L-aspartate was simultaneously infused with ammonia, the peak ammonia level was even lower (600 µg/dL). When L-ornithine-L-aspartate was infused with the ammonia, the peak only reached about 400 µg/dL. Thus, the antiammonia effect of aspartate is greater than that of ornithine, but the combination of the two amino acids is better than either alone. (*From* Shioya [67]; with permission.)

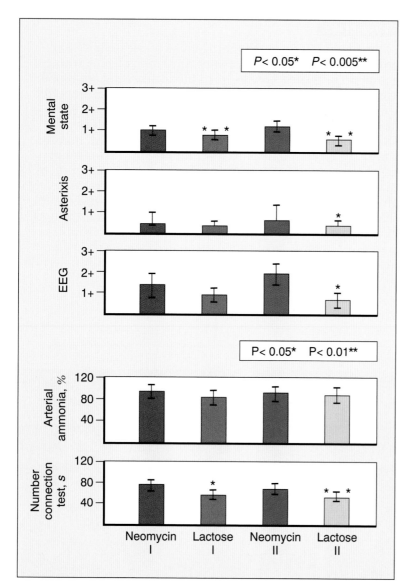

FIGURE 11-48.

Efficacy of lactose therapy in chronic portal systemic encephalo-pathy (PSE) in lactase-deficient cirrhotic patients [68]. Each of the components of the PSE Index—the mental state, the degree of asterixis, the degree of electroencephalographic (EEG) abnormality, the arterial ammonia concentration, and the Number Connection Test (NCT)—is expressed in arbitrary terms (0 to 4+). The *height of the bars* represents the mean value for each component in 10 patients. In the first and third columns, the effects of therapy for 2 weeks with neomycin (3 g/d plus milk of magnesia) are shown. In the second and fourth columns the effects of therapy for 2 weeks with lactose (100 g/d) are shown. The mean mental state improved to a greater degree after lactose than after neomycin ($P < 0.01$) [68]. Similarly, the mean EEG grade and the mean NCT time were signif-icantly more normal after lactose than after neomycin ($P < 0.05$ to $P < 0.01$). The mean arterial ammonia level was lower after lactose, but this difference is not statistically significant. The PSE Efficacy Index, which integrates the components of the PSE I [48], is highly significant in favor of lactose. (*From* Conn *et al.* [47]; with permission.)

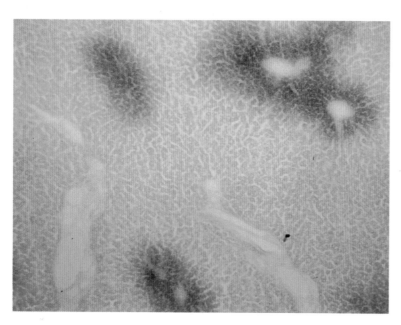

FIGURE 11-49.

Lobular localization of ammonia-disposing enzymes in the liver. Urea synthesis and glutamine synthesis are the two predominant biochemical pathways for removing ammonia from the blood stream. Ureagenesis, which is catalyzed by the five urea cycle enzymes, occurs almost exclusively in the peri-portal hepatocytes that make up more than 75% of the hepato-cytes [69]. Glutamine synthetase, the ubiquitous enzyme that combines ammonia with glutamate to form glutamine, is restricted to a small fraction of hepatocytes (about 7%), which are found in the two to five rings of hepatocytes around the central hepatic veins. This localization can be demonstrated by histoautoradiography in which gluterate and 3-H glutamate are infused into rat livers either antegrade (portal to hepatic) or retrograde (hepatic to portal) [70]. These cells, which are also known as perivenous scavenger cells, also take up vascular glutamate, aspartate, and α-ketoglutarate. Lobular distribution of these enzymes and the uptake of these substrates is identical. (*From* Stoll *et al.* [70]; with permission.)

■ REFERENCES AND RECOMMENDED READING

1. Beppu K, Inokuchi K, Koyanagi N, *et al.*: Prediction of variceal hemorrhage by esophageal endoscopy. *Gastrointest Endosc* 1981, 27:213–218.

2. McCormack TT, Rose JD, Smith PM: Perforating veins and blood flow in esophageal varices. *Lancet* 1983, 2:1442–1444.

3. Conn HO, Helzberg J: Complications of portal hypertension. *Current Hepatology* 1986, 6:133–140.

4. Goldman ML, Freeny PC, Tallman JM, *et al.*: Transcatheter vascular occlusion therapy with isobutyl 2-cyanoacrylate (bucrylate) for control of massive upper-gastrointestinal bleeding. *Radiology* 1978, 129:41–49.

5. Sadler MA, Shapiro RS: Transjugular portosystemic shunt. *N Engl J Med* 1994:330:182.

6. Beppu K, Inokuchi K, Koyanagi N, *et al.*: Prediction of variceal hemorrhage by esophageal endoscopy. *Gastrointest Endosc* 1981, 27:213–218.

7. Ponce J, Froufe A, Morena E, *et al.*: Morphometric study of esophageal mucosa in cirrhotic patients with variceal bleeding. *Hepatology* 1981, 1:641–646.

8. Parra *et al.*: Classificacao de varizes esofagicas port un sistema metrico. *Rev Assoc Med Brazil* 1980, 26:264–269.

9. Lebrec D, Poynard T, Bernuau J, *et al.*: Randomized controlled study of propranolol for prevention of recurrent gastrointestinal bleeding in patients with cirrhosis: A final report. *Hepatology* 1984, 4:355–358.

10. Conn HO: Propranolol in portal hypertension. Problems in paradise. *Hepatology* 1984, 4:560–564.

11. Van Steigmann G, Cambre T, Sunn JH: A new endoscopic elastic band ligating device. *Gastrointest Endosc* 1986, 32:230–233.

12. Hou M-C, Lin H-C, Kuo B I-T, *et al.*: Comparison of endoscopic variceal injection sclerotherapy and ligation for the treatment of esophageal variceal hemorrhage: A prospective randomized trial. *Hepatology* 1995, 21:1517–1522.

13. Orloff JM, Bell RH, Hyde PV, Skivolocki WP: Long-term results of emergency portacaval shunt for bleeding esophageal varices in unselected patients with alcoholic cirrhosis. *Ann Surg* 1980, 192:325–340.

14. McCormick PA, Dick R, Irving JD, *et al.*: Transjugular intrahepatic portosystemic stent-shunt. *J Hosp Med* 1993, 49:28–32.

15. Bosch J, Mastai R, Kravetz D, *et al.*: Measurement of azygos venous blood flow in the evaluation of portal hypertension in patients with cirrhosis: Clinical and hemodynamic correlations in 100 patients. *J Hepatol* 1985, 1:125–139.

16. Bosch J, Groszmann RI: Measurement of azygos venous blood flow by a continuous thermal dilution technique: An index of blood flow through gastroesophageal collaterals in cirrhosis. *Hepatology* 1984, 4:424–429.

17. Vinel JP, Cassigneul J, Levade M, *et al.*: Assessment of short-term prognosis after variceal bleeding in patients with alcoholic cirrhosis by early measurement of portohepatic gradient. *Hepatology* 1986, 6:116–117.

18. Conn HO: The varix-volcano connection. *Gastroenterology* 1980, 79:1333–1337.

19. Garcia-Tsao G, Grace HD, Groszmann RJ, *et al.*: Short-term effects of propranolol on portal venous pressure. *Hepatology* 1986, 6:101–106.

20. Gimson AES, Westaby D, Hegarty J: A randomized trial of vasopressin and vasopressin plus nitroglycerin in the control of acute variceal hemorrhage. *Hepatology* 1986, 6:410–413.

21. Groszmann R, Kravetz D, Bosch J: Nitroglycerin improves the hemodynamic response to vasopressin in portal hypertension. *Hepatology* 1982, 3:757–762.

22. Gibson PR, McLean AJ, Dudley FJ: The hypotensive effect of oral nitroglycerin on portal venous pressure in patients with cirrhotic portal hypertension. *J Gastroenterol Hepatol* 1986, 201–206.

23. Zimmon DS, Kessler RE: Effect of portal venous blood flow diversion on portal pressure. *J Clin Invest* 1980, 65:1388–1397.

24. Sarfeh IJ, Rypins EB: Partial versus total portacaval shunt in alcoholic cirrhosis. *Ann Surg* 1994, 219:353–361.

25. Graham DY, Smith JL: The course of patients after variceal hemorrhage. *Gastroenterology* 1981, 80:800–809.

26. Smith JL, Graham DY: Variceal hemorrhage. A critical evaluation of survival analysis. *Gastroenterology* 1982, 82:968–973.

27. Conn HO: Theoretic influence of surgical intervention on survival. Effects of early, intermediate and late shunt surgery. *Current Hepatology* 1984, 4:152–154.

28. Conn HO, Ramsby GR: Aneurysm of the inferior vena cava after portacaval anastomosis. *Surgery* 1972, 71:828–833.

29. Castell DO, Conn HO: The determination of portacaval shunt patency: A critical review of methodology. *Medicine* 1972, 51:315–336.

30. Goldberg BB, Patel J: Ultrasonic evaluation of portacaval shunts. *J Clin Ultrasound* 1978, 5:304–306.

31. Yamamoto S, Hidemura R, Sawada M, *et al.*: The late result of terminal esophago-proximal gastrectomy (TEPG) with extensive devascularization and splenectomy for bleeding varices in cirrhosis. *Surgery* 1976, 80:106–114.

32. Inokuchi K, Cooperative Study Group of Portal Hypertension of Japan: Improved survival after prophylactic portal nondecompression surgery for esophageal varices: A randomized clinical trial. *Hepatology* 1990, 12:1–6.

33. Conn HO, Grace ND, Bosch J, *et al.*: Propranolol in the prevention of the first hemorrhage from esophageal varices: A multicenter, randomized clinical trial. *Hepatology* 1991, 13:902–912.

34. Sarin SK, Lahoti D, Saxena SP: Prevalence, classification and natural history of gastric varices. A long-term follow-up study in 568 portal hypertension patients. *Hepatology* 1992, 16:1343–1349.

35. Leavitt S, Tyler HR: Studies in asterixis. *Arch Neurol* 1964, 10:360–368.

36. Conn HO, Lieberthal MM: *The Hepatic Coma Syndromes and Lactulose.* Baltimore: Williams & Wilkins; 1978:49.

37. Conn HO, Bircher J: Quantifying the severity of hepatic encephalopathy. In *Hepatic Encephalopathies: Syndromes and Therapies.* Bloomington: Medi-Ed Press; 1994:13–26.

38. Fessel JM, Conn HO: An analysis of the causes and prevention of hepatic coma [Abstract]. *Gastroenterology* 1972, 62:191.

39. Stahl J: Studies of the blood ammonia in liver disease. Its diagnostic, prognostic and therapeutic significance. *Ann Intern Med* 1963, 58:1–24.

40. Lockwood AH, McDonald JM, Reiman RE, *et al.*: The dynamics of ammonia metabolism in man: Effects of liver disease and hyperammonemia. *J Clin Invest* 1979, 63:449–460.

41. Rosenspire KC, Schwaiger M, Manger TJ, *et al.*: Metabolic fate of [^{13}N] ammonia in human and canine blood. *J Nucl Med* 1990, 31:163–167.

42. Rosen HM, Yoshimura N, Hodgman JM, Fischer JE: Plasma amino acid patterns in hepatic encephalopathy of differing etiology. *Gastroenterology* 1977, 72:483–487.

43. Eriksson LS, Conn HO: Branched-chain amino acids in the management of hepatic encephalopathy: An analysis of variants. *Hepatology* 1989, 10:228–246.

44. Naylor CD, O'Rourke K, Detsky AS, Baker JP: Parenteral nutrition with branched-chain amino acids in hepatic encephalopathy. *Gastroenterology* 1989, 97:1033–1042.

45. Haussinger D, Kaiser S, Stehle T: Liver carbonic anhydrase and urea synthesis. The effect of diuretics. *Biochem Pharmacol* 1986, 35:3317–3322.

46. Conn HO: The trailmaking and number connection tests in assessing mental state in portal systemic encephalopathy. *Am J Dig Dis* 1977, 22:541–550.

47. Conn HO, Leevy CM, Vlahcevic ZR, *et al.*: A comparison of lactulose and neomycin in the treatment of portal-systemic encephalopathy: A double-blind controlled trial. *Gastroenterology* 1977, 72:573–583.

48. Tannen RL: Ammonia and acid base homeostasis. *Med Clin North Am* 1983, 67:781–798.

49. Zavagli G, Ricci G, Bader G, *et al.*: The importance of the highest normokalemia in the treatment of early hepatic encephalopathy. *Miner Electrolyte Metab* 1993, 19:362–367.

50. Zeneroli ML, Cioni G, Ventura P: The number connection test: Corrections for age and education [Letter]. *J Hepatol* 1992, 15:263–264.

51. Lockwood AH: *Hepatic Encephalopathy*. Boston: Butterworth-Heinemann; 1992:36.

52. Adams RD, Foley JM: The neurological disorder associated with liver disease. In *Metabolic and Toxic Diseases of the Nervous System*. Edited by Merritt HH, Hare C. Baltimore: Williams & Wilkins; 1953: 298–347.

53. Lockwood AH: Ammonia-induced encephalopathy. In *Cerebral Energy Metabolism and Metabolic Encephalopathy*. Edited by McCanless DW. New York: Plenum; 1985:203–228.

54. Jones EA, Ferenci P: Hepatic encephalopathy, gabaergic neurotransmission and the benzodiazepines. In *Hepatic Encephalopathy: Syndromes and Therapies*. Edited by Conn HO, Bircher J. Bloomington: Medi-Ed Press; 1994:75–100.

55. Paul SM, Manangos PJ, Skolnick P: The benzodiazepine-GABA chloride ionophore receptor complex: common site of minor tranquilizer action. *Biol Psychiatry* 1981, 16:213–229.

56. Basile AS, Hughes RD, Harrison PM: Elevated brain concentrations of 1,4-benzodiazepines in fulminant hepatic failure. *N Engl J Med* 1991, 325:473–478.

57. Ferenci P, Grimm G, Meryn S, *et al.*: Successful long-term treatment of portal-systemic encephalopathy by the benzodiazepine antagonist flumazenil. *Gastroenterology* 1989, 96:240–243.

58. Zieve L, Doizaki WM, Zieve FJ: Synergism between mercaptans and ammonia or fatty acids in the production of coma; a possible role for mercaptans in the pathogenesis of hepatic coma. *J Lab Clin Med* 1974, 83:16–28.

59. Conn HO, Bircher J: *Hepatic Encephalopathy: Management with Lactulose and Related Carbohydrates*. East Lansing: Medi-Ed Press; 1988:370.

60. Weber FL Jr, Banwell JG, Fresard KM, *et al.*: Nitrogen in fecal bacterial, fiber and soluble fractions of patients with cirrhosis: Effects of lactulose and lactulose plus neomycin. *J Lab Clin Med* 1987, 110:256–263.

61. Uribe M, Marquez MA, Garcia-Ramos G, *et al.*: Treatment of chronic portal-systemic encephalopathy with lactose in lactase-deficient patients. *Dig Dis Sci* 1980, 25:924–928.

62. Mortensen PB, Holtug K, Bonnen H: The degradation of amino acids, proteins and blood to short-chain fatty acids in the colon is prevented by lactulose. *Gastroenterology* 1990, 98:353–360.

63. Conn HO, Lieberthal MM: *The Hepatic Coma Syndromes and Lactulose*. Baltimore: Williams & Wilkins; 1978:340–345.

64. Young LS, Hewitt WL: Activity of five aminoglycoside antibiotics in vitro against gram-negative bacilli and staphylococcus aureus. *Antimicrob Agents Chemother* 1973, 4:617–636.

65. Bucci L, Palmieri GC: Double-blind, double-dummy comparison between treatment with rifaximin and lactulose in patients with medium to severe degree hepatic encephalopathy. *Curr Med Res Opin* 1993, 13:109–118.

66. Schultz SG: Coupled transport of sodium and organic solutes. *Physiol Rev* 1970, 50:637–643.

67. Shioya A: Pharmacological study on L-ornithine-L-aspartate. *Jap J Pharmacol* 1964, 14:201–214.

68. Uribe M: Management of portal-systemic encephalopathy with lactose in patients with lactase deficiency. In *Hepatic Encephalopathy: Syndromes and Therapies*. Edited by Conn HO, Bircher J. Bloomington: Medi-Ed Press; 1994:311–327.

69. Haussinger D: Liver glutamine metabolism. *JPEN J Parenter Enteral Nutr* 1990, 14:56S–62S.

70. Stoll B, McNelly S, Buscher HP, Haussinger D: Functional hepatocyte heterogeneity in glutamate, aspartate and α-keto-glutarate uptake: A histoautoradiographic study. *Hepatology* 1991, 13:247–253.

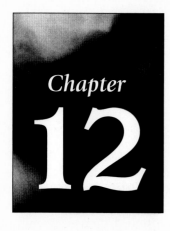

Chapter 12

Vascular Diseases, Abscesses, and Cysts

■ VASCULAR DISEASES

Vascular diseases of the liver can affect either large vessels or the microvasculature of the organ. The liver receives approximately one quarter of the cardiac output with one third of that total flow provided by the hepatic artery. The dual blood supply of the liver reduces the likelihood of infarction, although under certain circumstances, ischemic injury to the liver occurs. Because of the anatomic relationship between the hepatic veins and right atrium, systemic venous hypertension results in the congestion of the liver and the development of portal venous hypertension.

Occlusion of the hepatic veins, the Budd-Chiari syndrome, results in painful hepatomegaly and ascites. The portal vein may occasionally become occluded by thrombosis, thus resulting in presinusoidal portal hypertension. Recanalization of a thrombosed portal vein may occur but is seldom complete. Cavernous transformation of the portal vein may occur after infection or catheterization of the umbilical vein in neonates, this is because the umbilical vein drains directly into the portal circulation.

The clinical manifestations of hepatic venoocclusive disease (VOD) are similar to those seen with the Budd-Chiari syndrome. Thrombosis occurs in the terminal hepatic venules, usually following an inflammatory and fibrotic reaction that begins in the endothelial lining. VOD may occur following both allogeneic and autologous bone marrow transplantation, suggesting that the preoperative regimens of total body irradiation and high-dose chemotherapy are more important in the pathogenesis of VOD than are immunologic mechanisms.

Hemangiomas are the most common benign tumors of the liver, found in 3% to 5% of autopsies. Although seldom

IGNACIO AIZA
EUGENE R. SCHIFF

symptomatic, hemangiomas are frequently identified during radiographic evaluation of suspected gallbladder pathology.

CYSTIC DISEASES

Simple hepatic cysts are common, patients presenting with them are, for the most part, asymptomatic. Biliary cysts may involve both the extrahepatic or the intrahepatic bile ducts. The origin of both hepatic and biliary cysts remains subject to controversy. Many investigators believe that hepatic and biliary cysts are congenital, although some suggest that anomalous arrangement of the pancreaticobiliary tree leading to cholangitis followed by cystic dilatation is responsible. Biliary cysts have been classified into five major types according to their location. Although simple hepatic cysts do not usually require treatment unless patients become symptomatic. Biliary cysts are more frequently treated either by surgical excision or internal drainage into a Roux-en-Y loop. A higher incidence of cholangiocarcinoma is present in patients with biliary cysts. These malignancies occur throughout the biliary tree and are not confined to the site of the cyst. Polycystic liver disease is a congenital abnormality associated, in 50% of cases, with renal cysts and less frequently with pancreatic and splenic cysts. These cysts are not connected to the biliary tree. Rupture, hemorrhage into the cyst, and infection are rare complications.

Biliary cystadenomas appear almost exclusively in middle-aged women. They are most commonly found in the right lobe, are frequently pedunculated, and rarely obstruct the biliary tree. Echinoccocal cysts arise from infestation with larvae of the cestode *Ecchinococcus granulosis*. Formation of daughter cysts from the innermost or granular layer of the cyst and calcification of the wall are characteristics commonly found in these lesions.

ABSCESS

The majority of liver abscesses seen in developed countries are pyogenic in origin. Pyogenic abscesses may be solitary or multiple depending on etiology. Multiple abscesses occur in patients with systemic bacterial infections and decreased immunity, such as intravenous illicit drug users, whereas a solitary pyogenic liver abscess is usually a complication of diverticulitis, or other intra-abdominal infections, or of ascending cholangitis with poor biliary drainage. Multiple liver abscesses are sometimes treated with surgical drainage but may also resolve with prolonged antibiotic treatment. A solitary abscess may be drained surgically or percutaneously with radiographic guidance.

Amebic liver abscesses are almost always solitary. The course of an amebic abscess is usually indolent and may not be accompanied by diarrhea or other evidence of intestinal amebiasis. After definitive diagnosis of amebic abscess, the preferred drug therapy is metronidazole or chloroquine. Both are equally effective in resolving the infection.

NORMAL VASCULAR ANATOMY

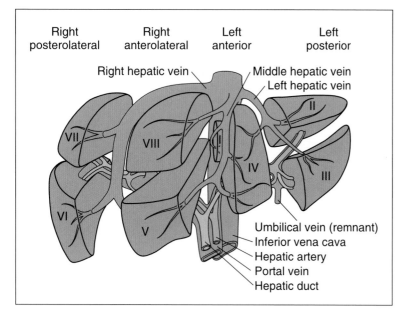

Right posterolateral   Right anterolateral   Left anterior   Left posterior

Right hepatic vein   Middle hepatic vein   Left hepatic vein

VII   VIII   II   IV   III   VI   V

Umbilical vein (remnant)
Inferior vena cava
Hepatic artery
Portal vein
Hepatic duct

FIGURE 12-1.

Normal vascular anatomy of the liver. The liver receives one third of its blood supply from the hepatic artery, which is a branch of the celiac trunk arising from the aorta superior to the superior mesenteric artery. The major branches of the hepatic artery are the gastroduodenal artery, the right gastric artery, and the cystic artery, which supplies the gallbladder. The common portal vein receives blood from the superior mesenteric vein and the splenic vein. Esophageal veins may drain either into the azygous system or into the coronary branch of the gastric veins, which in turn enter the portal system, depending on the pressure in the two systems. Beyond the hepatic sinusoid, the mixed portal venous and hepatic arterial blood drains into the hepatic veins. There are several branches that separately enter the inferior vena cava before returning to the heart. The caudate lobe of the liver has a separate venous drainage. (*From* Rappaport and Wanless [1]; with permission.)

RADIOGRAPHIC ANATOMY

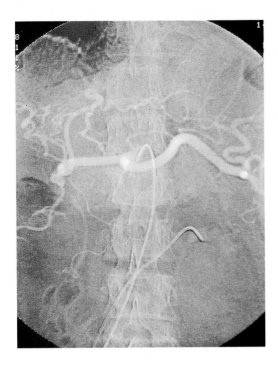

FIGURE 12-2.

Radiographic anatomy of the arteries of the liver. The arteries of the liver are best imaged by selective catherization of the celiac trunk or the hepatic artery itself.

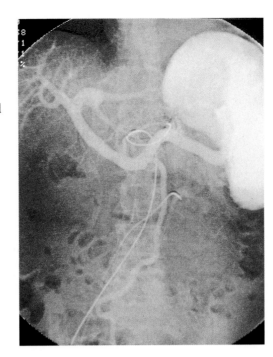

FIGURE 12-3.

Radiographic anatomy of the portal veins. The portal venous system is best seen after selective injection of contrast dye into the superior mesenteric or splenic arteries followed by delayed images to visualize the venous phase.

BUDD-CHIARI SYNDROME

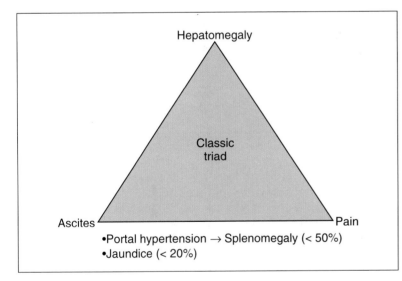

FIGURE 12-4.

Clinical manifestations of Budd-Chiari syndrome. The classic triad of abdominal pain, hepatomegaly, and ascites is present in the majority of patients with Budd-Chiari syndrome. Of these, pain is the least constant finding. Jaundice is rare, occurring in less than 20% of patients. Splenomegaly is found in almost 50%. In some instances, splenomegaly is a consequence of an underlying hematologic disorder, such as polycythemia rubra vera, whereas in others it results from portal hypertension. The remaining clinical signs are those associated with portal hypertension per se.

TABLE 12-1. BUDD-CHIARI SYNDROME

PREDISPOSING FACTORS

Hematologic	Phlebitis
Polycythemia rubra vera	**Trauma**
Paroxysmal nocturnal hemoglobinuria	**Infectious**
Myeloproliferative disorders	Amebic abscess
Chronic myelogenous leukemia	Aspergillosis
Hypercoagulable states (lupus anticoagulant, antithrombin III deficiency protein C/protein S deficiency)	Hydatid cysts
	Oral contraceptives
	Pregnancy and postpartum
	Venal caval web
Tumors	**Radiation**
Hepatocellular carcinoma	**Behcet's disease**
Renal cell carcinoma	**Rare causes**
Adrenal cell carcinoma	Inflammatory bowel disease
Leiomyosarcoma	Protein-losing enteropathy
Choriocarcinoma	Syphilitic gummas
Right atrial myxoma	Sarcoidosis
	? Cirrhosis
	? Previous episodes of hepatitis

TABLE 12-1.

Etiology of Budd-Chiari syndrome. This table lists the disorders that predispose patients to the development of Budd-Chiari syndrome. The majority of underlying disorders are hematologic with a thrombotic diathesis.

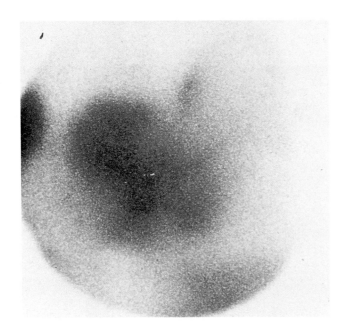

FIGURE 12-5.

Use of liver scintiscan for diagnosis of Budd-Chiari syndrome. ^{99}Technetium liver spleen scans often provide clues for making a positive diagnosis of Budd-Chiari syndrome. There is usually decreased uptake of tracer in the right and left lobes of the liver, corresponding to occlusion of the right and left hepatic veins. By contrast, the caudate lobe, which has a separate venous drainage, is often hypertrophied and has increased tracer uptake.

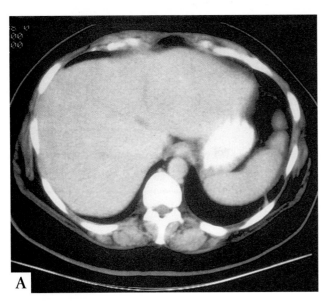

A

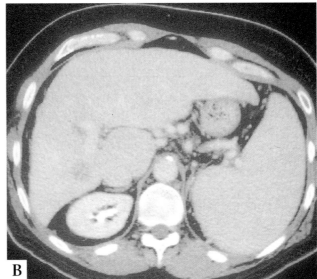

B

FIGURE 12-6.

A, Computerized tomography in diagnosis of Budd-Chiari syndrome. The use of contrast computed tomographic scans can often identify hepatic veins. The failure to visualize hepatic veins is highly suggestive of Budd-Chiari syndrome, although not reliable enough to exclude anatomic variants or other causes. **B**, A characteristic finding on computed tomography in patients with Budd-Chiari syndrome is hypertrophy of the caudate lobe, which occurs because of its independent venous drainage.

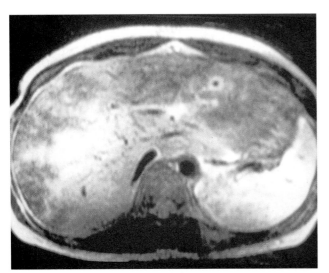

FIGURE 12-7.

Magnetic resonance imaging with pulsed sequences allows visualization of flow within the hepatic veins. This figure illustrates absence of flow in the hepatic veins in a patient with Budd-Chiari syndrome. Portal blood flow and direction can be determined using magnetic resonance imaging. In addition, other problems such as focal defects within the hepatic parenchyma can be excluded.

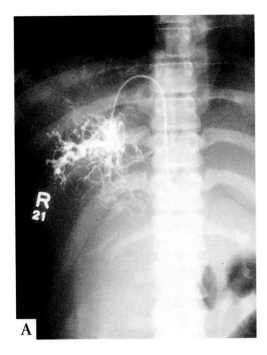

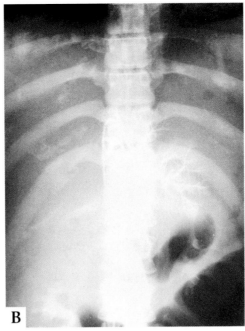

FIGURE 12-8.

A, The spider web pattern illustrates collateral flow from the small hepatic veins directly into the systemic circulation. Although seen infrequently, the spider web pattern of hepatic venography is almost definitely diagnostic of Budd-Chiari syndrome. This pattern is speculated to result from the formation of collateral anastomoses between the small hepatic veins and the systemic circulation. (This pattern confirms the obstruction to venous outflow has existed for a prolonged period.) **B,** A normal venogram in the patent left hepatic vein of the same patient. (*Courtesy of* K. R. Reddy, Miami, FL)

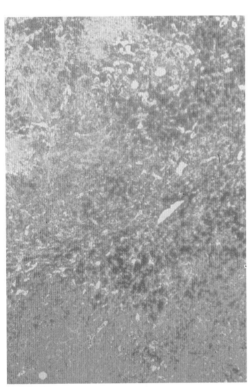

FIGURE 12-9.

Liver biopsy is often needed to establish duration of Budd-Chiari syndrome and to exclude the existence of cirrhosis before making decisions about therapy. Acute obstruction of the hepatic veins leads to severe sinusoidal dilatation often associated with congestion and necrosis of hepatocytes in the centrilobular perivenular zone. These hepatocytes are replaced by erythrocytes within the space of Disse. The periportal zone is affected much less than the centrilobular zone.

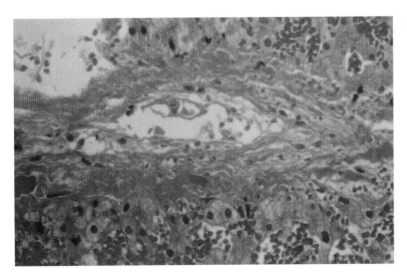

FIGURE 12-10.

Prolonged obstruction of the hepatic veins eventually leads to perivenular fibrosis that may be associated with bridging between perivenular zones. High-grade obstruction stimulates collagen deposition. There is usually a distinct absence of inflammation. Because occlusion of hepatic veins may occur at different times, the age of the lesions may vary within different areas of the liver. In the most extensive and prolonged cases, cirrhosis similar to that seen in congestive heart failure may occur.

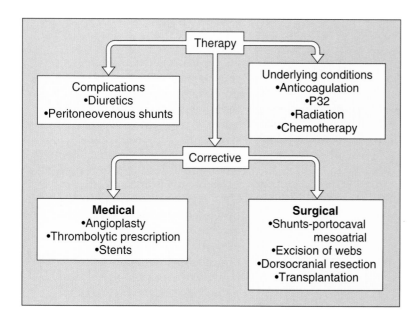

FIGURE 12-11.

Treatment modalities for patients with Budd-Chiari syndrome (BCS). The natural history of patients with BCS who are untreated is not known with certainty. Early reports suggested that the majority of affected individuals developed severe complications of liver disease or died within several months of diagnosis. More recent reports, however, suggest that the prognosis may not be as ominous, particularly in patients with BCS resulting from oral contraceptive use. Severity of symptoms most often demands treatment for relief of intractable ascites, pain, or to preserve hepatic function. Decisions regarding the type of treatment depend on duration of the symptoms, extent of hepatic fibrosis, and presence of underlying diseases. Despite the theoretical attractiveness of thrombolytic therapy, relatively few patients present early enough to benefit from this therapy. Routine anticoagulation with heparin, warfarin sodium, or both combined does not relieve acute obstruction but may be used as therapeutic adjunct following surgery.

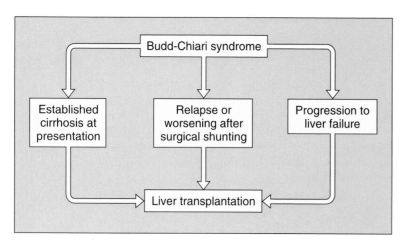

FIGURE 12-12.

Liver transplantation for Budd-Chiari syndrome. In those patients who have established cirrhosis at the time of presentation, liver transplantation is the most desirable therapeutic option. Liver transplantation can also be considered in patients who relapse or worsen following placement of mesoatrial or mesocaval shunts. In younger patients who may later require liver transplantation, mesocaval shunts are preferred over side-to-side portacaval shunts for technical reasons. If obstruction of the inferior vena cava is present, the anastomosis may be more difficult. Some investigators have argued that transplantation should be used more often as primary surgical treatment. The long-term success of transplantation for Budd-Chiari syndrome is uncertain. Most patients do not, however, experience a higher rate of thrombosis if maintained adequately anticoagulated.

ALTERNATIVES TO SURGERY

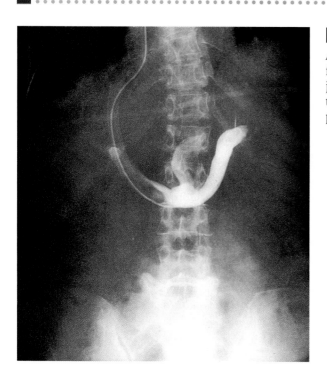

FIGURE 12-13.

A nonsurgical alternative is transjugular portosystemic shunt, which may be feasible in some patients. A radiographically placed shunt is placed through the jugular vein into the one of the hepatic veins and then creates a bridge between the hepatic vein and a branch of the portal vein. This produces a decrease in portal pressure and hepatic congestion. (*Courtesy of* K. R. Reddy, Miami, FL)

ISCHEMIC HEPATITIS

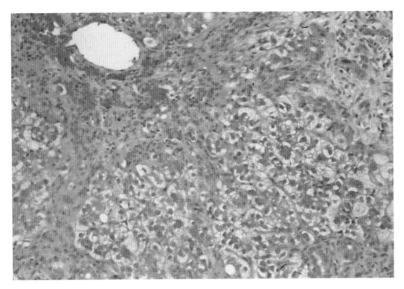

FIGURE 12-14.

Ischemic hepatitis. Transient decreases in arterial flow to the liver may result in ischemic necrosis of the centrilobular perivenular zone of the liver. In some patients, even a brief episode of hypotension is sufficient to cause ischemic injury. Patients with severe heart failure often develop ischemic hepatitis during episodes of ventricular tachycardia. The most common setting for ischemic hepatitis is following or during cardiac bypass. Those patients with preexisting elevation in right atrial pressures, such as is seen in patients with tricuspid regurgitation, appear to be at greatest risk for developing ischemic hepatitis.

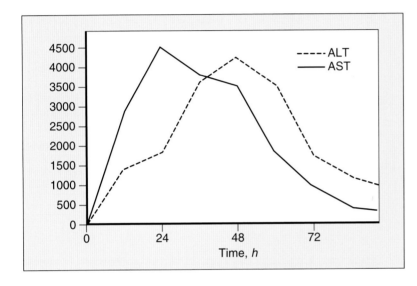

FIGURE 12-15.

Laboratory features of ischemic hepatitis. The most characteristic feature is extreme elevations of the aminotransferase levels. The enzymes usually rise within 12 to 24 hours after the ischemic episode and peak within 48 hours. Thereafter, the levels decline logarithmically. The decreases reflect clearance of the enzymes from the circulation, which is a first-order process. In the majority of instances, the level of aspartate aminotransferase (AST) is higher than the level of alanine aminotransferase (ALT) in the first 2 to 3 days but declines at a more rapid rate, as a result of differences in the serum half-lives of the two proteins.

HEPATIC VENOOCCLUSIVE DISEASE

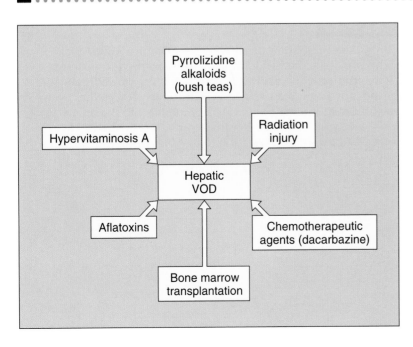

FIGURE 12-16.

Hepatic venoocclusive disease (VOD). Hepatic VOD was initially reported in association with consumption of herbal teas made from the leaves of *Crotalaria* and *Senecio* that contain pyrrolizidine alkaloids. Today chemotherapeutic and radiotherapeutic preoperative regimens for bone marrow transplantation are the most common causes. VOD may occur after autologous as well as allogeneic transplants. Risk factors for development of VOD are indicated in this figure.

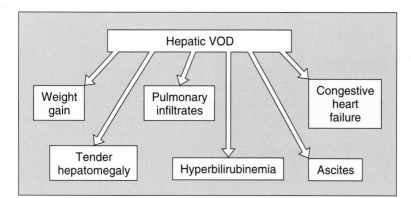

FIGURE 12-17.

Clinical manifestations of hepatic venoocclusive disease (VOD). The syndrome of VOD involves multiple organs including the liver. Typically, patients experience rapid weight gain, tender hepatomegaly, and early development of ascites. Pulmonary infiltrates and clinical signs of congestive heart failure are also observed in the most severe cases. Severe jaundice is a poor prognostic sign, although mild elevation of levels of bilirubin and alkaline phosphatase are common.

BILIARY CYSTS

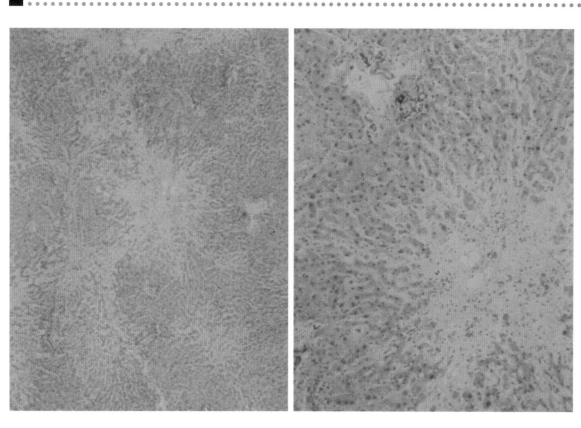

FIGURE 12-18.

Histologic manifestations of hepatic venoocclusive disease. In the early stages, endotheliitis associated with proliferative changes is present. Progressively, there is more fibrotic reaction in the endothelial space, eventually leading to obliteration of the terminal hepatic venules. The portal areas are spared. Sinusoids are dilated; often atrophy of hepatocytes in the surrounding perivenular zone exists. (*Courtesy of K. R. Reddy, Miami, FL*)

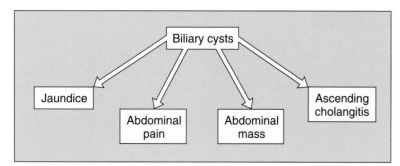

FIGURE 12-19.

Clinical manifestations of biliary cysts. Obstructive jaundice, abdominal pain, and abdominal masses are often considered classic features of biliary cysts. Many patients have recurrent episodes of ascending cholangitis, particularly if there has been previous instrumentation or injection of dye into the biliary tree without surgical drainage. For this reason, most patients are considered for surgical resection if possible.

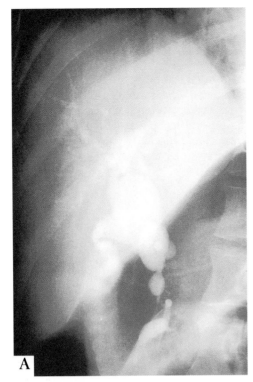

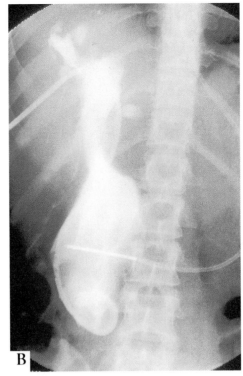

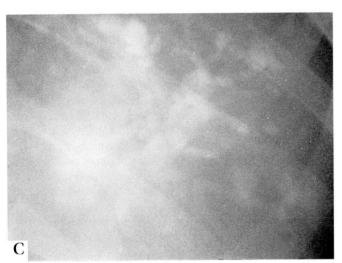

FIGURE 12-20.

Classification of biliary cysts and choledochoceles. Todani and coworkers [2] have classified biliary cysts into five types. Type I cysts are segmental dilatations of the common bile duct (choledochal cysts) (**A**). These are the most common variety. Type II are diverticula occurring anywhere along the extrahepatic bile ducts. Type III are choledochoceles occurring at the ampulla of Vater. These have been subclassified into A1, in which both the pancreatic and bile ducts join before opening into the cyst, A2 with distinct openings into the cyst, A3, in which the choledochocele is small and intramural, and B, in which the choledochocele is joined to the ampulla which opens separately into the duodenum. Type IV cysts are multiple cysts involving both intrahepatic and extrahepatic bile ducts (**B**). Type V (Caroli's disease) cysts are intrahepatic bile duct cysts (**C**).

■ INTRAHEPATIC CYSTS

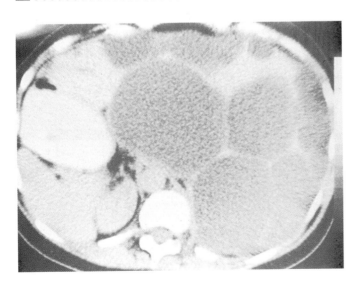

FIGURE 12-21.

Noncommunicating intrahepatic cysts (polycystic liver). Intrahepatic cysts that do not communicate directly with the biliary tree are much more common than biliary cysts. It is likely that the pathogenesis of these cysts differs from that of biliary cysts. Many investigators have speculated that these cysts are related to the failure of the development of Meyenburg's complexes leading to noncommunication with the biliary tree. Unlike biliary cysts, these cysts lack a true epithelial lining. They are lined by hepatocytes rather than columnar-type epithelium. Treatment by surgical resection is only necessary if the cyst produces symptoms.

HEPATIC CYSTS

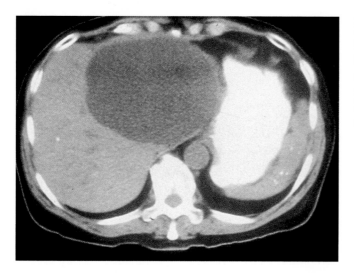

FIGURE 12-22.

Computed tomographic imaging of an hepatic cyst. Intrahepatic cysts are seen on computed tomographic scans as a low-attenuation space-filling lesion. The attenuation coefficient is usually similar to water and always lower than blood. They do not fill with administration of intravenous contrast dye.

HEMANGIOMAS

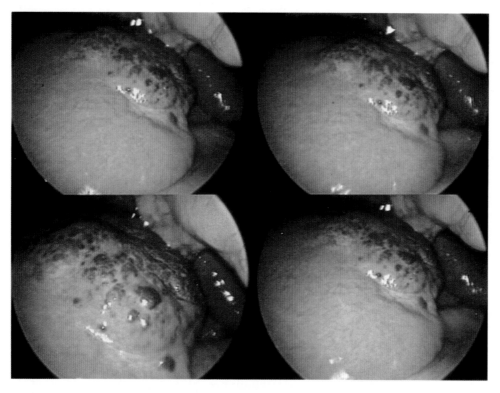

FIGURE 12-23.

Hepatic cavernous hemangioma. This tumor is the most common benign hepatic tumor, found in 3% to 5% of all autopsies. Hemangiomas are usually single and small, but may be multiple and large. The majority of patients are asymptomatic and have normal liver chemistries. Large lesions (larger than 4 cm) may cause symptoms such as a sensation of a mass and abdominal pain. (*Courtesy of* K. R. Reddy, Miami, FL)

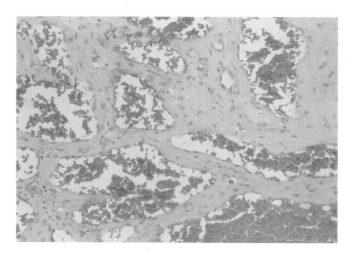

FIGURE 12-24.

Histologic characteristics of hepatic hemangiomas. The lesion is composed of endothelium-lined areas surrounded by fibrous stroma. Hemangiomas have no malignant potential. Histologic diagnosis is rarely necessary because the diagnosis can usually be made by its radiologic imaging appearance. (*Courtesy of* K. R. Reddy, Miami, FL)

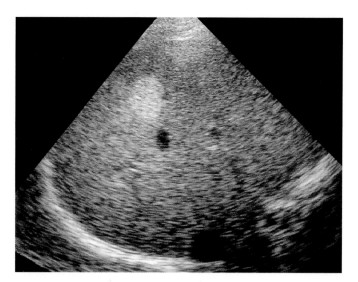

FIGURE 12-25.

FIGURE 12-25.

Ultrasound in the diagnosis of hepatic hemangiomas. On imaging with ultrasound, hemangiomas appear as single echogenic lesions with well-defined borders. Posterior acoustic enhancement is characteristic.

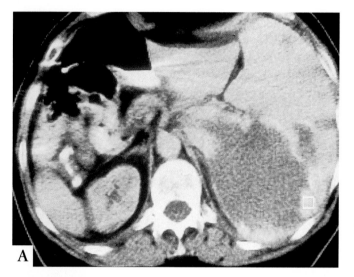
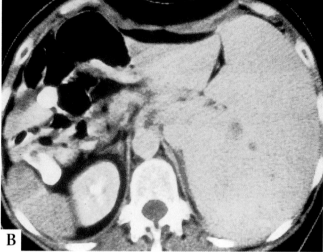

FIGURE 12-26.

Dynamic computed tomographic scanned hemangiomas typically show early peripheral opacification (**A**) and delayed central enhancement with sinusoidal pudding (**B**). These characteristics, however, may also be seen in primary and metastatic tumors, which can make the distinction between these lesions sometimes difficult by computed tomographic scan.

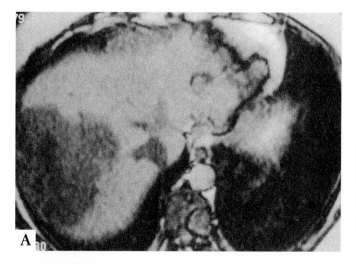
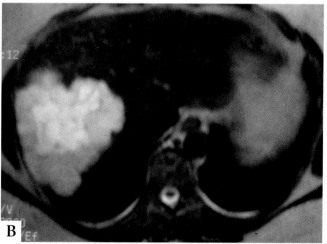

FIGURE 12-27.

Magnetic resonance imaging is very useful in characterizing hemangiomas, especially those measuring less than 5 cm. On magnetic resonance imaging, hemangiomas appear as well-circumscribed homogeneous lesions with low signal intensity in T_1-weighted images (**A**) and a characteristic high intensity in T_2-weighted images (**B**).

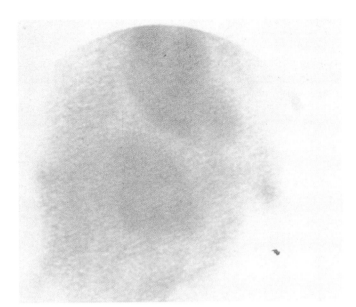

FIGURE 12-28.

Large hemangiomas may also be differentiated from other hepatic lesions by a ^{99}Technetium-labeled erythrocyte-pooled study. The labeled erythrocytes will characteristically fill the lesion from the periphery to the center, with prolonged retention of the isotope in the tumor. A *hot spot* representing a hemangioma is present. Uptake by the heart is also noted. (*Courtesy of* K. R. Reddy, Miami, FL)

■ HEPATOBILIARY CYSTADENOMAS

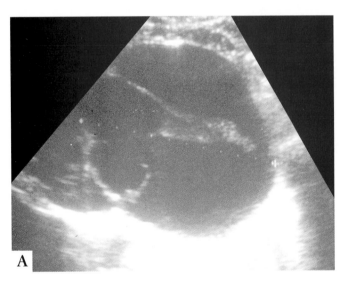

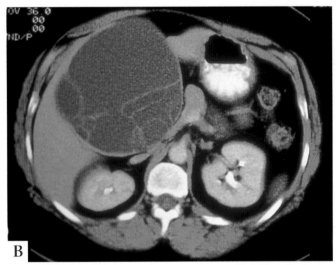

FIGURE 12-29.

Hepatobiliary cystadenomas almost always occur in middle-aged women. Abdominal pain is the most common presenting symptom. Cystadenomas may rupture, necrose, or calcify. They may undergo malignant transformation to papillary adenocarcinoma in 20% of patients, although these rarely metastasize. Both ultra-sound and computed tomography are useful tools in the diagnosis of these lesions. **Panels A** and **B** show the characteristic septation by ultrasound and computed tomographic scan, respectively, possessed by cystadenomas. These septations distinguish them from simple hepatic cysts.

AMEBIC ABSCESSES

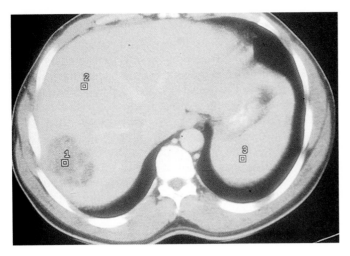

FIGURE 12-30.

Amebic abscesses are the most common type of liver abscesses worldwide. They are more frequently localized in the right lobe superoanteriorly, near the diaphragm. They are usually single, but may also be multiple and involve both lobes. Computed tomographic scan is very sensitive in the detection of amebic abscesses. It is also very useful in detecting extrahepatic involvement such as in the pleural space or lung. Amebic abscesses appear as a hypodense round or oval lesions with irregular borders. Approximately 20% of amebic abscesses may be superinfected by bacteria. Both ultrasound and computed tomographic scan may be used when drainage is indicated and as follow-up after institution of medical therapy.

PYOGENIC ABSCESSES

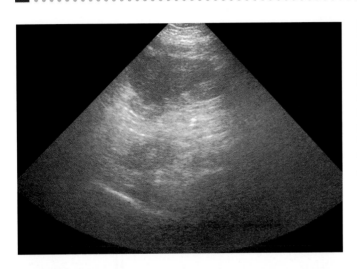

FIGURE 12-31.

Pyogenic abscesses are the most common type found in the United States. They may arise from biliary or hematogenous sources, may be single or multiple, and are more frequently found in the right lobe. The abscess cavities are variable in size and when multiple may coalesce to give a honeycomb appearance. By ultrasound they appear as round or oval hypoechoic lesions with a well-defined border and a variable number of internal echoes.

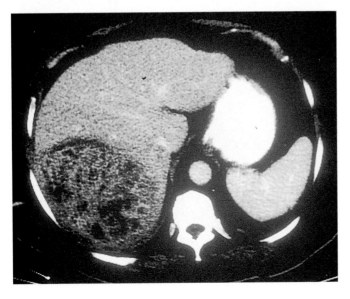

FIGURE 12-32.

Computed tomographic scan is highly sensitive in the localization of pyogenic liver abscesses. These lesions are hypodense areas that may sometimes show an air-fluid level indicating a gas-producing organism. Both computed tomography and ultrasound may be used in the aspiration of pyogenic abscesses, which can be done for both diagnostic and therapeutic purposes.

■ ECHINOCOCCUS GRANULOSIS

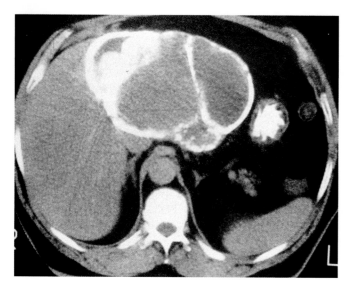

FIGURE 12-33.

Echinococcal or hydatid cysts arise from the infestation with the larval stage or cysts of the cestode *Echinococcus granulosis*. Man acts as an intermediate host. The larva of this tapeworm penetrates the intestinal wall, reaching the liver through the portal system. They are more common in the right lobe. Presenting symptoms include low-grade fever, tender hepatomegaly, and eosinophilia. The cysts may rupture into the pleural space or abdomen, and sometimes may produce a severe anaphylactic reaction. Segmentation of the innermost, or granular, layer of the cyst gives rise to daughter cysts. Calcification of the wall of the cyst is common. Hydatid cysts may be treated surgically with complete resection being the therapeutic goal. Puncture of the cyst for either diagnostic or therapeutic purposes is contraindicated. (*Courtesy of* K. R. Reddy, Miami, FL)

■ REFERENCES AND RECOMMENDED READING

1. Rappaport AR, Wanless JR: *Diseases of the Liver*, edn 7. Edited by Schiff, Schiff. Philadelphia: JB Lippincott; 1993.

2. Todani T, Watanabe Y, Narvse M, *et al.*: Congenital bile duct cysts: Classification, operative procedures, and review of thirty-seven cases including cancer arising from choledochal cysts. *Am J Surg* 1977, 134:263–269.

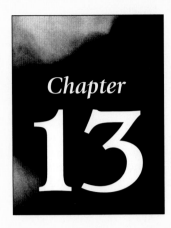

Chapter 13

Tumors of the Liver

Tumors of the liver may be classified as benign or malignant, adult or pediatric, or more relevant clinically as tumors with and without cirrhosis. In adults, malignant tumors are more common than benign tumors, and among the malignant tumors, metastases to the liver are most frequently encountered, particularly in the developed western world. The diagnosis of tumors of the liver relies largely on imaging studies and histopathology. Imaging studies confirm the presence of a neoplasm, indicate its location, and give some idea of its extent. In addition, typical and sometimes diagnostic features may be noted on imaging studies. However, making a specific diagnosis often requires obtaining liver tissue for histopathologic analysis. Liver tissue may be obtained by needle biopsy (guided by ultrasound or computed tomography in some cases) or at the time of resection. This chapter concentrates on those tumors most likely to be encountered rather than reviewing all tumors of the liver.

ADRIAN M. DI BISCEGLIE
PETER C. BUETOW

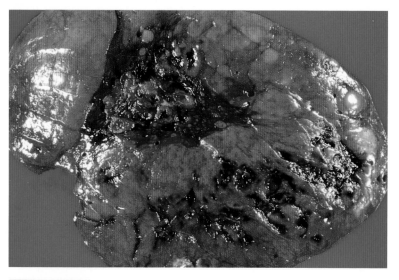

FIGURE 13-1.

Cut surface of a large hepatocellular adenoma. Hepatocellular adenoma is a benign neoplastic condition of hepatocytes. Although relatively rare, its incidence seems to have increased over the past few decades since the introduction and widespread use of oral contraceptives (incidence 3 to 4/100,000 long-term oral contraceptive users) [1].

It has also been associated with the use of anabolic steroids and is a complication of some types of glycogen storage disease. This tumor occurs almost exclusively in adult women. Most female patients with adenoma have a history of oral contraceptive use, either current or remote. The duration of oral contraceptive use in such patients is variable and may even have been as short as 1 to 2 years.

The most common presenting symptom is right upper quadrant abdominal pain or discomfort. The most feared complication of hepatocellular adenoma is free intra-abdominal rupture related to hemorrhage and necrosis within the tumor. This complication may be life threatening and requires urgent resuscitation and surgery. Liver biopsy is almost always required for confirmation of the diagnosis of adenoma. If this diagnosis is suspected in advance, biopsy may be best done at the time of surgical resection.

The histologic appearance of hepatocellular adenoma is of benign-looking hepatocytes often arranged in cords. Evidence of bile production may be noted. Surgical resection is usually recommended because of the risks of rupture. Possible exceptions to this recommendation are very small adenomata or in those where the patient is not fit for surgery. Shrinkage of these tumors has been noted in some cases with discontinuation of oral contraceptive use; although this maneuver may be attempted in some cases, it should not replace the need for resection in most instances. (*From* Di Bisceglie [2]; with permission.)

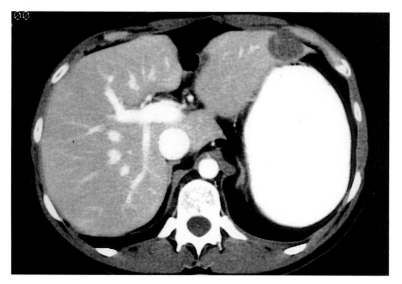

FIGURE 13-2.

Small hepatocellular adenoma in left lobe of the liver. Occasionally, adenomata may be found incidentally when an imaging procedure is done for some other reason. Such incidental tumors tend to be much smaller.

BENIGN TUMOR-LIKE LESIONS OF THE LIVER

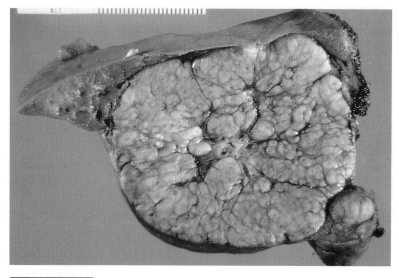

FIGURE 13-3.

A heterogenous group of lesions occurring in the liver may give a neoplastic appearance. Some of them may also cause diagnostic confusion with cirrhosis. This figure shows the cut surface of a focal nodular hyperplasia (FNH), approximately 5 to 6 cm in diameter.

Note the cirrhosis-like appearance (pseudocirrhosis) around a central area of fibrous tissue. This lesion represents a focal benign proliferation of hepatocytes occurring around an abnormal artery within the liver [3]. These lesions rarely cause symptoms and are most often found incidentally at the time of abdominal surgery (often at cholecystectomy). They are usually smaller than 5 cm in diameter. The cut surface typically shows a central stellate scar that contains the abnormal artery within it. As with hepatocellular adenoma, features of bile production and cholestasis may be seen both macroscopically and microscopically. The presence of central scar tissue may sometimes give the appearance of cirrhosis with regenerating nodules surrounded by fibrosis. This lesion is localized, however, rather than being throughout the liver and no bile ducts are seen within the lesions, whereas they would be present in most cases of cirrhosis. Interpretation of needle biopsy specimens obtained from FNH may be particularly difficult. Usually no treatment is required because these lesions rarely cause symptoms and are not prone to rupture or malignant transformation. In fact, they are very often removed at the time of excision biopsy. The differential diagnosis includes nodular regenerative hyperplasia, which is a diffuse nodular condition of the liver with no significant fibrosis and partial nodular transformation, a rare nodular condition usually confined to the hilar area of the liver.

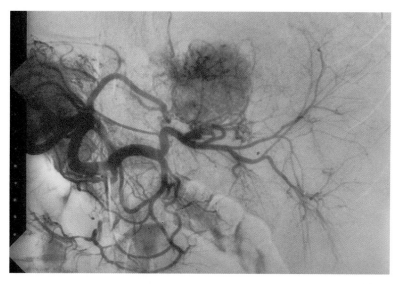

FIGURE 13-4.

Hepatic arteriogram from the same patient with focal nodular hyperplasia shown in Figure 13-3. Note the presence of hypervascularity with a single prominent artery in the center of the tumor.

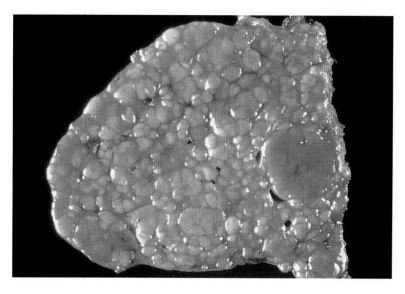

FIGURE 13-5.

Macroscopic appearance of a liver specimen at autopsy showing presence of cirrhotic nodules with one large dominant nodule representing an area of adenomatous hyperplasia approximately 2 cm in diameter. This condition occurs in the presence of established cirrhosis and appears to be related to excessive or uncontrolled proliferation of hepatocytes within regenerating nodules. Generally, areas of adenomatous hyperplasia are greater than 1 cm in diameter [4]. This lesion is of significance because it may cause diagnostic confusion by giving the appearance of a mass in the liver in a patient with cirrhosis, prompting an evaluation to exclude hepatocellular carcinoma (HCC). This diagnostic confusion is made more troublesome by the recent observation that areas of atypia may develop within the large nodules, and it has been suggested that these lesions are precursors for the development of HCC [5]. (*Courtesy of* M. Kojiro, Kurume, Japan)

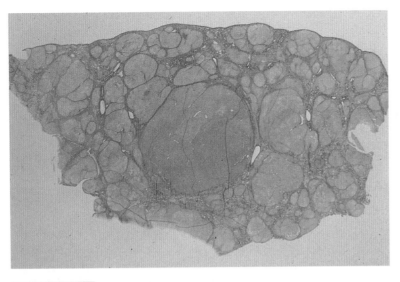

Low-power photomicrograph of a liver specimen stained for reticulin showing, against a background of smaller cirrhotic nodules, a cluster of three areas of adenomatous hyperplasia. (*Courtesy of* M. Kojiro, Kurume, Japan)

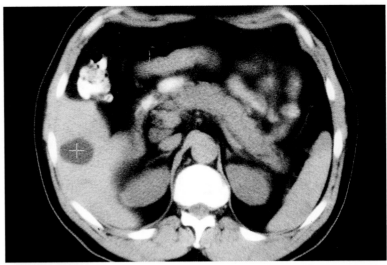

FIGURE 13-7.

Computed tomographic scan of the abdomen showing a single, fluid-filled lesion within the liver. This lesion had been observed over a period of several years, had not changed in size, and was therefore presumed to represent a benign simple cyst of the liver. Other benign cystic lesions of the liver include polycystic disease, choledochal cysts, and hydatid disease [6].

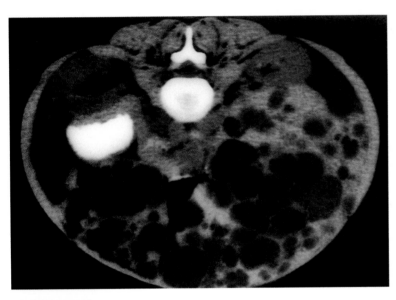

FIGURE 13-8.

Computed tomographic scan of the abdomen showing massive hepatomegaly related to multiple cysts of varying diameter, some as large as 4 to 5 cm. Interestingly, no cysts can be seen in the kidney.

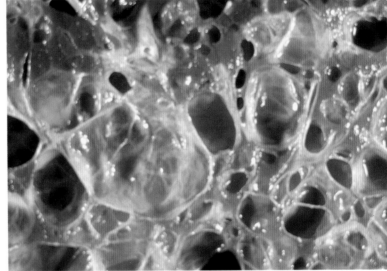

FIGURE 13-9.

Macroscopic appearance of polycystic disease of the liver from the same patient shown in Figure 13-8. Note the presence of innumerable cysts, some filled with clear fluid. Small amounts of normal hepatic parenchyma are noted between cysts. Adult polycystic disease is an autosomally dominant inherited disease associated with multiple cysts within the liver, pancreas, and spleen. Hepatic cysts are sometimes associated with abdominal discomfort. Rarely, they may be complicated by infection [7]. Hepatocellular function is rarely compromised. No specific treatment is available. Liver transplantation has occasionally been performed for polycystic disease because of the patient's intolerable abdominal discomfort.

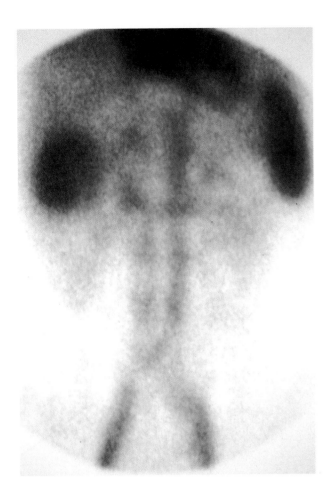

FIGURE 13-10.

Tagged erythrocyte study in a patient with a single large hemangioma in the right lobe of the liver. This scan was taken approximately 1 hour after injection of tagged erythrocytes. Note the rounded area of blackness within the liver related to the hemangioma. Tracer can also be seen within the heart, spleen, and major blood vessels.

Hemangiomata are the most common neoplasms of the liver, being found in up to 10% of individuals. In almost all cases, they are asymptomatic. They are usually single and smaller than 5 cm in diameter. Occasional, multiple hemangiomata may be found; and if very large, they may be associated with hyperdynamic circulation because of the large arteriovenous communications represented by the hemangiomata. Disseminated intravascular coagulation with thrombocytopenia may rarely occur with massive hemangiomata (Kasabach-Merritt syndrome). Hemangiomata may grow slowly but have little or no malignant potential [8]. Needle biopsy should be avoided because of the risk of intra-abdominal bleeding.

Hemangioma of the liver may be detected by several imaging modalities including ultrasound, computed tomographic scan, and radioisotope scan. Some imaging techniques take advantage of the characteristic slow flow of blood through hemangiomata to make the diagnosis with some certainty. These techniques include tagged erythrocyte scan, in which the patient's own erythrocytes are tagged with a radioisotope and injected back into the patient. The area over the liver is then scanned periodically for up to several hours. Characteristically, hemangioma will be associated with slow uptake and clearance of tagged erythrocytes.

The technique of dynamic sequential computed tomographic scanning is also useful for the diagnosis of hemangioma. In this procedure, water-soluble contrast material is infused constantly intravenously and the area of interest within the liver is scanned repeatedly at intervals of 30 to 60 seconds. Contrast enhancement of hemangioma can be seen progressively over time from the periphery of the lesion towards the center over a period of between 15 and 20 minutes.

■ MALIGNANT TUMORS OF THE LIVER

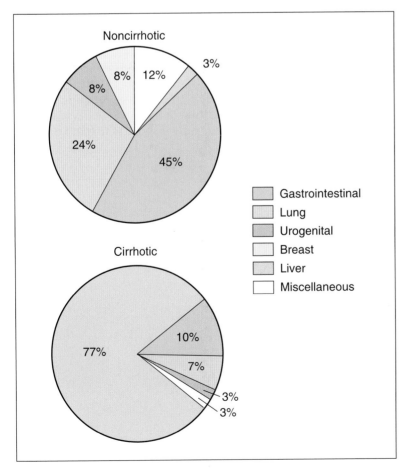

Noncirrhotic

Cirrhotic

Gastrointestinal
Lung
Urogenital
Breast
Liver
Miscellaneous

FIGURE 13-11.

The relative frequency of various tumors of the liver. Note that metastases are by far the most frequent, particularly in the developed western world. Among the primary malignant tumors, hepatocellular carcinoma is the most frequent.

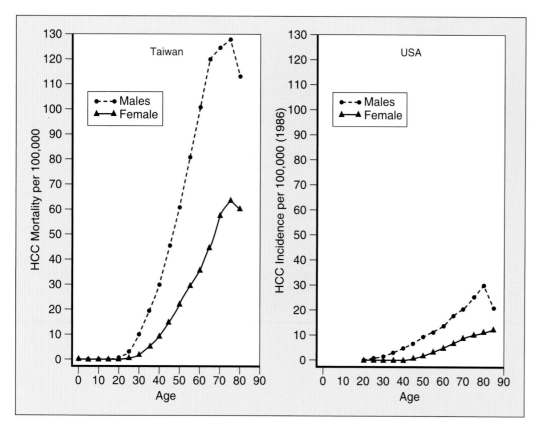

FIGURE 13-12.

Age-specific incidence of hepatocellular carcinoma (HCC) in Taiwan and the United States. HCC is one of the most common malignant tumors worldwide. It occurs most commonly in the Far East and in sub-Saharan Africa where it accounts for the greatest number of cancer deaths. In the United States, the incidence is generally much lower and the mean age at presentation is higher [9].

Hepatocellular carcinoma occurs against the background of cirrhosis. The underlying liver disease is most often caused by viral hepatitis or by alcohol, although the exact form of liver injury may vary in different areas. Thus, in countries such as China, Taiwan, Hong Kong, North and South Korea, and Vietnam and in sub-Saharan Africa, most cases are related to chronic infection with hepatitis B virus whereas in southern Europe and Japan, hepatitis C is more of a problem [10,11]. In the United States, both of these forms of hepatitis are related to HCC as well as to alcoholic cirrhosis. (*Adapted from* Beasley [12]; with permission.)

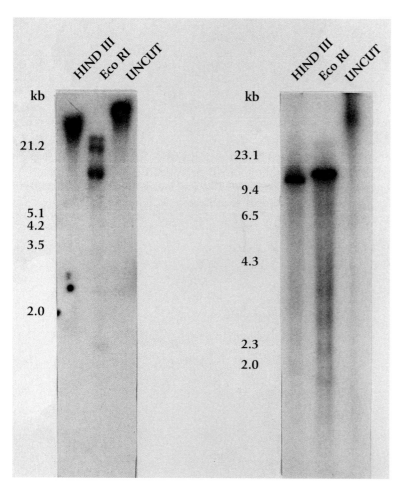

FIGURE 13-13.

Southern blot analysis of hepatitis B virus (HBV) DNA from tumor tissue taken from two patients with hepatocellular carcinoma (HCC). DNA was extracted from tumor tissue, electrophoresed in agarose after digestion with restriction enzymes (Eco 1, Hind III, UNCUT) hybridized to a radioactive HBV DNA probe, and subjected to autoradiography. In both cases, the presence of integrated viral DNA can be found as a dark band greater than 3.2 kb in size. It is thought that such viral integration may be an important factor in the pathogenesis of HCC [9]. Other evidence linking HBV infection to the development of HCC include the finding of hepatitis B surface antigen (HBsAg) in the large majority of patients with HCC in certain geographic areas. Patients with chronic HBV infection are much more likely to develop HCC on follow-up than control subjects that are negative for HBsAg.

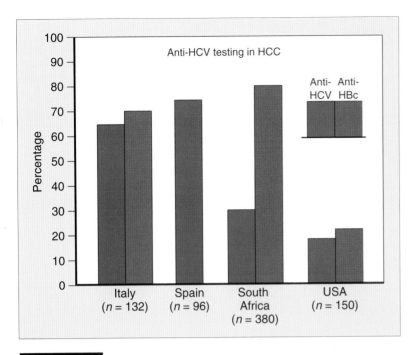

FIGURE 13-14.

Relative contributions of hepatitis B virus (HBV) and hepatitis C virus (HCV) to pathogenesis of hepatocellular carcinoma (HCC). It has only relatively recently become recognized that chronic infection with HCV plays a major role in the development of HCC in some areas. Thus, in southern Europe, nearly three-quarters of patients with HCC have antibodies to HCV (Anti-HCV) in serum. In sub-Saharan Africa and China, where HBV infection is more prevalent, HCV–related HCC is less common [13]. Most patients with HCC and Anti-HCV in serum also have HCV RNA present in serum, liver, and sometimes, even within tumor tissue. The development of HCC has been observed in patients with chronic HCV followed over time. Typically, this development occurs over intervals of more than 20 years, but it may occasionally happen in less time [11,13–17]. Anti-HBc—antibodies to hepatitis B core antigen.

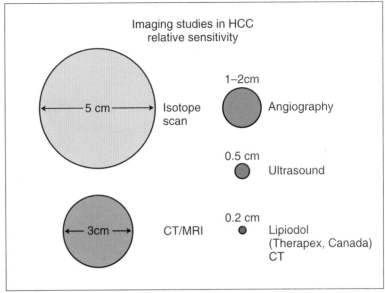

FIGURE 13-15.

Relative sensitivity of various imaging modalities in diagnosis of hepatocellular cancer (HCC). Some of the typical clinical features of HCC include abdominal swelling, right upper quadrant pain, weight loss, and apparent worsening of liver disease in patients known to have cirrhosis. This tumor only becomes clinically apparent, however, when it is far advanced. When patients present with these symptoms they usually have extensive tumor involvement within the liver as well as distant metastases. The use of radiologic imaging studies has allowed detection of HCC at an earlier stage, often before the development of symptoms. CT—computed tomography; MRI—magnetic resonance imaging. (*From* Di Bisceglie [2]; with permission.)

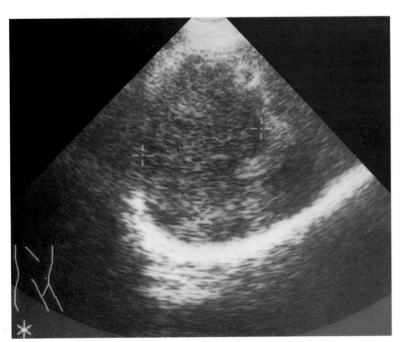

FIGURE 13-16.

Ultrasound examination of the liver showing a 5 × 10 cm hypoechoic mass (between markers). Ultrasound is one of the most sensitive methods for detecting tumors within the liver and is also relatively inexpensive and noninvasive [18]. Hepatocellular carcinoma often has echogenicity different from that in the remainder of the liver. Thus, small tumors are often hyperechoic with a thin hypoechoic rim. With time, and as the tumor grows, the whole tumor often becomes hypoechoic, and finally, when the tumor is large, it often has mixed echogenicity.

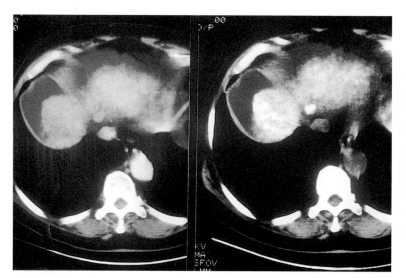

FIGURE 13-17.

Contrast-enhanced computed tomographic (CT) scan of the liver in a patient with hepatocellular carcinoma (HCC). *Left panel* shows a small, shrunken, irregular liver with no obvious tumor masses. *Right panel* shows CT scan repeated in the same subject 2 weeks after intra-arterial infusion of Lipiodol (Therapex, Canada). At that point, a small HCC can be seen in the posterior aspect of the right lobe because it continues to contain Lipiodol. CT scanning is relatively sensitive and, when combined with prior infusion of Lipiodol, is an extremely sensitive method of detecting HCC. The oily contrast medium Lipiodol, which is also used for lymphangiograms, appears to be selectively retained within HCC tissue for several weeks. Thus, if CT scan is done 2 to 3 weeks after intra-arterial infusion of Lipiodol, very small tumors may sometimes be viewed [19].

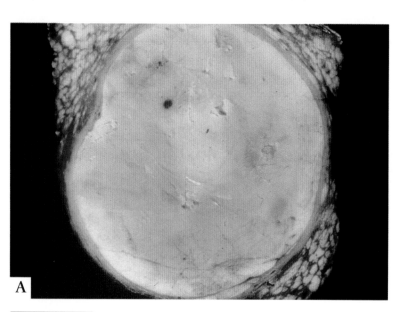

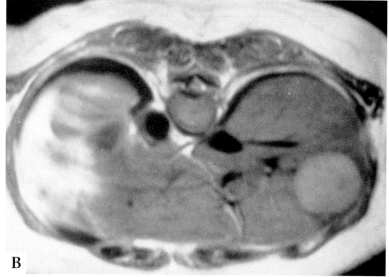

FIGURE 13-18.

A and B, A small resected hepatocellular carcinoma (HCC) and the corresponding magnetic resonance imaging (MRI) scan from a patient with hepatitis C–related cirrhosis and HCC. The role of MRI in diagnosing HCC remains uncertain. However, in some cases, these tumors may be readily detected by MRI. (*Courtesy of* T.G. Brewer, Washington, D.C.)

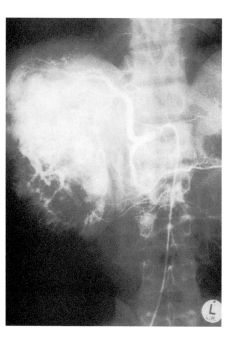

FIGURE 13-19.

Massive involvement of the right lobe of the liver by hepatocellular carcinoma (HCC) extensive tumor "blushing". Arteriography is a relatively invasive means of imaging tumors of the liver but is very useful in showing vascular tumors such as HCC. A catheter is passed, using the Seldinger technique, into the hepatic artery before infusion of the contrast medium. This procedure is often done before surgery to evaluate the full extent of the tumor and to study its vascular supply in order to better plan surgery [20].

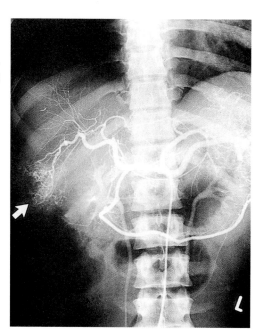

FIGURE 13-20.

A smaller hepatocellular carcinoma (*arrow*) that is marked by a small area of neovascularization on hepatic arteriography. Here the arteriogram may be useful in planning surgical resection.

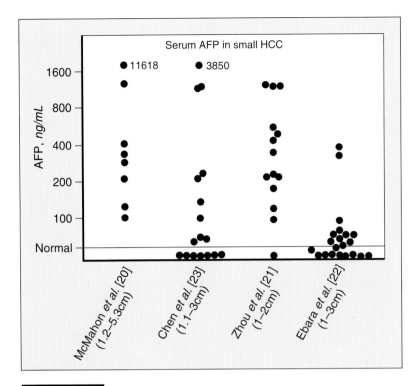

FIGURE 13-21.

Serum α-fetoprotein (AFP) levels among patients with small hepatocellular carcinoma (HCC) [21–26]. Serologic tumor markers are a valuable aid in the diagnosis of HCC. AFP is a glycoprotein normally found in fetal serum that disappears soon after birth. It may become detectable again in association with several diseases of the liver and other organs but is particularly useful in the diagnosis of HCC. Among patients with large HCC, AFP values in serum may be elevated in as many as 80% of cases, often to very high levels. However, in patients with small tumors, levels are less likely to be elevated, and they are often not even markedly elevated. Unfortunately, similarly elevated values may be seen in association with cirrhosis and active hepatitis, and this elevation may lead to diagnostic confusion.

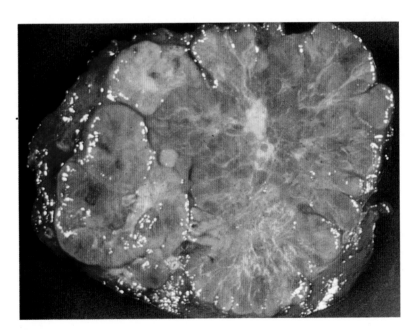

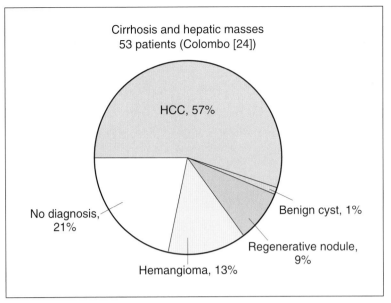

FIGURE 13-22.

Differential diagnosis of a mass found within the liver among cirrhotic patients [26]. Because of the poor prognosis for hepatocellular carcinoma (HCC) and the recognition that this tumor occurs against a background of chronic viral hepatitis and liver disease, attempts have been made to screen for the tumor in asymptomatic patients. In this way, small tumors may be found that are more amenable to therapy. Unfortunately, the presence of a mass within the liver of a patient with cirrhosis is not necessarily synonymous with HCC. This figure indicates that whereas most such masses turn out to be HCC, they may also represent cysts, angiomata, and regenerative nodules. In some cases, no obvious pathology can be found. The significance of regenerative nodules is uncertain, but it seems that the larger ones (greater than 1 cm, macroregenerative nodules) may sometimes lead to the development of HCC. (*Adapted from* Columbo *et al.* [27]; with permission.)

FIGURE 13-23.

Characteristic fibrotic lamellae coursing throughout a fibrolamellar hepatocellular carcinoma (HCC). This tumor is a variant with distinct morphologic features and is also associated with a better prognosis than other forms of HCC [26]. Thus, the surrounding nontumorous liver is usually not cirrhotic. (*Courtesy of* Z. Goodman, Washington, D.C.)

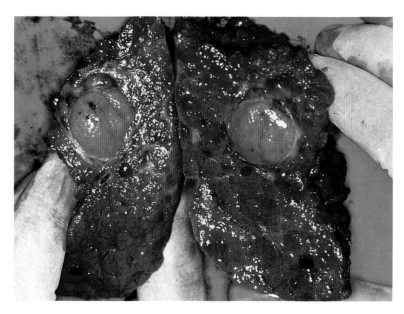

FIGURE 13-24.

Resected specimen of cirrhotic liver with a small (2.5 cm diameter) hepatocellular carcinoma (HCC). Therapy of HCC is difficult and

the prognosis is poor. The best chance of cure or long-term survival appears to be with resection. Because of the associated cirrhosis, extensive resection is usually not possible and the usual operation is a "segmentectomy" or enucleation of the tumor. Even so, a high rate of tumor recurrence exists within the first few years after surgery. Recently there have been some interest in liver transplantation for HCC that is confined to the liver, but is not otherwise resectable [29]. Again, there is a high rate of recurrence and attempts to prevent this complication have used adjuvant chemotherapy before and after transplantation. The value of this approach is currently being evaluated.

Other approaches that may be used for small tumors include ablation by injection with absolute alcohol or cryoablation. For large unresectable tumors, chemoembolization has been used in an attempt to shrink the tumor. The rationale for this approach is based on the fact that whereas the liver as a whole has a dual blood supply (from the hepatic artery and portal vein), HCC derives its supply exclusively from the hepatic artery. Thus, when this blood supply is cut off, tumor necrosis and shrinking can be seen. The use of systemic chemotherapy and external radiation appear to be of little benefit in HCC. Chemotherapy directed to the tumor by intra-arterial infusion of targeting with Lipiodol (Therapex, Canada) may be more helpful. (*From* Di Bisceglie [2]; with permission.)

Cholangiocarcinoma

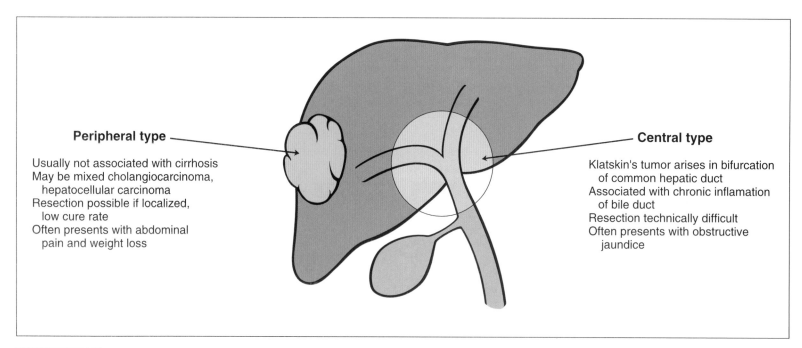

Peripheral type

Usually not associated with cirrhosis
May be mixed cholangiocarcinoma, hepatocellular carcinoma
Resection possible if localized, low cure rate
Often presents with abdominal pain and weight loss

Central type

Klatskin's tumor arises in bifurcation of common hepatic duct
Associated with chronic inflamation of bile duct
Resection technically difficult
Often presents with obstructive jaundice

FIGURE 13-25.

A comparison of the features of central and peripheral type of cholangiocarcinoma [30,31]. It is the next most common form of hepatic malignancy after HCC and does not usually occur against a background of cirrhosis but, rather, in patients who have long-standing inflammation and injury to the biliary system. Predisposing factors include sclerosing cholangitis [32], intrahepatic calculi, congenital anomalies such as Caroli's disease, and infestation with the liver fluke *Clonorchis sinensis*.

Clinical and presenting features of cholangiocarcinoma vary, depending on the location of the tumor. Thus, tumors that are located within the periphery of the liver (peripheral type) often grow to quite large dimensions before presenting with symptoms such as pain and weight loss. However, tumors that originate within the larger bile ducts (central type) often result in biliary obstruction and jaundice at a much earlier stage.

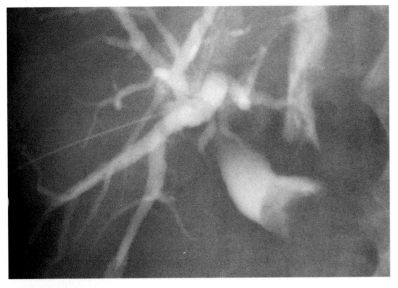

FIGURE 13-26.

Endoscopic retrograde cholangiopancreatography (ERCP) scan from a patient with long-standing primary sclerosing cholangitis (PSC) and cholangiocarcinoma. Note the convex upwards obstruction at the lower end of the common bile duct and the changes of PSC in the peripheral branches of the biliary tree. Such tumors may be very difficult to detect. Their presence may be signaled by sudden worsening in jaundice in a patient with PSC or may be found incidentally at the time of diagnostic ERCP or liver transplantation for PSC.

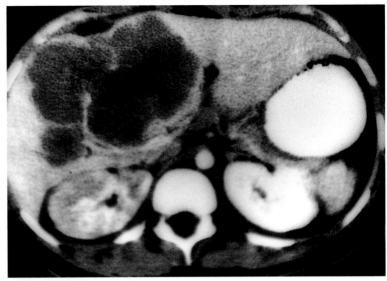

FIGURE 13-27.

Computed tomographic scan of liver of peripheral type cholangiocarcinoma. Note the large hypodense mass occupying most of the right lobe of the liver.

■ PEDIATRIC LIVER TUMORS

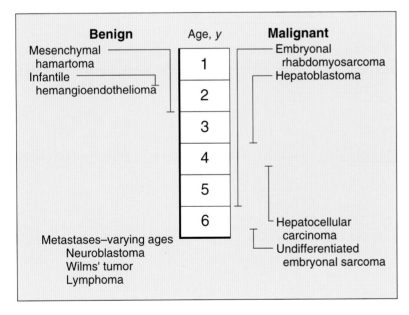

FIGURE 13-28.

The spectrum of tumors occurring in the liver in children is significantly different from those in adults [33]. Whereas hepatocellular carcinoma has been reported to occur in children as young as 2 years, its incidence rises from the age of 4. Hepatoblastoma rarely occurs in children over 3 years of age and certain other primary hepatic tumors are confined to the pediatric years.

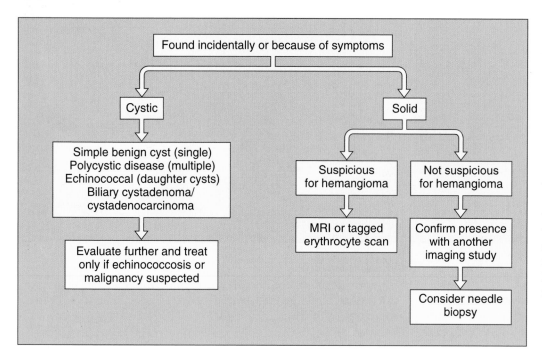

FIGURE 13-29.

Algorithm for evaluation of patients found to have a mass in noncirrhotic liver. The most likely etiology varies depending on whether the masses are found incidentally or if the patient presents with some symptoms referable to the liver. Thus cysts of the liver and hemangiomata are often found incidentally at the time of imaging studies for some other purpose, whereas patients with right upper quadrant pain or discomfort are more likely to have hepatic metastases, hepatocellular adenoma, or some unusual primary malignancy of the liver such as fibrolamellar hepatocellular carcinoma, angiosarcoma, or epithelioid hemangioendothelioma. MRI—magnetic resonance imaging.

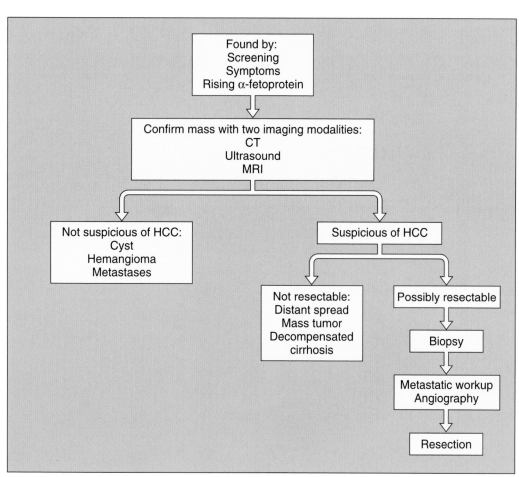

FIGURE 13-30.

An algorithm for evaluating masses in patients known to have cirrhosis where the possibility of hepatocellular carcinoma (HCC) is very much higher. The approach involves confirming the presence of the mass by using at least two imaging modalities which gives some idea of the extent of the tumor and also some preliminary idea of whether it is resectable or not. Definitive therapy usually requires a biopsy of the lesion—this may be done under direction by ultrasound or computed tomography (CT) or at the time of exploratory surgery. MRI—magnetic resonance imaging.

REFERENCES AND RECOMMENDED READING

1. Kerlin P, Davis GL, McGill DB, *et al.*: Hepatic adenoma and focal nodular hyperplasia: Clinical, pathologic, and radiologic features. *Gastroenterology* 1983, 84:994–1002.

2. DiBisceglie AM: Tumors of the liver. In *Current Practice of Medicine*. Edited by Bone R. Philadelphia: Current Medicine; in press.

3. Stromeyer FW, Ishak KG: Nodular transformation (nodular "regenerative" hyperplasia) of the liver. *Hum Pathol* 1981, 12:60–71.

4. Furuya K, Nakamura M, Yamamoto Y, *et al.*: Macroregenerative nodule of the liver. *Cancer* 1988, 61:99–105.

5. Theise ND, Schwartz M, Miller C, Thung SN: Macroregenerative nodules and hepatocellular carcinoma in forty-four sequential adult liver explants with cirrhosis. *Hepatology* 1992, 16:949–955.

6. Harris KM, Morris DL, Tudor R, *et al.*: Clinical and radiologic features of simple and hydatid cysts of the liver. *Br J Surg* 1986, 73:835–838.

7. Telenti A, Torres VE, Gross JB, *et al.*: Hepatic cyst infection in autosomal dominant polycystic kidney disease. *Mayo Clin Proc* 1990, 65:933–942.

8. Trastek VF, Van Heerden JA, Sheedy PF, Adson MA: Cavernous hemangioma of the liver: Resect to observe? *Am J Surg* 1983, 145:153.

9. DiBisceglie AM, Rustgi VK, Hoofnagle JH, *et al.*: Hepatocellular carcinoma. *Ann Intern Med* 1988, 108:390–401.

10. Nishioka K, Watanabe J, Furuta S, *et al.*: A high prevalence of antibody to the hepatic C virus in patients with hepatocellular carcinoma in Japan. *Cancer* 1991, 67:429–433.

11. Bruix J, Barrera JM, Calvet X, *et al.*: Prevalence of antibodies to hepatitis C virus in Spanish patients with hepatocellular carcinoma and hepatic cirrhosis. *Lancet* 1989, 2:1004–1006.

12. Beasley RP: Hepatitis B virus as the etiologic agent in hepatocellular carcinoma: Epidemiologic considerations. *Hepatology* 1982, 2:21S–26S.

13. Bukh J, Miller RH, Kew MC, Purcell RH: Hepatitis C virus RNA in southern African blacks with hepatocellular carcinoma. *Proc Natl Acad Sci U S A* 1993, 90:1848–1851.

14. Colombo M, Kuo G, Choo Q-L, *et al.*: Prevalence of antibodies to hepatitis C virus in Italian patients with hepatocellular carcinoma. *Lancet* 1989, 2:1006–1008.

15. Kew MC, Houghton M, Choo Q-L, Kuo G: Hepatitis C virus antibodies in southern African blacks with hepatocellular carcinoma. *Lancet* 1990, 335:873–884.

16. Yu MC, Tong MJ, Coursaget P, *et al.*: Prevalence of hepatitis B and C viral markers in black and white patients with hepatocellular carcinoma in the United States. *J Natl Cancer Inst* 1990, 82: 1038–1041.

17. DiBisceglie AM, Order SE, Klein JL, *et al.*: The role of chronic viral hepatitis in hepatocellular carcinoma in teh United States. *Am J Gastroenterol* 1991, 86:335–338.

18. Kobayashi K, Sugimoto T, Makino H, *et al.*: Screening methods for early detection of hepatocellular carcinoma. *Hepatology* 1985, 5:1100–1105.

19. Kuroda C, Sakurai M, Monden M, *et al.*: Limitation of transcatheter arterial embolization using iodized oil for small hepatocellular carcinoma. *Cancer* 1991, 67:81–86.

20. Okuda K: Radiologic imaging of hepatocellular carcinoma in Japan. In *Etiology, Pathology and Treatment of Hepatocellular Carcinoma in North America*. Edited by Tabor E, DiBisceglie AM, Purcell RM. Houston: Portfolio; 1991:273–286.

21. Chen D-S, Sung J-L, Sheu J-C, *et al.*: Serum alpha-fetoprotein in the early stage of human hepatocellular carcinoma. *Gastroenterology* 1984, 86:1404–1409.

22. McMahon BJ, Lanier AP, Wainwright RB, Kilkenny SJ: Hepatocellular carcinoma in Alaska Eskimos: Epidemiology, clinical features, and early detection. In *Progress in Liver Disease*, vol IX. Edited by Popper H, Schaffner F. Philadelphia: WB Saunders; 1990:643–656.

23. Zhou X-D, Tang Z-Y, Yu Y-Q, *et al.*: Solitary minute hepatocellular carcinoma. *Cancer* 1991, 67: 2855–2858.

24. Ebara M, Ohto M, Shinagawa T, *et al.*: Natural history of minute hepatocellular carcinoma smaller than three centimeters complicating cirrhosis. *Gastroenterology* 1986, 90: 289–298.

25. Chen D-S, Sung J-L, Shen J-C: Serum alpha-fetoprotein in the early stage of human hepatocellular carcinoma. *Gastroenterology* 1984, 86:1404–1409.

26. Colombo M, de Franchis R, Del Ninno E, *et al.*: Primary hepatocellular carcinoma. *N Engl J Med* 1991, 325:729–731.

27. Columbo M, de Franchis R, Del Ninno E, *et al.*: Hepatocellular carcinoma in Italian patients with cirrhosis. *N Engl J Med* 1991, 325:675–680.

28. Craig JR, Peters RL, Edmundson HA, Omata M: Fibrolamellar carcinoma of the liver. A tumor of adolescents and young adults with distinctive clinicopathologic features. *Cancer* 1980, 46:372–379.

29. Altaee MY, Johnson PJ, Farrant JM, Williams R: Etiologic and clinical characteristics of peripheral and hilar cholangiocarcinoma. *Cancer* 1991, 68:2051–2055.

30. Stone MJ, Klintmalm GBG, Polter D, *et al.*: Neoadjuvant chemotherapy and liver transplantation for hepatocellular carcinoma: A pilot study in 20 patients. *Gastroenterology* 1993, 104:196–200.

31. Bosma A: Surgical pathology of cholangiocarcinoma of the liver hilus (Klatskin tumor). *Semin Liver Dis* 1990, 10:85–90.

32. Rosen CB, Nagorney DM, Wiesner RH, *et al.*: Cholangiocarcinoma complicating primary sclerosing cholangitis. *Ann Surg* 1991, 213:21–25.

33. Boechat MI, Kangarloo H, Gilsanz V: Hepatic masses in children. *Semin Roentgen* 1988, 23:185–193.

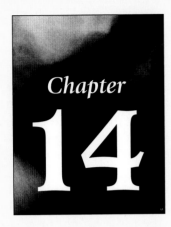

Chapter

14

Liver Transplantation

Robert S. Brown, Jr.
John R. Lake

Liver transplantation, once thought of only as a last desperate measure for patients sure to die, has come of age over the past decade. With improvements in pretransplant care of patients with severe liver disease, surgical technique, organ preservation, immunosuppression, and infectious prophylaxis, orthotopic liver transplantation (OLT) has become an accepted mode of therapy for end-stage liver disease (ESLD) of all types with survival rates approaching 90%. Thus, the field has experienced rapid changes and will continue to evolve throughout the 1990s.

As the efficacy of OLT improved, indications for it became broader. Patients with chronic hepatitis and alcoholic liver disease began to replace patients with malignancy in whom survival rates were lower. With marked increases in the success rate, the number of transplantation centers, and the number of total transplants, the awareness of OLT and number of referrals for OLT have increased logarithmically. Waiting time has become progressively longer and mortality of those on the waiting list is now an issue. One of the challenges for transplantation physicians and society in the future is the timing of transplant and how to allocate organs equitably in a time where demand is exceeding supply and costs are mounting.

Careful pretransplant evaluation is key to selection for OLT. Patients need to be rigorously screened for appropriate indications and all contraindications need to be excluded. This evaluation should be multidisciplinary, involving hepatologists, surgeons, and social workers. Those patients with significant cardiopulmonary disease need to be excluded, and those with coexisting renal disease should be evaluated for the possibility of combined liver-kidney transplant. Psychiatrists, cardiologists, pulmonologists, anesthesiologists, and nephrologists are also important members of the transplantation team.

Before transplant, management of the complications of ESLD has markedly improved. Sclerotherapy and transjugular intrahepatic portacaval shunts (TIPS) have evolved into highly effective treatments to arrest and prevent variceal hemorrhage. TIPS are also beginning to be used for refractory ascites. Mounting evidence exists for the use of prophylactic antibiotics for spontaneous bacterial peritonitis. For patients with fulminant hepatic failure (FHF), improvements in continuous arteriovenous hemofiltration and continuous venovenous hemofiltration for fluid management and intracranial pressure monitoring have increased the ability to appropriately select and manage patients prior to transplantation. Though the mortality rate in FHF still exceeds that of transplantation for other forms of liver disease, prospects for extracorporeal liver assistance and other improvements in management of complications keeps clinicians hopeful that transplant success rates for FHF will continue to improve over the next decade.

After transplant, immunosuppression and infectious prophylaxis have improved to a point that patients who survive 1 year post-OLT have an approximate 90% 5-year survival rate. Cyclosporine has probably had the single largest impact on the success of transplantation. Newer immunosuppressives including FK506 (tacrolimus) have decreased the rate of graft loss to acceptable levels. Prophylaxis, not only for opportunistic infections (*eg*, cytomegalovirus) but for recurrent hepatitis B, have also decreased post-OLT morbidity rates. Challenges still remain for finding improved and less costly prevention strategies for rejection and infection, including decreasing the risk of malignancy and lymphoproliferative disorders following transplantation.

This chapter reviews the history of liver transplantation, patient selection criteria, and pre- and posttransplant management strategies. Because the topic cannot be covered exhaustively, we have emphasized the most recent changes and advances in liver transplantation. The past decade has been one of great changes and the following decade promises far more, both in terms of patient management and allocation of resources.

HISTORY OF LIVER TRANSPLANTATION IN THE UNITED STATES

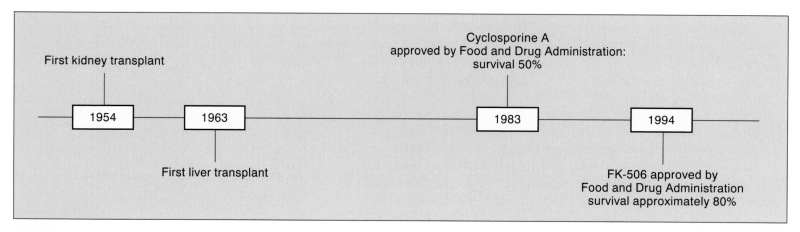

FIGURE 14-1.

Solid organ transplantation in the United States began as a clinical reality in 1954 when Joseph Murray at the Peter Bent Brigham Hospital in Boston performed the first human kidney transplant. Less than a decade later, the first liver transplant was first performed by Starzl and coworkers [1] in Denver in 1963. Throughout the 1970s and 1980s, survival rates were poor, approximately 30% after a 1-year period. Thus, liver transplantation was considered a life-saving maneuver, but it was only performed when death was imminent. In the 1980s, improved surgical techniques, immunosuppressive regimens,

patient selection, and treatments for opportunistic infections all contributed to substantially improved survival rates. With some programs now reporting survival rates of 90% at 1 year, orthotopic liver transplantation has become standard therapy for almost all forms of end-stage liver disease. With this, the number of liver transplants performed throughout the 1980s increased from less than 100 to approximately 3000 per year. Currently, more than 100 liver transplantation programs are registered with the United Network for Organ Sharing.

SURVIVAL AND CYCLOSPORINE A USE

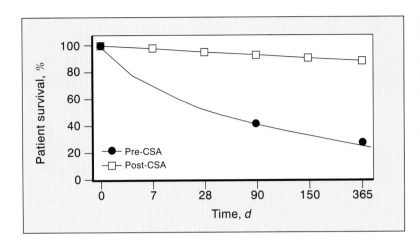

FIGURE 14-2.

Patient survival after liver transplantation, before and after introduction of cyclosporine A (CSA). In a review of 540 patients receiving a transplantation before 1983 at four centers, the 1- and 3-year patient survival rate was 26% and 12%, respectively [2]. The use of CSA has, in part, assisted the improved patient survival rate. Other factors also contributing include patient selection, surgical techniques, better liver preservation solutions, and improved treatments for posttransplantation complications.

INDICATIONS FOR TRANSPLANTATION

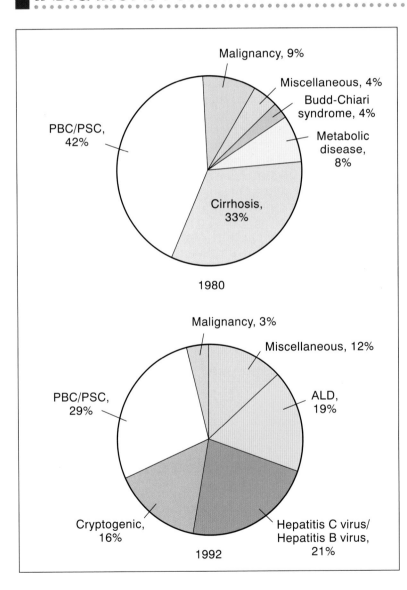

FIGURE 14-3.

Changing indications for orthotopic liver transplantation (OLT) over the past decade. In 1980, the most common diseases for which OLT was performed were the cholestatic liver diseases, primary biliary cirrhosis (PBC), and primary sclerosing cholangitis (PSC), followed by postnecrotic cirrhosis and primary hepatic malignancies. At present, the most common indication for OLT is postviral cirrhosis (usually hepatitis C) followed by alcoholic liver disease (ALD). Malignant disease represents a relatively uncommon indication for OLT. OLT was rarely performed for fulminant hepatic failure in 1980, but currently fulminant hepatic failure represents the indication for OLT in approximately 8% of transplantations. The decrease in the percentage of patients with cholestatic liver disease is caused by 1) an increase in the total number of liver transplants performed, and 2) relatively constant numbers of patients with PBC and PSC available for OLT.

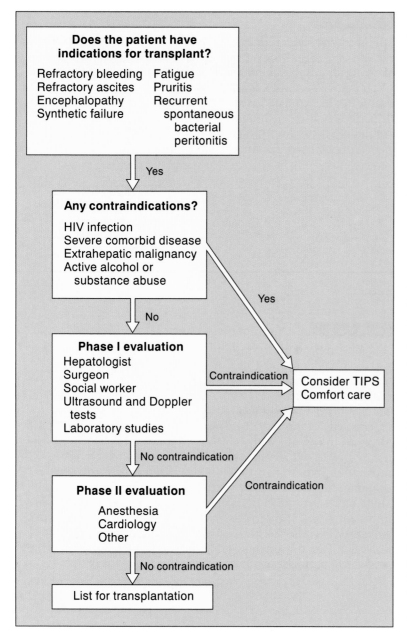

Does the patient have indications for transplant?

Refractory bleeding	Fatigue
Refractory ascites	Pruritis
Encephalopathy	Recurrent
Synthetic failure	spontaneous
	bacterial
	peritonitis

Yes ↓

Any contraindications?

HIV infection
Severe comorbid disease
Extrahepatic malignancy
Active alcohol or
substance abuse

→ Yes

No ↓

Phase I evaluation

Hepatologist
Surgeon
Social worker
Ultrasound and Doppler
tests
Laboratory studies

Contraindication →

**Consider TIPS
Comfort care**

No contraindication ↓

Phase II evaluation

Anesthesia
Cardiology
Other

Contraindication →

No contraindication ↓

List for transplantation

FIGURE 14-4.

The evaluation of patients for liver transplantation represents team efforts including hepatologists, transplantation surgeons, social workers, and consultants. The initial evaluation involves assessing whether indications for orthotopic liver transplantation (OLT) are present, including refractory variceal bleeding, encephalopathy, ascites, and marked impairment of synthetic function. Other unusual indications representing impaired quality of life include pruritus, metabolic bone disease, and xanthomatous neuropathy (seen in cholestatic diseases). Relatively uncommon indications are for correction of metabolic disorders that may (*ie*, α_1-antitrypsin deficiency, Wilson's disease, and tyrosinemia) or may not (hereditary oxalosis, familial hypercholesterolemia, and Crigler-Najjar syndrome) produce liver disease. If the patient has appropriate indications for OLT, comorbidities need to be evaluated. Severe cardiopulmonary disease, severe neurologic disease, extrahepatic malignancy, and HIV infection represent absolute contraindications. A careful cardiac evaluation is particularly important in patients over 50 years of age, who have alcoholic liver disorder or hemochromatosis as the cause of their end-stage liver disease, or if pulmonary hypertension is considered. Psychosocial contraindications include active illicit drug use, active alcohol abuse, and a lack of appropriate social support. Patients need considerable assistance after OLT. Compliance with medical therapy following OLT is also important. Portal vein thrombosis can make OLT technically more difficult but represents a contraindication only if a suitable blood vessel cannot be identified to connect a new liver, or if the thrombosis is secondary to tumor. Hepatitis B viremia (HBV) indicated by the presence of hepatitis B e antigen or HBV-DNA in serum represents a contraindication for many programs because of the high risk of HBV re-infection. The use of high-dose hepatitis B immunoglobulin to prevent re-infection in this group (*see* Fig. 14-26) represents an area of active clinical investigation. Selection criteria for patients with a history of substance abuse varies from program to program. In a recent study [3], only 6 months of abstinence was found to predict a low risk of post-OLT recidivism. This process of patient selection is dynamic. Patients may be placed on the waiting list or removed as complications or contraindications develop and are treated. TIPS—transjugular intrahepatic portacaval shunts.

WAITING TIMES AND MORTALITY

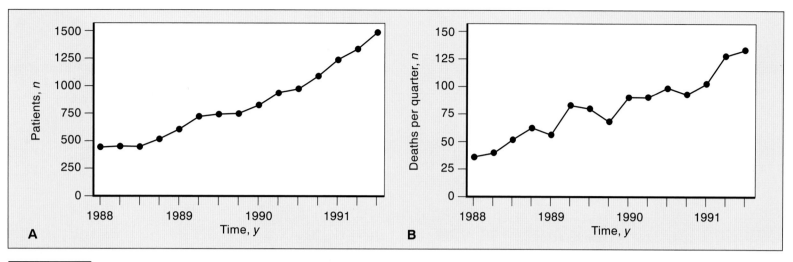

A and **B**, The number of patients on the United Network for Organ Sharing waiting list for orthotopic liver transplantation (OLT) has increased logarithmically over the past 7 years from 449 in January, 1987 to 3492 in June, 1994. The number of liver donors has increased only marginally during this same period. The result of this difference is a marked increase in waiting time, greater than 1 year for patients with blood groups O or B in certain parts of the United States. This waiting period has contributed to the mortality rate on the waiting list, with the number of patients dying while on the list having increased from 35 in 1988 to 171 in 1992. The increase in waiting list mortality rates has also led to a reexamination of the donor organ allocation process. (*From* Wiesner *et al.* [4]; with permission.)

TIMING OF TRANSPLANTATION

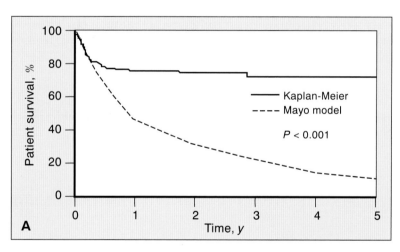

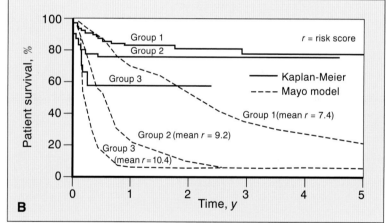

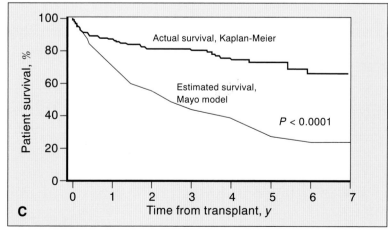

A, **B**, and **C**, To optimize the timing of transplantation, a clear understanding of the natural history of the disease is needed. This understanding has been accomplished for primary biliary cirrhosis (PBC) and primary sclerosing cholangitis (PSC); the Mayo models make it possible to calculate the probability of survival at differing time points based on certain clinical features. Using this model as a simulated control, Wiesner and coworkers [4] performed Kaplan-Meier analyses of survival with and without transplantation in 161 patients with PBC (*panel A*) and 216 patients with PSC (*panel C*) who underwent orthotopic liver transplantation (OLT) at the Mayo Clinic. Overall, long-term survival improved for both diseases with transplantation. In addition, patients in the low and moderate risk groups (groups 1 and 2 in *panel B*) derived the largest survival benefit. This fact provides evidence that performing transplantation earlier in the disease has a more profound impact on long-term patient survival. In addition, Wiesner and coworkers [4] showed that OLT in low and moderate risk patients was less costly. Thus, such a policy may represent a more cost-effective use of a limited resource. (**A** and **B**, *From* Markus *et al.* [5]; with permission.) (**C**, *From* Wiesner *et al.* [4]; with permission.)

TRANSJUGULAR INTRAHEPATIC PORTACAVAL SHUNTS

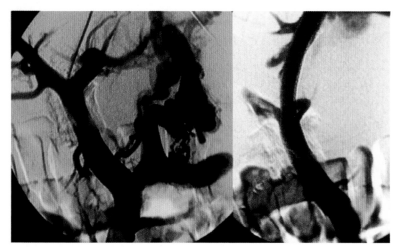

FIGURE 14-7.

Transjugular intrahepatic portacaval shunts (TIPS) represent an important advance in the management of complications of portal hypertension in patients awaiting orthotopic liver transplantation (OLT). TIPS function like side-to-side portacaval shunts and allow for a nonoperative reduction in portal hypertension. In the hands of experienced interventional radiologists, shunting can be achieved with high rates of success and low complication rates. TIPS avoid the morbidity and mortality associated with surgical shunts. They also avoid anatomic disruption of the portal vein before OLT and are removed at the time of transplantation. TIPS represent the treatment of choice for variceal bleeding refractory to sclerotherapy in patients on the waiting list. They may also benefit patients with diuretic refractory ascites.

Rebleeding

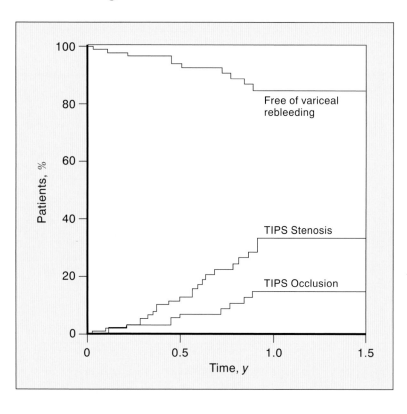

FIGURE 14-8.

The use of transjugular intrahepatic portacaval shunts (TIPS) is highly successful in prevention of rebleeding from gastro-esophageal varices. This figure shows rebleeding rates in 93 patients following TIPS. Rebleeding occurred in less than 20% of patients with at least 18 months of follow-up. Rebleeding is rare with a well-functioning TIPS. Thus, in a patient with recurrent gastrointestinal bleeding post-TIPS, ultrasound with Doppler or hepatic angiography (TIPS venogram) should be performed to assess TIPS patency. The other common complication of TIPS is new or worsened encephalopathy, seen in approximately 25% of patients. Encephalopathy is usually easily managed with lactulose but occasionally requires TIPS occlusion if severe. Rapid deterioration of liver function can occur after TIPS and may require urgent transplantation. The exact etiology of this complication and which patients are at risk is unknown. (*From* Röossle *et al.* [6]; with permission.)

Restenosis

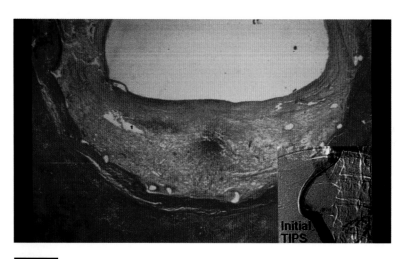

FIGURE 14-9.

Histologic examination of a transjugular intrahepatic portacaval shunt removed at transplantation shows a stenosis caused by neointimal hyperplasia. Rebleeding generally reflects shunt stenosis or occlusion. This rebleeding can usually be managed either by balloon dilatation of the stenosis or by placing a second shunt in parallel.

TABLE 14-1. TRANSJUGULAR INTRAHEPATIC PORTACAVAL SHUNTS FOR ASCITES

	University of California, San Francisco	Medical College of Virginia	Freiberg	Pamplona	Paris
Patients, n	5	7	6	7	7
Urine volume, %	>	> 15–25	>	>	>
Urinary Na+, %	> 530*	> 40†	—	> 340*	>*
Glomerular filtration rate/CrCl, %	> 33	> 5–35	>	No change	No change
Ascites improved, %	100	100	100	100	67
Ascites resolved, %	60	71	83	—	33
Diuretics decreased, %	40	57	—	—	—

*Urinary Na+ in mEq/24h
†Urinary Na+ in mEq/L

TABLE 14-1.

Another use for transjugular intrahepatic portacaval shunts (TIPS) is in the management of intractable ascites. TIPS increases central venous volume and renal perfusion leading to natriuresis. Several small studies have shown consistent increases in urine volume, urine sodium, and free-water excretion with improvement or resolution of ascites. As yet, no controlled studies of TIPS versus peritoneovenous shunting or large volume paracentesis have been done.

FULMINANT HEPATIC FAILURE

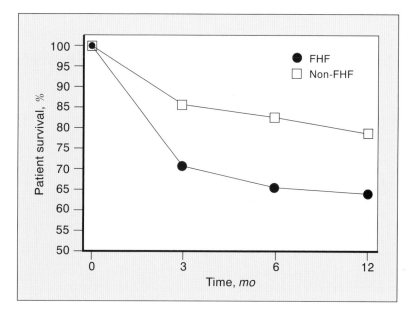

FIGURE 14-10.

Fulminant hepatic failure (FHF) requires a substantial multidisciplinary effort to support patients before and after orthotopic liver transplantation (OLT). The most common causes of FHF in patients undergoing OLT are hepatitis A, B, non-A, non-B, non-C, and drugs or toxins. As yet, however, the outcome of OLT for FHF lags behind other indications with a reported 1-year survival rate of 63% compared with 80% for patients with other diseases [7]. Factors leading to decreased survival in FHF include the prevalence of renal failure, prolonged post-OLT mechanical ventilation, and post-OLT infection. (*From* Detre *et al.* [7]; with permission.)

COMPLICATIONS OF FULMINANT HEPATIC FAILURE

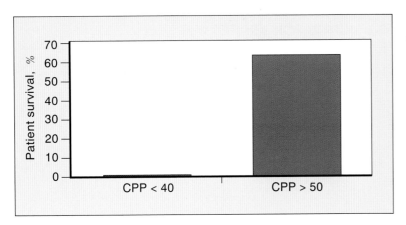

The most serious complication of fulminant hepatic failure (FHF) is cerebral edema leading to intracranial hypertension. Its pathogenesis is unknown. Physical examination and computed tomographic scanning are unreliable in identifying patients with early intracranial hypertension. The neurologic outcome of patients with moderate-severe intracranial hypertension with or without orthotopic liver transplantation is poor. As this figure shows, patients with a cerebral perfusion pressure (CPP) (defined as intracranial pressure (ICP)–mean arterial pressure) of less than 40 mm Hg for more than 2 hours have a survival rate of 0 as compared with a 60% survival in patients with CPP consistently more than 50 mm Hg. Thus, ICP monitoring appears useful in patients with FHF and coma, not only to diagnose and treat increased ICP with mannitol and barbiturates but also to exclude patients with prolonged, uncontrolled intracranial hypertension from undergoing transplantation. (*From* Inagaki *et al.* [8]; with permission.)

INTRACRANIAL PRESSURE MONITORING

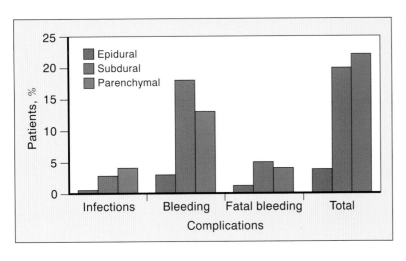

FIGURE 14-12.

The major complication of intracranial pressure monitoring is intracranial bleeding. As this graph shows, the use of epidural transducers are associated with bleeding or infection in less than 5% of cases, which is an acceptable risk. The required correction of coagulopathy removes one of the better indicators of the return of liver function. Thus, placement of an intracranial pressure monitor should be viewed as a commitment to transplantation if a donor organ becomes available and no contraindications are present. (*From* Blei *et al.* [9]; with permission.)

LIVER ASSIST DEVICES

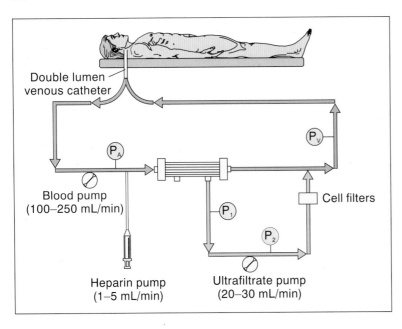

FIGURE 14-13.

The schematic diagram depicts an extracorporeal liver assist device. This device functions in a fashion similar to veno-venous hemofiltration and uses a well-differentiated hepatocyte cell line to provide temporary support. It is hoped that such devices will produce sufficient metabolic support for a long enough time to either allow for adequate liver regeneration or to serve as a bridge to successful liver transplantation.

■ LIVING RELATED DONOR TRANSPLANTATION

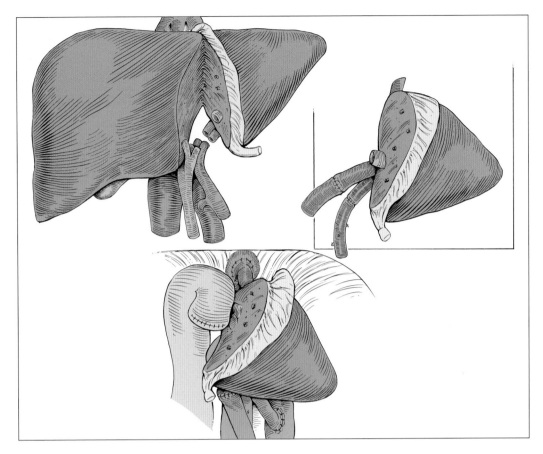

FIGURE 14-14.

Live donor liver transplantation is a process in which a partial hepatectomy is performed on a compatible family member. This part of the liver is then used for transplantation. The procedure has been used almost exclusively for pediatric patients because of the small amount of liver needed to provide adequate hepatic support. The use of live donors increases the donor pool, decreases waiting time for patients, and may provide an immunologic benefit because a family member is used. A careful evaluation of donors, including a psychosocial evaluation, is important before considering whether to use a live donor.

■ VASCULAR COMPLICATIONS

Hepatic artery thrombosis

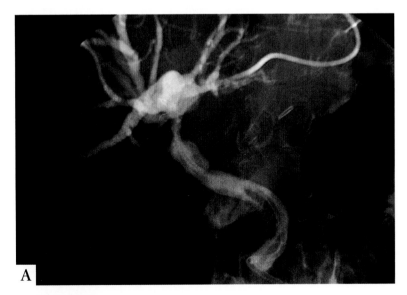

A   B

FIGURE 14-15.

Vascular complications of liver transplantation include hepatic artery thrombosis, portal vein thrombosis, and portal vein stenosis. Hepatic artery thrombosis is a serious postorthotopic liver transplantation (post-OLT) complication that may result in liver failure. Because the bile duct is supplied solely by the hepatic artery, hepatic artery ischemia can also result in biliary strictures (*see* cholangiogram in **panel A**), though these strictures can be managed by dilatation or stenting as is seen in **panel B**. However, recurrent cholangitis, liver abscesses, and the development of secondary biliary cirrhosis may result in the need for retransplantation.

Portal vein thrombosis

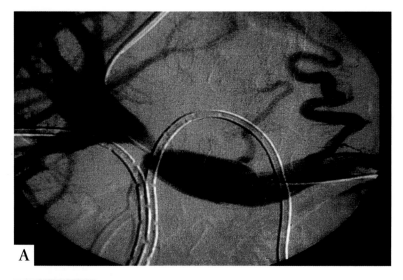

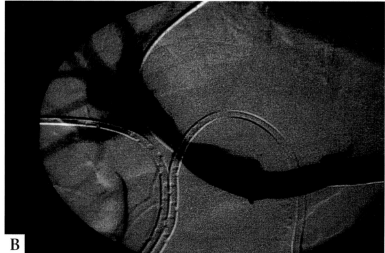

A

B

FIGURE 14-16.

Portal vein thrombosis or stenosis manifested by recurrent portal hypertension with ascites and gastrointestinal bleeding usually requires retransplantation. There also are a few reports of radiologic dilatation and portal vein stenting being used to treat this complication. An example of such treatment is seen in this figure. **Panel A** depicts pre-angioplasty, and **panel B** depicts decreased stenosis after angioplasty.

■ IMMUNOSUPPRESSION

Immunology

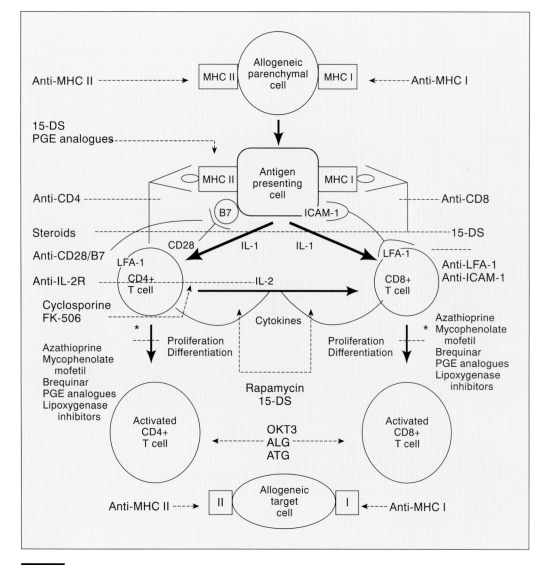

FIGURE 14-17.

This figure illustrates the immunologic pathways leading to allograft rejection and points where various pharmacologic agents act to disrupt the process. Antigen-presenting cells present donor antigens to CD4+ and CD8+ T cells in association with major histocompatibility complex (MHC) class II and I antigens, respectively. Activated CD4 cells stimulate a B-cell response. Activated CD8+ cells differentiate to cytotoxic T cells. Both CD4 and CD8 cells can then infiltrate and damage the graft. Steroids act early and nonspecifically at the level of interleukin (IL)-1 induced stimulation of CD4 and CD8 cells. Cyclosporine and FK-506 (tacrolimus) interfere with IL-2 production blocking the self-amplification from stimulated CD4 cells. Azathioprine and RS61443 (mycophenolate mofetil) inhibit proliferation or differentiation of T cells. Polyclonal and monoclonal antibody preparation-like antithymocyte globulin (ATG) and muromonob (OKT3) act on activated T cells to cause cell lysis or inactivation. Newer monoclonals directed specifically against IL-2, IL-2 receptor, and various cell-surface markers offer the hope for more specific prevention or treatment against rejection with less general immunosuppression. ALG—antilymphocytic globulin; ICAM—intracellular adhesion molecule; LFA—lymphocyte function-associated antigen; PGE—prostaglandin E. (*From* Baumgardner and Roberts [10]; with permission.)

Tacrolimus and cyclosporine A

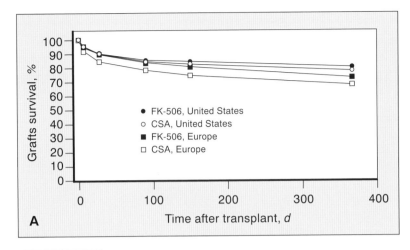

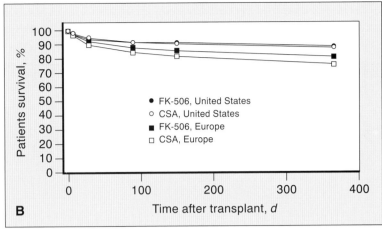

FIGURE 14-18.

A and **B**, The introduction of tacrolimus (FK-506) has been the first major improvement in maintenance immunosuppression since cyclosporine A (CSA). It was initially hoped that FK-506 would be more effective than CSA but with less nephrotoxicity. Though FK-506 can rescue some patients with refractory rejection on CSA–based immunosuppression, two recent trials comparing tacrolimus against CSA–based immunosuppression showed no advantage in terms of 1-year graft or patient survival in both Europe and the United States [11,12]. The incidence of nephrotoxicity and serious neuro-toxicity was similar. Tacrolimus therapy was associated with less hirsutism, hypertension, and lower serum cholesterol levels at 1 year. CSA therapy was associated with less diarrhea, hair loss, and diabetes. One advantage of FK-506 is that it does not require bile salts for absorption. This advantage allows for earlier conversion from intravenous to per os therapy and may provide more reliable drug levels in patients who are cholestatic. It has been suggested that the incidence of lymphoproliferative disorders in children less than 2 years of age may be higher with FK-506.

■ BILIARY COMPLICATIONS

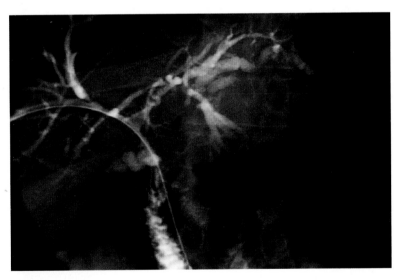

FIGURE 14-19.

Biliary complications develop in up to one-third of patients following liver transplantation. Anastomotic strictures at the choled-ochocholedochostomy are the most common. T-tube exit site leaks occurring at the time the T tube is pulled are manifested by pain with or without fever and can usually be treated with a naso-biliary drain for 24 hours or with endoscopic stenting or sphinc-terotomy. More extensive stricturing is seen following hepatic artery thrombosis, with long cold ischemia times or recurrent primary sclerosing cholangitis (PSC). The radiologic picture of recurrent PSC, as this cholangiogram demonstrates, is difficult to distinguish from that of a cpatient with hepatic artery ischemia. Recurrent PSC has been reported, but rarely causes graft failure. Treatment is symptomatic with endoscopic or radiologic dilatation or stenting of significant strictures.

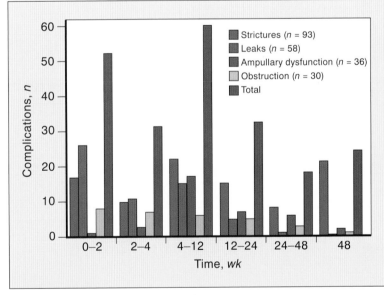

FIGURE 14-20.

This graph illustrates the timing of biliary complications. Leaks are the most common problem in early postorthotopic liver transplan-tation (post-OLT) period. Strictures can occur at any time post-OLT and are the only significant complication seen beyond 1 year. Ampullary dysfunction (usually papillary stenosis) is also seen with a peak incidence at 1 to 3 months post-OLT. Obstruction usually by stones or foreign bodies (ie, T tubes) can occur at any time throughout the 1st year but rarely after 1 year. (*From* Greif *et al.* [13]; with permission.)

TABLE 14-2. DEFINITIONS OF GRADES FOR CHRONIC REJECTION AND FOR REJECTION INDEFINITE FOR CHRONICITY (INDEFINITE FOR BILE DUCT LOSS)*

REJECTION INDEFINITE FOR CHRONICITY (INDEFINITE FOR BILE DUCT LOSS)	CHRONIC (DUCTOPENIC) REJECTION†
No complicating lobular changes Lobular changes including one of the three findings—centrilobular cholestasis, perivenular sclerosis, or hepatocellular ballooning or necrosis or dropout	Bile duct loss without centrilobular cholestasis, perivenular sclerosis, or hepatocyte ballooning or necrosis and dropout Bile duct loss with one of the following four findings—centrilobular cholestasis, perivenular sclerosis, or hepatocellular ballooning or necrosis and dropout Bile duct loss with at least two of the following four findings—centrilobular cholestasis, perivenular sclerosis, or hepatocellular ballooning or centrilobular necrosis and dropout

*Definition provided by the National Institute of Diabetes and Digestive and Kidney Disease
†Bile duct loss in > 50% of triads

TABLE 14-2.

Acute cellular rejection in liver transplantation patients is manifested by mixed but prominently mononuclear periportal inflammation, bile duct injury, and endothelitis. These histologic findings are also seen in patients with postorthotopic liver transplantation hepatitis C and recurrence of primary biliary cirrhosis. Chronic ductopenic rejection is histologically manifested by arteriopathy and loss of intralobular bile ducts. The pathogenesis of this lesion is unclear but the vasculopathy may be primary. In general, chronic rejection responds poorly to medical treatment. Some patients have responded successfully to treatment with tacrolimus. A working group of pathologists, physicians, and surgeons recently developed a consensus statement on the classification and accepted histologic diagnosis of rejection. (*From* Demetris *et al.* [14]; with permission.)

DIFFERENTIATION OF REJECTION OF HEPATITIS POSTTRANSPLANTATION

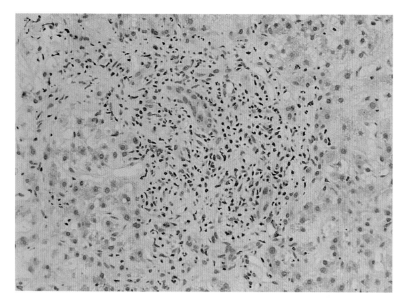

FIGURE 14-21.

Often the most difficult differentiation to make on liver biopsy is between acute allograft rejection and posttransplant hepatitis C virus (HCV). This figure shows a postorthotopic liver transplantation (post-OLT) biopsy from a patient transplanted for HCV cirrhosis. She developed both acute rejection and recurrent HCV after transplantation. Her liver dysfunction progressed despite intensive treatment of the rejection and resulted in graft loss. In this histologic section, the prominent bile duct damage and mixed cell (*ie*, eosinophils) infiltrate suggest rejection, whereas the piecemeal necrosis and acidophil bodies suggest HCV. None of these findings taken alone is specific for either diagnosis. Serologies can often be negative. Although all patients post-OLT HCV will be HCV-RNA positive, most HCV-RNA–positive patients will not have hepatitis. If rejection and hepatitis coexist on the biopsy, it might be reasonable to treat the rejection in difficult to distinguish cases. If there is no response, post-OLT HCV is likely and the immunosuppression should be brought down to the lowest possible levels.

RECURRENT HEPATITIS C AFTER TRANSPLANTATION

HCV Pretransplant infection	Posttransplant serum HCV Positive, %	Posttransplant serum HCV Negative, %
Positive, n = 41	39 (95%)*	2 (5%)
Negative, n = 48	17 (35%)*	31 (65%)

*P = 0.0001

A

HCV Pretransplant infection	Posttransplant hepatitis Definite or possible, %	Posttransplant hepatitis Absent, %
Positive, n = 41	17 (41%)*	24 (59%)
Negative, n = 48	9 (19%)*	39 (81%)

*P = 0.02

B

FIGURE 14-22.

A, Chronic hepatitis C virus (HCV) is currently the most common disease for which orthotopic liver transplantation (OLT) is performed in the United States. Posttransplant HCV infection is not accurately diagnosed using only serologic assays. Using polymerase chain reaction (PCR) testing for HCV-RNA, Wright and coworkers [15] found that 95% of these patients who were positive for HCV-RNA by PCR pretransplant developed recurrent HCV infection post-transplant. Of 48 HCV–negative controls (defined by antibodies to HCV [Anti-HCV] negative pretransplant), 35% developed apparently new HCV infections. Whether this latter group reflects occult pre-OLT HCV infection or infection acquired from the donor organ or blood products remains unclear. **B**, Post-OLT HCV causes severe allograft damage and graft loss less frequently than post-OLT hepatitis B virus. As shown here, post-OLT hepatitis is more common in patients who were Anti-HCV positive than Anti-HCV negative before transplantation (41% versus 19%). Most patients who are Anti-HCV positive before transplantation do not develop posttransplant hepatitis, however, HCV infection is present in 96% of cases of noncytomegalovirus-related post-OLT hepatitis. (*From* Wright *et al.* [15].)

RECURRENT HEPATITIS C—TREATMENT

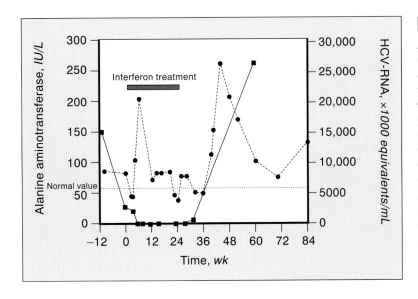

FIGURE 14-23.

Although postorthotopic liver transplantation (post-OLT) hepatitis C virus (HCV) usually leads to fairly mild disease, it can lead in some cases to severe allograft damage and graft loss. α-Interferon can lead to a normalization of serum transaminase activity and loss of HCV viremia in approximately 25% of patients with chronic HCV in the nontransplant setting. Whether therapy with α-interferon can alter the course of posttransplant HCV is certainly of great interest to transplantation physicians. Impediments to successful interferon therapy include the high level of HCV viremia post-OLT and potential precipitation of rejection by the up-regulation of human lymphocyte antigens. A pilot study of 18 patients at the University of California, San Francisco [16] treated with α-interferon 3×10^6 units three times a week for 26 weeks found a complete response rate of 28% (defined by normalization of serum transaminases). Both responders and nonresponders experienced significant decreases in levels of HCV-RNA. Posttreatment liver function tests remained normal in four of five responders, but HCV-RNA levels returned to pretreatment levels in all patients. Allograft rejection was seen in one patient. The response of HCV-RNA levels and alanine transaminase concentrations over time are shown in this figure. Clinical factors predictive of a biochemical response to therapy included lower serum HCV-RNA levels, lower serum bilirubin concentrations, and a longer interval between transplant and initiation of therapy. (*From* Wright *et al.* [16]; with permission.)

RECURRENT HEPATITIS B

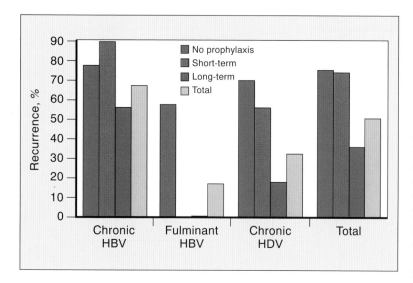

FIGURE 14-24.

Recurrence of hepatitis B virus (HBV) infection and post-transplant hepatitis occurs in the vast majority of untreated patients transplanted for chronic HBV. Re-infection leads to far more aggressive disease than is seen in the nontransplant setting. Passive immunization with high-dose hepatitis B immune globulin (HBIg) can reduce risk of re-infection. HBIg is usually given monthly and some investigators base the need for redosing on the titres of antibodies to hepatitis B surface antigen. In a study by Samuel and coworkers [17], the impact of prophylaxis with HBIg on outcome was investigated. No prophylaxis or short-term immunoprophylaxis with HBIg produced equivalent rates of re-infection. Long-term immunoprophylaxis lowered the recurrence rate to 35%. HBV re-infection rates were higher with chronic HBV than acute HBV or hepatitis D virus (HDV) co-infection. Long-term prophylaxis in this study was defined as longer than 6 months of therapy and was not always life-long administration. Patients who were hepatitis B e antigen negative or HBV-DNA negative in serum also carried a lower risk of HBV infection. The survival of patients with long-term prophylaxis was approximately 75% as compared with 45% in the other two groups (*ie*, no or short-term prophylaxis). The current protocol used to transplant patients with HBV is to give HBIg at high doses and for life. The impact of HBIg administration on the outcome of HBV-DNA–positive patients is currently being investigated. (*From* Samuel *et al.* [17]; with permission.)

LYMPHOPROLIFERATIVE DISEASE POSTORTHOTOPIC LIVER TRANSPLANTATION

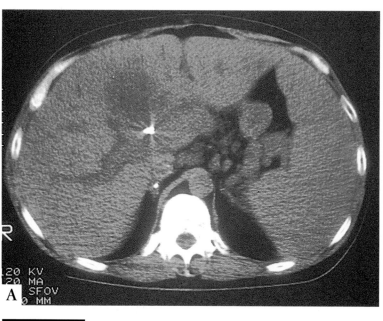

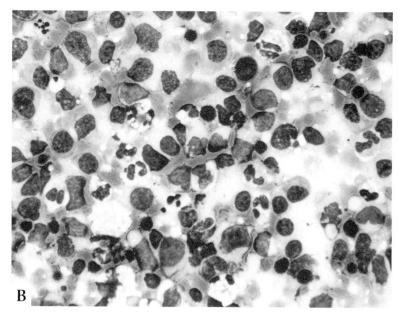

FIGURE 14-25.

Posttransplant lymphoproliferative disease (PTLD) is an uncommon but serious complication following liver transplantation. Seen in 1% to 3% of patients, it is associated with the use of greater amounts of immunosuppression and, thus, is usually seen in patients who have had multiple episodes of rejection. A reported association of this disorder with FK-506 use in children less than 2 years of age may also be due to the fact that FK-506 was used predominantly as rescue therapy for persistent rejection in this group. PTLD may occur anywhere in the body; they frequently are multicentric and often involve the liver. PTLD is associated with Epstein-Barr virus

(EBV) infection with EBV genome demonstrable in the tumors. Therapy involves lowering immunosuppression levels and some programs give high-dose intravenous acyclovir or gancyclovir. This therapy has reported success rates of approximately 30% to 50%. However, some patients do develop progressive disease and death. Predictors of response to therapy are not currently well defined. **A,** This computed tomographic scan demonstrates findings of a mass in the porta hepatis and retroperitoneal and para-aortic adenopathy. The diagnosis of PTLD can be made by fine needle aspiration revealing nests of atypical lymphocytes, as seen in **B.**

EVALUATION OF POSTTRANSPLANTATION PROBLEMS—INCREASED LIVER FUNCTION TESTS

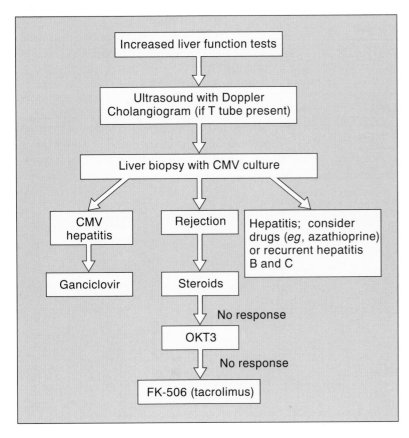

FIGURE 14-26.

This algorithm is an approach to the evaluation of increased liver tests after transplantation. A cholangiogram, if a T tube is present, and ultrasound with Doppler to rule out vascular thrombosis are typically the first steps. If the patient is more than 6 months postorthotopic liver transplantation (post-OLT), these two steps are frequently not needed. Liver biopsy is critical to the evaluation as the clinical presentation of rejection, cytomegalovirus (CMV) hepatitis, biliary obstruction, and posttransplant hepatitis all overlap. Rejection occurs early (peak incidence on day 8). CMV hepatitis, by contrast, is not usually seen within the first 30 days post-OLT. CMV hepatitis is the most common reason for increased liver function tests after rejection during the period of 1 to 6 months after transplantation and usually responds to a 2-week course of intravenous ganciclovir. OKT3—muromonab.

EVALUATION OF POSTTRANSPLANTATION PROBLEMS—FEVER

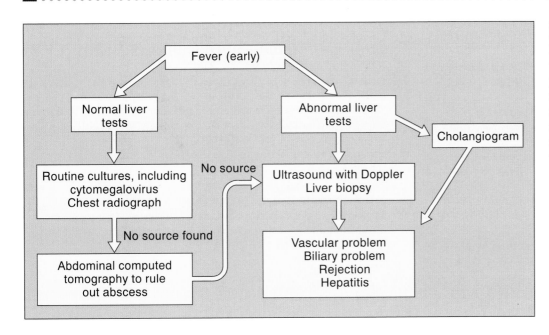

FIGURE 14-27.

Fever early after orthotopic liver transplantation (OLT) usually represents technical problems related to surgery (*eg*, wound infections), intravenous lines, pulmonary infections, or rejection. Most opportunistic infections occur between 6 weeks and 6 months post-OLT. A diagnostic approach to fevers is outlined here.

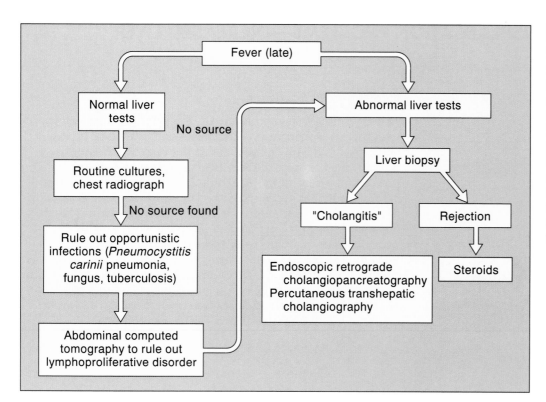

FIGURE 14-28.

Fevers occurring more than 4 months after transplantation most commonly result from rejection or bile duct obstruction with cholangitis or community-acquired infections. Other considerations include opportunistic infections (including *Pneumocystis carinii* pneumonia, tuberculosis, and fungi). Lymphoproliferative syndromes are seen during this period. The diagnostic approach should include routine cultures of blood, urine, and a liver biopsy. Further evaluation should be done based on the findings of those initial evaluations and on symptoms.

■ REFERENCES AND RECOMMENDED READING

1. Starzl TE, Demetris AJ, Van Thiel D: Liver transplantation. *N Engl J Med* 1989, 329:1013–1022, 1092–1099.

2. Scharschmidt BF: Human liver transplantation: Analysis of data on 540 patients from four centers. *Hepatology* 1984, 4:95S–101S.

3. Osario RW, Ascher NL, Avery M, *et al.*: Predicting recidivism after orthotopic liver transplantation for alcoholic liver disease [Part 1]. *Hepatology* 1994, 20:105–110.

4. Wiesner RH, Porayko MK, Dickson ER, *et al.*: Selection timing of liver transplantation in primary biliary cirrhosis and primary sclerosing cholangitis. *Hepatology* 1992, 16:1290–1299.

5. Markus BH, Dickson ER, Grambsch PM, *et al.*:Efficiency of liver transplantation in patients with primary biliary cirrhosis. *N Engl J Med* 1989, 320:1709–1713.

6. Röossle M, Kaag K, Ochs A, *et al.*: The transjugular intrahepatic portosystemic stent-shunt procedure for variceal bleeding. *N Engl J Med* 1994, 330:165–209.

7. Detre K, Belle S, Berginer K, Daily OP: Liver transplantation for fulminant hepatic failure in the United States: October 1987 through December 1991. *Clin Transpl* 1994, 8:274–280.

8. Inagaki M, Shaw B, Schafer D, *et al.*: Advantages of intracranial pressure monitoring in patients with fulminant liver failure. *Gastroenterology* 1992, 102:A826.

9. Blei AT, Olafsson S, Webster S, Levy R: Complications of intracranial pressure monitoring in fulminant hepatic failure. *Lancet* 1993, 341:157–158.

10. Baumgardner GL, Roberts JP: New immunosuppressive agents. *Gastroenterol Clin North Am* 1993, 22:421–449.

11. The U.S. Multicenter FK506 Liver Study Group: A comparison of tacrolimus (FK506) and cyclosporine for immunosuppression in liver transplantation. N Engl J Med 1994, 331:1110–1115.

12. European FK506 Multicenter Liver Study Group: Randomised trial comparing tacrolimus (FK506) and cyclosporin in prevention of liver allograft rejection. *Lancet* 1994, 34:423–428.

13. Greif F, Bronsther OL, Van Thiel DH, *et al.*: The incidence, timing, and management of biliary tract complications after orthotopic liver transplantation. *Ann Surg* 1994, 219:40–45.

14. Demetris AJ, Seaberg EC, Batts KP, *et al.*: Reliability and predictive value of the National Institute of Diabetes and Digestive and Kidney Diseases Liver Transplantation Database nomenclature and grading system for cellular rejection of liver allografts. *Hepatology* 1995, 21:408–416.

15. Wright TL, Donegan E, Hsu HH, *et al.*: Recurrent and acquired hepatitis C viral infection in liver transplant recipients. *Gastroenterology* 1992, 103:317–322.

16. Wright TL, Combs C, Kim M, *et al.*: Interferon-α therapy for hepatitis C virus infection after liver transplantation. *Hepatology* 1994, 20:1–7.

17. Samuel D, Muller R, Alexander G, *et al.*: Liver transplantation in European patients with the hepatitis B surface antigen. *N Engl J Med* 1993, 329:1842–1847.

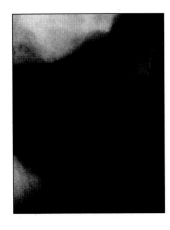

Index

Page numbers followed by *t* or *f* indicate tables or figures, respectively.

G

Gallstones, imaging, 1.12*f*
Gamma-glutamyl transpeptidase, in alcoholism, 1.13*f*
Ganciclovir, for CMV hepatitis, 14.15*f*
Gastroesophageal varices. *See* Varices
Germander, hepatotoxicity, 6.19*t*, 6.21*f*
Gilbert's syndrome, 1.4*f*
   characteristics, 1.6*t*, 1.7*f*
    serum bilirubin level
      phenobarbital administration and, 1.6*t*, 1.8*f*
      reduced caloric intake and, 1.7*f*
Glutathione, protective effect in liver, 6.12*f*
Glutathione-*S*-transferase, 1.3*f*
GOR-47 antibodies, in type 2 autoimmune hepatitis, 3.14*f*
Gordoloba, hepatotoxicity, 6.19*t*

H

Halothane
   hepatitis, 6.16*f*
   hepatotoxicity, 6.11*f*
    histopathology, 7.13*f*, 7.14*f*–7.15*f*
HAV. *See* Hepatitis A virus
HBcAg. *See* Hepatitis B virus, core antigen
HBeAg. *See* Hepatitis B virus, e antigen
HBsAg. *See* Hepatitis B virus, surface antigen
HBV. *See* Hepatitis B virus
HCV. *See* Hepatitis C virus
HDV. *See* Hepatitis D virus
HELLP syndrome, 1.10*t*
   liver biopsy in, 1.11*f*
Hemangioma, hepatic, 12.1–12.2, 12.10–12.12, 13.5*f*
   cavernous, 12.10*f*
   diagnosis, 13.12*f*
    by dynamic computed tomography, 12.11*f*, 13.5*f*
    by ultrasound, 12.11*f*
   histology, 12.10*f*
   magnetic resonance imaging, 12.11*f*
   technetium-99m labeled erythrocyte study, 12.12*f*
Heme, catabolism, 1.1, 1.2*f*
Hemochromatosis, hereditary, 8.1–8.11
   arthritis in, 8.4*t*, 8.5*f*
   with cirrhosis, survival, 8.10*f*
   clinical manifestations, 8.4*f*, 8.4–8.5, 8.5*f*
   computed tomography in, 8.8*f*
   diagnosis, 8.5–8.8
   differential diagnosis, 8.8–8.9
   excess iron removal in, 8.10*f*
    survival and, 8.11*f*
   family screening for, 8.11*t*
   genetics, 8.3*f*
   heart in, 8.7*f*
   hepatic cirrhosis in, 8.5*f*
   hepatic iron index in, 8.9*t*
   historical aspects, 8.2*f*
   iron absorption in, 8.3*f*
   liver biopsy in, 8.6*f*, 8.7*f*
   magnetic resonance imaging in, 8.8*f*
   magnetic susceptibility in, 8.8*f*
   micronodular cirrhosis in, 8.7*f*
   pancreas in, 8.7*f*
   pathogenesis, 8.3*t*
   pathophysiology, 8.3–8.4
   phlebotomy therapy, 8.10*f*, 8.10*t*
   physical findings in, 8.4*t*, 8.5*f*
   prognosis for, 8.10–8.11
   signs and symptoms, 8.4*t*
   survival, 8.10*f*
   treatment, 8.10–8.11
Hemolysis, hyperbilirubinemia with, 1.4*f*, 1.5*t*
   evaluation, 1.6*t*
Hepadnavirus, 4.1, 4.2*f*
Hepatic arteries
   radiographic anatomy, 12.3, 12.3*f*
   thrombosis, postorthotopic liver transplantation, 14.9*f*
Hepatic coma, 7.8*f*
Hepatic encephalopathy, 7.8*f*, 11.12–11.22. *See also* Portal
      systemic encephalopathy
   abnormal astrocytes in, 11.18*f*
   blood ammonia concentration in, 11.14*f*
   branched chain amino acid therapy for, 11.15*f*
   carbonic anhydrase inhibition and, 11.15*f*
   cerebral blood flow and cerebral metabolic rate for
      ammonia in, 11.17*f*
   nonabsorbed carbohydrate therapy, 11.19*f*, 11.20*f*
   Number Connection Test in, 11.16*f*
   L-*ORNITHINE*-L-aspartate for, 11.21*f*
   pathogenesis
    gamma-aminobutyric acid hypothesis, 11.18*f*
    multifactorial, 11.18*f*
Hepatic iron index
   calculation, 8.9*t*
   development, 8.8*t*
   in hemochromatosis, 8.9*t*
Hepatic portoenterostomy, 1.10*f*
Hepatic sinusoidal bed
   pathophysiology, in ascites, 10.9*f*
   physiology, 10.9*f*
Hepatic venooclusive disease. *See* Venoocclusive disease
Hepatitis
   acute viral, 2.1–2.21, 5.2*f*. *See also* Hepatitis A virus;
      Hepatitis B virus; Hepatitis C virus; Hepatitis D
      virus; Hepatitis E virus
    epidemiology, 2.2*f*
    non-A,B,C, prevalence, 2.2*f*
    proportion, by agent, 2.2*f*
   alcoholic. *See* Alcoholic hepatitis
   autoimmune. *See* Autoimmune hepatitis
   chronic, differential diagnosis, 4.13*t*, 5.6*f*
   chronic active, Wilson's disease and, 8.13*f*
   chronic nonviral, Wilson's disease and, 8.13*f*
   chronic viral
    autoantibody titers in, 3.8*f*
    proportion, by agent, 2.2*f*
   cytomegalovirus, posttransplant, 14.15*f*
   hepatocellular carcinoma and, 2.20
   ischemic, 12.7
   lobular, in type 1 autoimmune hepatitis, 3.10*f*
   non-A, non-B, hepatocellular carcinoma and, 2.20*f*
   periportal, in type 1 autoimmune hepatitis, 3.9*f*, 3.10*t*
    prognosis for, 3.11*f*
   toxic, 6.18